Embracing Complexity in Health

Joachim P. Sturmberg
Editor

# Embracing Complexity in Health

## The Transformation of Science, Practice, and Policy

Springer

*Editor*
Joachim P. Sturmberg
School of Medicine and Public Health
University of Newcastle
Wamberal, NSW, Australia

International Society for Systems
and Complexity Sciences for Health
Waitsfield, VT, USA

ISBN 978-3-030-10939-4 ISBN 978-3-030-10940-0 (eBook)
https://doi.org/10.1007/978-3-030-10940-0



This Springer imprint is published by the registered company Springer Nature Switzerland AG.
The registered company address is: Gewerbestrasse 11, 6330 Cham, Switzerland

*A social movement that only moves people is merely a revolt. A movement that changes both people and institutions is a revolution.*

*Martin Luther King Jr.*

*I dedicate this book to the foundation members of the International Society for Systems and Complexity Sciences for Health for their tireless efforts to promote systems and complexity thinking and change the people and their institutions—David Aron, Jeanette Bennett, Curt Lindberg, Gaetano Lotrecchiano, Paige McDonald, Jennifer Potts, John Scott, Andrew Seely, Chad Swanson, Randy Thompson, and Peter Tsasis.*

# Preface

*We neither fear complexity nor embrace it for its own sake, but rather face it with the faith that simplicity and understanding are within reach.*
Frederick R. Adler, Department of Mathematics, University of Utah

In November 2017, the *3rd International Conference for Systems and Complexity Sciences for Health* was held at the *Virginia Science & Technology Campus* of *The George Washington University*, Ashburn, VA. The conference theme—*Embracing Complexity in Health: The Transformation of Science, Practice, and Policy*—highlighted the urgent need to promulgate systems and complexity thinking as a pragmatic way to enhance the health of our patients, the effectiveness of our health professionals, and the affordability and sustainability of our health systems at large.

The 19 chapters in this book demonstrate how embracing complexity sciences has transformed approaches and understandings of health problems from a foundational philosophical perspective as much as in pragmatic terms in relation to the physiological dynamics underpinning health and disease, the delivery of health care, education and leadership, and health system and policy planning and redesign. Readers will find many eye-opening examples to contemplate and to adapt for the context of their own work. As Adler said, lets not fear but embrace complexity approaches for the benefit of our patients and the health system at large.

I would like to thank my editors Janet Kim and Christina Tuballes for their assistance in compiling this book as well as their enthusiasm and support in promoting previously published books, in particular *Handbook of Systems and Complexity in Health* and *Health System Redesign: How to Make Health Care Person-Centered, Equitable, and Sustainable*. My thanks also go to the entire production team for their work on shaping the layout of *Embracing Complexity in Health: The Transformation of Science, Practice, and Policy*.

Holgate, NSW, Australia
October 2018

Joachim P. Sturmberg

# Acknowledgments

Drs. Paige McDonald and Gaetano Lotrecchiano from the School of Medicine and Health Sciences organized and convened the *3rd International Conference for Systems and Complexity Sciences for Health* at the *Virginia Science & Technology Campus* of *The George Washington University*, Ashburn, VA. Their enthusiasm and hospitality are greatly acknowledged.

# Contents

# Contributors

**Sarah Alemara** Center for Molecular Medicine and Genomics, Wayne State University School of Medicine, Detroit, MI, USA

**Zachary Armstrong** Center for Molecular Medicine and Genomics, Wayne State University School of Medicine, Detroit, MI, USA

**Jason H. T. Bates** Larner College of Medicine, University of Vermont, Burlington, VT, USA

**Johanna Becho** Department of Psychiatry, University of Texas Health Science Center San Antonio, San Antonio, TX, USA

**Sandra Burge** Department of Family and Community Medicine, University of Texas Health Science Center San Antonio, San Antonio, TX, USA

**Sergio G. Camorlinga** Department of Applied Computer Science, The University of Winnipeg, Winnipeg, MB, Canada

**Suzie Carmack** George Mason University, Washington, DC, USA

Adjunct Faculty School of Integrative Studies, George Mason University, Fairfax, VA, USA

**Leticia Mucci da Conceição** Department of Nutrition, University of São Paulo, São José dos Campos, São Paulo, Brazil

**Annette Sofie Davidsen** Section of General Practice and Research Unit for General Practice, Department of Public Health, University of Copenhagen, Denmark

**Elena A. Doty** Larner College of Medicine, University of Vermont, Burlington, VT, USA

**Robert Ferrer** Department of Family and Community Medicine, University of Texas Health Science Center San Antonio, San Antonio, TX, USA

**Andrea Ghazzawi** Telfer School of Management, University of Ottawa, Ottawa, ON, Canada

**Robert C. Hausmann** College of Education, The University of Houston, Houston, TX, USA

**James K. Hazy** Robert B. Willumstad School of Business Management, Adelphi University, Garden City, NY, USA

**Henry H. Heng** Center for Molecular Medicine and Genomics and Department of Pathology, Wayne State University School of Medicine, Detroit, MI, USA

**Emma Iriarte** Social Protection and Health, The Inter-American Development Bank, Washington, DC, USA

**Alonzo H. Jones** Common Sense Medicine, Plainview, TX, USA

**Alexandra B. R. Jønsson** Section of General Practice and Research Unit for General Practice, Department of Public Health, University of Copenhagen, Denmark

**David Katerndahl** Department of Family and Community Medicine, University of Texas Health Science Center San Antonio, San Antonio, TX, USA

**C. Matthew Kinsey** Larner College of Medicine, University of Vermont, Burlington, VT, USA

**Craig Kuziemsky** Telfer School of Management, University of Ottawa, Ottawa, ON, Canada

**Sung Young Lim** Department of Applied Computer Science, The University of Winnipeg, Winnipeg, MB, Canada

**Guo Liu** Center for Molecular Medicine and Genomics, Wayne State University School of Medicine, Detroit, MI, USA

**Gaetano R. Lotrecchiano** Department of Clinical Research and Leadership, George Washington University School of Medicine and Health Sciences, Washington, DC, USA

**Carmel Martin** Department of Medicine, Nursing and Allied Health, Monash University, and Monash Health, Clayton, VIC, Australia

**Shalini Misra** Virginia Tech School of Public and International Affairs, Alexandria, VA, USA

**Marlene C. R. Møller** Research Unit for General Practice, Department of Public Health, Aarhus University, Denmark

**Maria Del Pilar Montanez Villacampa** Department of Family and Community Medicine, University of Texas Health Science Center San Antonio, San Antonio, TX, USA

**Jennifer Nelson** Social Protection and Health, The Inter-American Development Bank, Washington, DC, USA

**Kevin E. Nortrup** Sugar Creek Solutions LLC, Fairland, IN, USA

**Line Olsen** Section of General Practice and Research Unit for General Practice, Department of Public Health, University of Copenhagen, Denmark

**James Caldwell Palmer** DMan, Denver, CO, USA

**Thomas Plochg** Netherlands Public Health Federation, Amersfoort, Netherlands

**Ferdinando Regalia** Social Protection and Health, The Inter-American Development Bank, Washington, DC, USA

**Sarah Regan** Center for Molecular Medicine and Genomics, Wayne State University School of Medicine, Detroit, MI, USA

**Susanne Reventlow** Section of General Practice and Research Unit for General Practice, Department of Public Health, University of Copenhagen, Denmark

**Keith Stockman** Operations Research and Projects, General Medicine Program, Monash Health, Clayton, VIC, Australia

**Joachim P. Sturmberg** School of Medicine and Public Health, University of Newcastle, Wamberal, NSW, Australia

International Society for Systems and Complexity Sciences for Health, Waitsfield, VT, USA

**Jan van der Kamp** Health Systems Innovations, Blaricum, Netherlands

**John Watkins** Centre for Population Medicine, Cardiff University and Public Health Wales, Cardiff, UK

**Bruce J. West** Information Science Directorate, Army Research Office, Research Triangle Park, NC, USA

**Tilo Winkler** Department of Anesthesia, Critical Care and Pain Medicine, Masschusetts General Hospital, and Harvard Medical School, Boston, MA, USA

**Robert Wood** Department of Family and Community Medicine, University of Texas Health Science Center San Antonio, San Antonio, TX, USA

**Christine J. Ye** Division of Hematology and Oncology, Department of Internal Medicine, University of Michigan, Ann Arbor, MI, USA

# Part I
# Introduction: A Systems and Complexity Science Understanding of Health

# *If You Change the Way You Look at Things, Things You Look at Change*. Max Planck's Challenge for Health, Health Care, and the Healthcare System

**Joachim P. Sturmberg**

Max Planck observed that 'If you change the way you look at things, things you look at change'. It is high time for healthcare professionals to embrace the challenge—the linear reductionist view of health and disease is failing our patients, our profession and our societies. These insights are not really new, Osler has coined many aphorisms to emphasise the need to understand the person with an illness over and above the diseases that might be responsible for his predicament. The challenges posited in this chapter are summarised in Fig. 1. So, let us look at what is health, health care and the healthcare system from a complex adaptive systems perspective and see how 'things we look at change'.

## 1 Looking Differently: At *Health, Dis-ease and Disease*

Does this person have a disease, what is the disease and what can we do about it—this is the prevailing way we look at those coming to us seeking health care. Accordingly, and consistent with our entrained way of thinking and seeing, we respond—reflex like—ordering tests to find the disease with the aim of 'removing it'.

There are at least three flaws inherent in this simplistic approach—the assumption that people who seek health care actually have a disease; that disease has a defined cause, and that disease is defined by its visualisable anatomical correlate.

J. P. Sturmberg (✉)
School of Medicine and Public Health, University of Newcastle, Wamberal, NSW, Australia

International Society for Systems and Complexity Sciences for Health, Waitsfield, VT, USA



J. P. Sturmberg (ed.), *Embracing Complexity in Health*,
https://doi.org/10.1007/978-3-030-10940-0_1

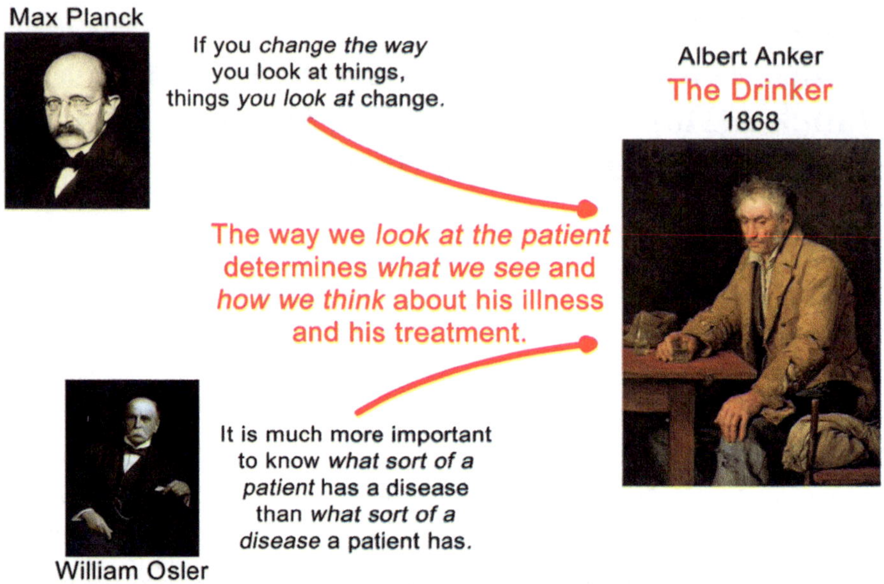


**Fig. 1** Are you aware which lens you use looking at a patient? 'If you change the way you look at things, things you look at change.' How much are we aware of the lenses we use to 'look at' particular patients, and how much are we aware how this influences the way we approach and manage their illnesses. Research has repeatedly shown subconscious biases in patient management based on age, gender and ethnicity

## *1.1 Most People Are Healthy Most of the Time*

Despite the widespread belief, propagated by sensationalism in the media, few people experiencing illness symptoms have a definable disease. The figures should speak for themselves [1–3]—at any time 80% of people are healthy or healthy enough not to perceive the need for health care, of the 20% seeking health care 80% (or 16% of the total) only require primary care, of the 20% requiring disease-specific care 80% (or 3.2% of the total) require secondary and only the remaining 20% (or 0.8% of the total) require tertiary care services. Equally, 80% of people have 20% of all diseases, and about 80% of all primary care consultations result in a nonspecific condition [4–6], i.e. most people seeking GP care do so for reasons other than specific diagnosis management (Fig. 2).

## *1.2 Dis-ease Versus Disease Versus Health*

Most of the things that cause dis-ease are not caused by disease. The experience of health and dis-ease are dynamic phenomena, and we feel healthy and/or ill in

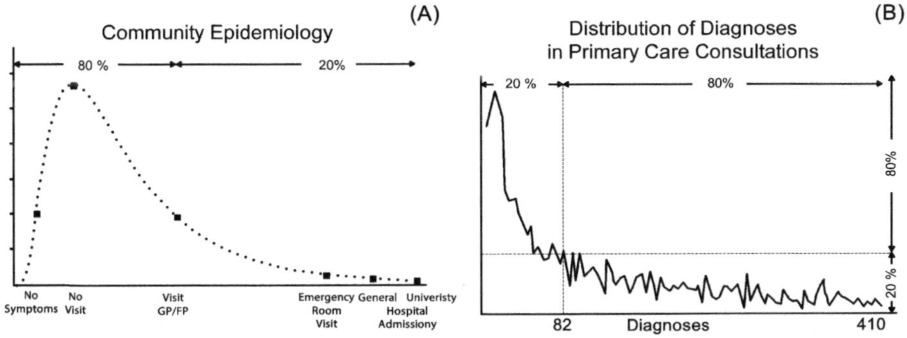


**Fig. 2** Epidemiology of health and disease in the community and in primary care. The 80/20 split or *Pareto distribution* is ubiquitous in natural phenomena. The experience of health and illness in the community shows that 80% of the population is healthy or healthy enough not to seek health care, 16% solely require primary care attention, 3.2% require specific disease-focused interventions and 0.8% care of a tertiary medical centre (**a**). The 80/20 split is also seen in the outcome of consultations—80% of consultations end without a 'specific diagnosis' being established (figure not shown), and 80% of patients have 20% of all different diagnoses, i.e. the majority of all different diseases effect only a small number of patients (**b**)

different ways at different points in time. The four main components contributing to our health and dis-ease experience are our somatic (or bodily) condition, our social connectedness, our emotional feelings and our semiotic (or sense-making) abilities—these four domains define the ***somato-psycho-socio-semiotic model*** of health and dis-ease [7].

While the definition of health remains contentious, almost all embrace its *experiential*, and to a lesser degree, its *semiotic* nature [7]. Health and dis-ease are personal and can be experienced both in the *presence* and *absence* of identifiable pathology (i.e. disease); hence, health and dis-ease are better defined in terms of 'complex adaptive states' (Fig. 3) [7, 8].

At this point, it needs to be emphasised that, over time, the term 'disease' has undergone a change in meaning; it no longer refers to its subjective experiential meaning of *dis-ease* and acquired the objective meaning of—principally visualisable—*pathology*.

## 1.3 The Cause of Disease

Historically, ailments were only observable at the macroscopic level, and thus classified by their observable characteristics based on morphological, emotional and cognitive experiences. This *phenomenological worldview* saw illness and disease arising from bad spirits, humoral imbalances or conflicts with the Gods. Accordingly, bad spirits needed to be set free (e.g. trephination), imbalances corrected with

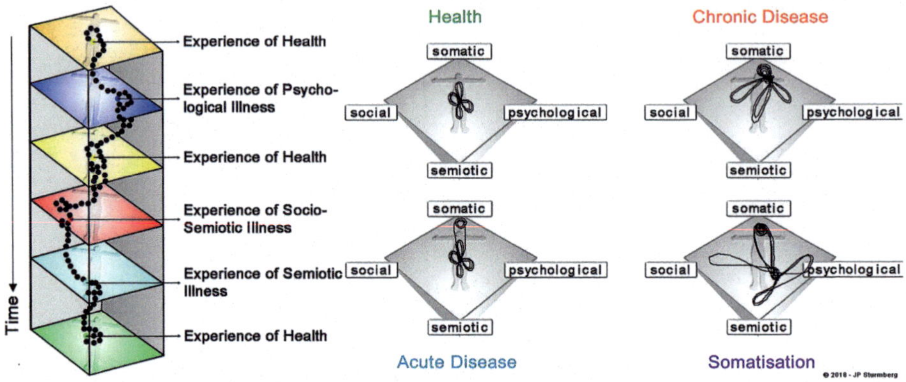


**Fig. 3** Dynamic picture of health and different disease states. The *experience of health and disease* varies over time—we are not 'healthy' exactly the 'same way' every morning we wake up. The left-hand side of the figure illustrates how the different components of health can shift our health experience over time, and how we generally regain our health experience in time. Collapsing the timeline onto a plain will show different patterns of our 'health dynamics'—minor variation around the *balanced state of health*, a shift in balance to the somatic component associated with a short episode of an acute illness (like the flu, pneumonia or a broken bone) resulting in a full recovery to health, a permanent shift of one's centre of health associated with chronic disease (like diabetes, osteoarthritis or melancholic depression) and the pattern of somatisation where a person 'jumps' between two states of health

remedies (e.g. herbs and magical potions) and conflicts with the Gods resolved with symbolic actions (e.g. dances and rituals) [9].

Not much has changed—we still follow the ancient patterns of visualising diseases, and then aim to correct this abnormal appearance to its 'pre-disease state', an approach holding well within the still prevailing mechanistic Newtonian worldview. While the techniques of visualisation have expanded and improved, therapeutic approaches have remained largely unchanged—*excising lesions*, *killing invaders* or *replacing broken parts* (Fig. 4). This visible 'cause-and-effect' mindset prevails, despite the emerging network physiological understandings of adaptive responses being able to maintain and restore 'healthy function'.

### 1.3.1 The Fallacy of 'Macroscopic Causation'

The fallacy of 'macroscopic causation'—or, these changes 'cause' this disease—goes back to Giambattista Morgagni who described the lesions he observed in an affected organ as the '*seat of disease*'. His understanding is holding well with the ancient ideas of disease understandings. Surprisingly, or maybe not so surprisingly, this notion persists into the present—the idea of the 'seat of disease' lives on in the International Classification of Disease (ICD) [10] and constantly reinforces the concept that the prime endeavour of medicine is the identification and treatment of 'macroscopic disease entities'.

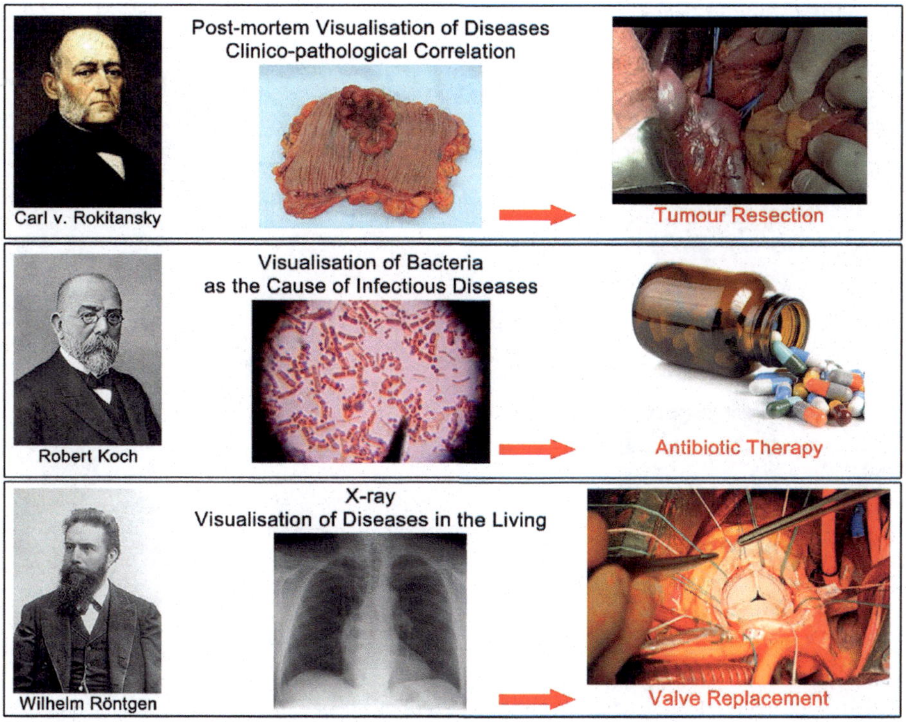


**Fig. 4** The macroscopic picture of disease and its 'therapeutic consequences'. Our understanding of disease is historically bounded by its visualisation—first, it was the post-mortem correlation of the symptoms of the patient with its pathological changes that caused them, and 'naturally' resulted in the therapeutic approach of removing those changes (top panel). The development of the microscope allowed the discovery of the 'disease-causing' organisms behind the dominant infectious diseases leading to premature mortality. The observation that the dyes used to visualise bacteria could also kill led to the emergence of the antibiotic area (middle panel). Finally, the discovery of X-rays allowed the visualisation of disease in the living person, and the correction of many abnormalities associated with the development of disabling or potentially life-threatening conditions

### 1.3.2 The Emergence of a Network Physiological Understanding of Health and Disease

The equation 'anatomical change = disease' is no longer a workable framework. This equation overlooks that the anatomical changes visible to the pathologist are the end-product of '*processes*', and thus the real question has to be: what have been the triggers in this person to trigger the pathways that 'created' this person's macroscopic lesion of disease (Fig. 5)?

Put differently, the preoccupation with the 'structural appearance' of disease detracts from the necessary focus on understanding HOW health and disease *emerge*, i.e. HOW the interconnected feedback loops of basic physiological inter-

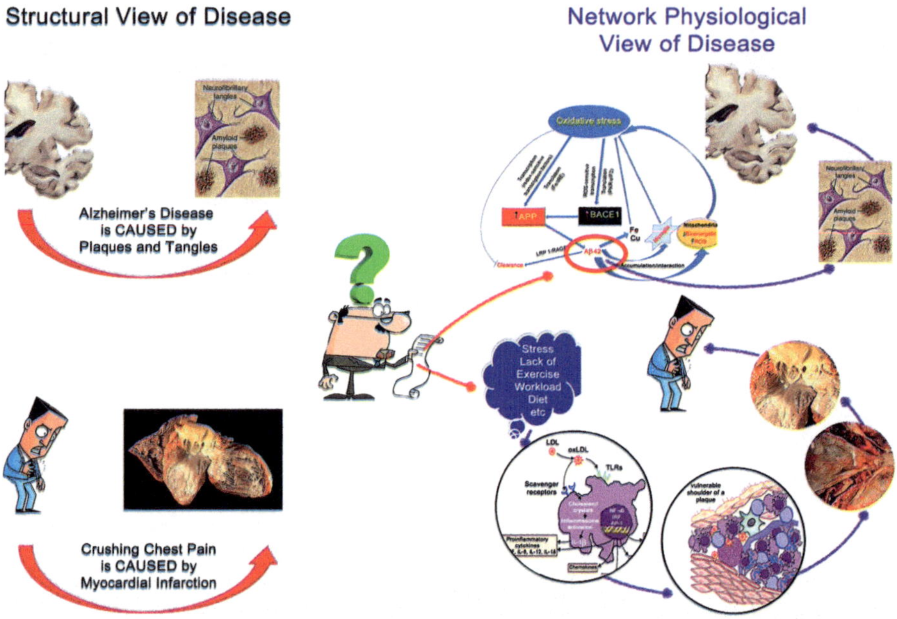


**Fig. 5** Shifting understanding of disease—no longer structural but rather functional. The still prevailing fallacy of "these changes 'cause' this disease"—as seen by the pathologist—is shown on the left of the figure. However, an increasing number of clinicians challenge this understanding and ask the questions: HOW did these change emerge? What is the dysfunction in the physiological mechanisms that created these changes? Network physiology has untangled the interdependent and circular pathways 'keeping us healthy' and their dysfunction 'making us sick'

actions regulate genomic, transcriptomic, metabolomic, proteomic and inflammasomic activities (Fig. 6)?

## *1.4 Disease: An Outcome of Mal-/Adaptive Regulatory Feedback*

Physiological pathways aim to maintain the organisms in a 'steady state', i.e. physiological parameters vary only slightly within a narrow 'normal range' (*homeostasis*). However, this is not always possible, and some dysfunction can result in temporary change outside the range resulting in 'reversible disease states'. If it is not possible to return to the 'normal range', the organism transitions to a new 'maintainable steady state', i.e. the physiological system and the organism as 'a whole' adapt (*homeokinesis*) [11, 12] (Fig. 7).

Thus, disease arises as an outcome of mal-/adaptive regulatory feedback amongst the interactions of multiple physiological networks—in particular, those that regulate gene networks [14, 15], activities of the autonomic nervous system [16] and

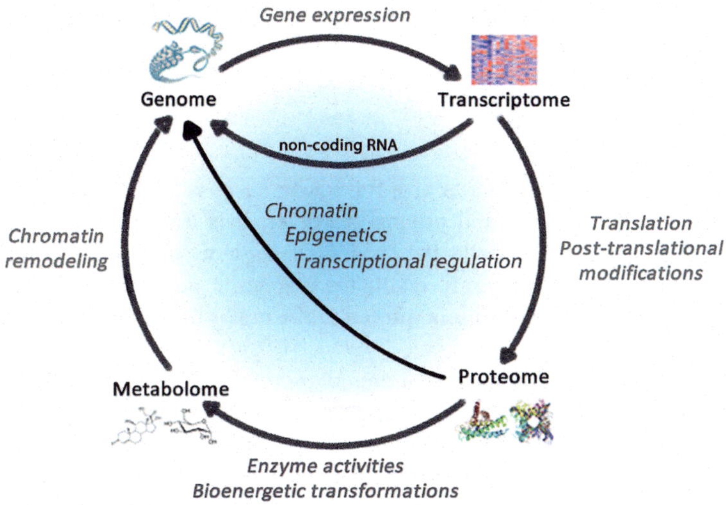


**Fig. 6** The 'Physiology of Life'. Regulatory cycle linking the omics of life. The genome comprises the totality of genes within an organism, which constitute the blueprint for the transcriptome, whose translation leads to proteins that accomplish enzymatic functions including bioenergetics transformations that consume and produce metabolites constituting the metabolome. In turn, gene transcripts, proteins and metabolites all impact expression genetic elements via dynamic processes subject to regulation. Reproduced from: Sturmberg et al. [13] (Creative Commons Attribution License (CC BY))

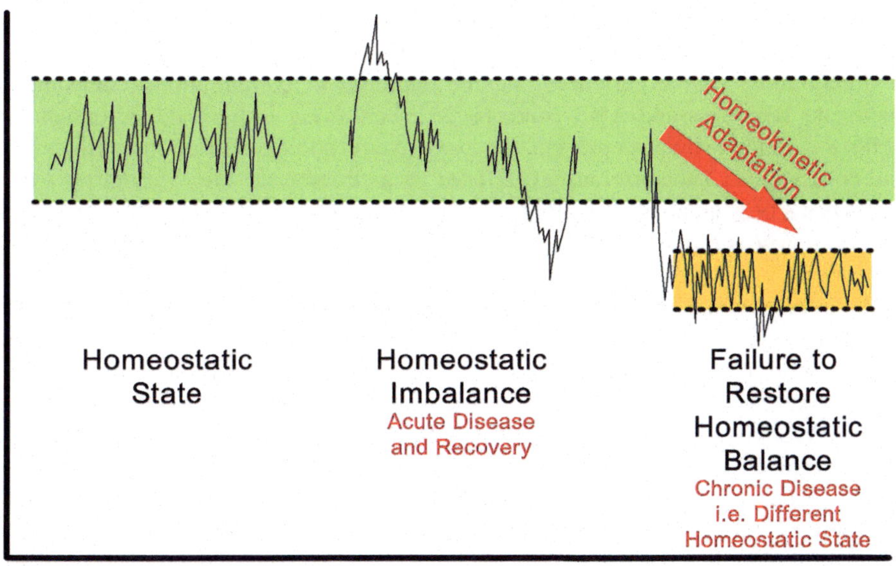


**Fig. 7** Homeostasis/Homeokinesis

the hypothalamic–pituitary–adrenal axis (HPA) [17, 18] as well as the bioenergetics within the mitochondrion [19, 20].

### 1.4.1 Genome Regulation

Genes provide the individual units of information necessary to produce the biological building blocks of cells and organs; however, it is the genome, i.e. the gene network interactions that encode the 'organism as a whole' [15]. Common and complex diseases appear to rarely result from specific gene mutations but rather from genome instability resulting in altered DNA methylation and changes in gene expression [15].

Furthermore, different cells may contain unique acquired genetic features in DNA sequence, DNA methylation and protein expression [21, 22] resulting in multiple cellular variants. These are essential for cellular adaptation during dynamic environmental change, but as a trade-off, they also contribute to disease [23].

### 1.4.2 Autonomous Nervous System and HPA-Axis Regulation

The overall function of the body is regulated by the fine-tuned HPA-axis and autonomous nervous system (ANS) regulatory pathways that jointly control the immune system responses to internal and external stressors.

HPA-axis perturbation influences gene expression via primary neuroendocrine mediators, neurotransmitters, hormones, and cytokines [18] which in turn influences the proteomic and metabolic network pathways. Dysregulated or perturbed beyond the adaptive capacity of the system, stressors may ultimately result in the emergence of diseases [24].

Importantly, past experiences and the appraisal of current life circumstances modulate HPA-axis and ANS controls [25]. Perceiving to have the resources or skills to handle a situation prevents an excessive physiological response. However, the conscious or subconscious experience of a stressor as 'loss of control'—the importance of which has been highlighted by Antonovsky [26, 27]—or threat to self results in over-stimulation of the stress systems and withdrawal of the calming ANS influence.

Short-term threatening situations activate the sympathetic nervous system resulting in the systemic release of high levels of epinephrine/norepinephrine which in turn promote immune system activity—in particular, the production of proinflammatory cytokine [28–30]. During recovery, cortisol and acetylcholine inhibit immune activity, thereby restoring the balance between the neuroendocrine and immune systems.

However, under chronic threat conditions [31], recovery of the calming nervous system may not occur, and immune cells become resistant to the constant presence of cortisol [32], leading to the removal/reduction of both anti-inflammatory pathways. Hence, proinflammatory cytokine production escalates and continues to fuel the stress systems—creating a vicious negative feedback cycle and multi-system perturbation.

### 1.4.3 Mitochondrial Regulation

Mitochondria are particularly sensitive to the effects of chronic stress and, as a consequence, interfere with the cellular energy production and other cell functions through intracellular signalling [33].

Chronic stress can result in mitochondrial damage [20] leading to pathogenic signalling cascades that can trigger systemic inflammation, alter the circulating metabolome, reduce energy production capacity and influence cellular gene expression [34]. These have wide-ranging effects on cell-specific parameters and the 'organism as a whole'. Mitochondrial dysfunction can cause organ-specific as well as multi-systemic disease resulting from increased oxidative stress [19, 35].

## *1.5 Diseases as Phenotypes*

Goh et al. first described the link between the disease *genome* and *disease phenome*—the observation resulted in the definition of the *diseasome* [14]. These findings challenge the historical understanding of 'phenotypical disease' as a result of specific dysfunctions; rather, they demonstrate that disease results from perturbations of complex intracellular and intercellular networks that link tissue and organ systems within a dynamic environmental context. This explains how and why diseases—as phenotypes—occur in clusters within the same person [14, 36].

## *1.6 Health, Dis-ease and Disease: A 'Whole of Person' Phenomenon*

All of the emerging evidence from diverse fields of studies indicate that health, dis-ease and disease are three different '*prototypical*' states arising from regulatory feedback between a person's interconnected physiological networks, i.e. they are a '*whole of person*' phenomenon [13, 37, 38]. Pro- and anti-inflammatory regulation—involving the immune, the autonomous nervous system and lipid-based mediators—are the main regulatory pathways mediating the *states* of health, dis-ease and disease [13, 39].

Physiological networks are constantly perturbated by internal (disease-causing agents) and external (social agents) disturbances—it is a person's physiological system's ability to maintain homeostatic stability that results in health; inability to maintain homeostasis results in dis-ease and/or disease. Mostly, the loss of homeostasis is temporary, and the system is able to return to a stable homeostatic state, i.e. restoring the 'state of health'. However, if unable to do so, the system aims to adapt to a 'new stable state' (*homeokinetic adaptation*)—fortunately, this new state is mostly associated with the experience of health despite objectively being associated with physical disease and/or disability (Fig. 7).

The understandings of health, dis-ease and disease as a '*whole of person*' phenomenon arising from network interactions across macro- to micro-scales can be summarised as depicted in Fig. 8. McEwen outlined the consequences of stressors on the brain and its physiological effects on the systems—quantified as allostatic load [40, 41]. Allostatic load determines acute and chronic responses leading to adaptive 'biological changes', especially in the brain[1] resulting in 'fixed changes' of emotional and physical disease [42]. Sturmberg et al. have outlined the consequences of chronic 'whole of person perturbation' on chronic disease development and its implications for disease prevention and health promotion [37, 38].

## *1.7 Detecting Physiological Dysregulation*

In the first instance, physiological dysregulation should be diagnosed based on the patient's complaints such as:

- Anxiety
- Low mood
- Irritability
- Low self-esteem
- Sleep disturbance and sleep deprivation
- Social isolation
- 'Being stressed out'
- Workplace issues—high workload, bullying and lack of support
- Physical and sexual abuse

and the presence of clinical conditions such as:

- Obesity
- Diabetes
- Heart disease—hypertension and ischaemic heart disease
- Frequent infections

These features are seen in many patients seeking health care and should alert the clinician to explore and manage the nature of the patient's increased allostatic load.

[1] Chronic stress results in brain remodelling:

- Atrophy of the ***prefrontal cortex***—impaired decision making, loss of working memory and loss of fear memory—impulse disorders, increased vigilance
- Atrophy of the ***hippocampus***—impaired contextual, temporal and spatial memory, and mood dysregulation
- Initial hypertrophy, later atrophy of the ***amygdala***—increased fear and anxiety, PTSD-like symptoms and impaired aggression control

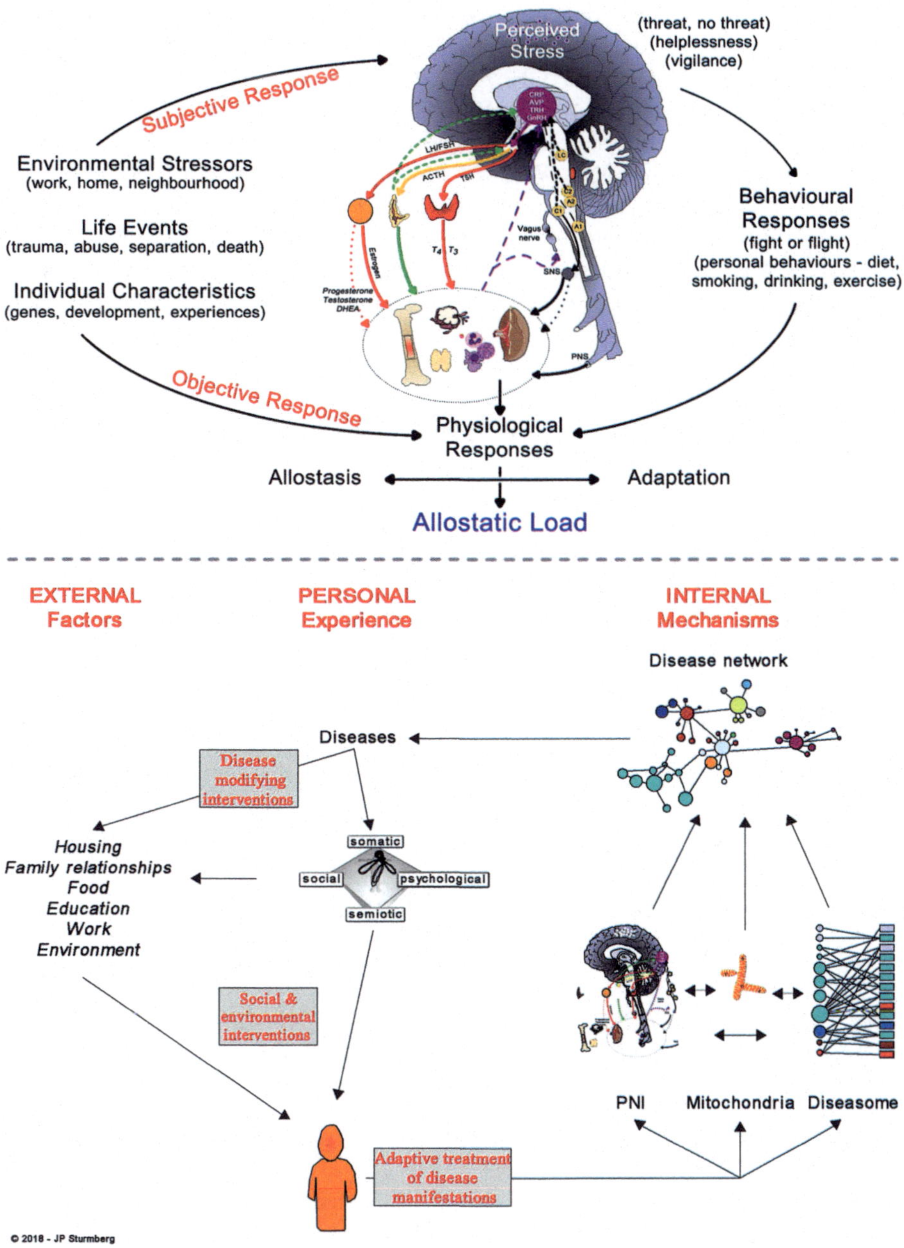


**Fig. 8** Physiological network understandings of health, dis-ease and disease. The central role of the brain in stress regulation and its effects on allostatic load (adapted from McEwan [43]) (top), and the system dynamics between external and internal mechanisms on the personal health experience (adapted from Sturmberg et al. [37]) (bottom)

Scientific endeavours demand that one should measure physiological dysregulation—proposed measures based on its neuroendocrine (cortisol, dehydroepiandrosterone-sulfate (DHEA-S), dopamine, epinephrine, norepinephrine and TSH), metabolic (BMI, cholesterol, glucose, $HbA_{1c}$, HDL, insulin resistance, insulin, insulin-like growth factor 1 (IGF-1), LDL, triglycerides, waist circumference, waist-hip-ratio (WHR)), cardiovascular (albumin, BP, heart rate variability (HRV), pulse pressure and resting heart rate), immune (CRP, E-selectin, ESR, fibrinogen, intracellular adhesion molecule 1 (ICAM-1), interleukin-6 (IL-6), percentage of neutrophils, tumour necrosis factor alpha (TNF-$\alpha$) and WBC count) and pulmonary (FEV1 and PEFR) and excretory (creatinine and homocysteine) consequences [44].

### 1.7.1 Biomarkers of Physiological Dysregulation Have Limited Application in Clinical Practice

As yet, there is no consensus which combination of biomarkers should be included in an allostatic load score—the most frequently used ones are systolic and diastolic blood pressure, BMI and waist-hip-ratio, triglyceride, HDL/TC ratio, HDL, $HbA_{1c}$, norepinephrine, epinephrine, cortisol DHEA-S and CRP [45]—and there are no clear cut-off points to guide clinical practice [46]. In addition, the experts' advice needs to be heeded—*biomarkers are frequently an imperfect measure of actual physiological processes* [47].

Overall, while allostatic load predicts future morbidity and mortality, as a measure it currently has promising but limited application in clinical practice [48–50]. Research has shown that allostatic load predicts successful ageing—high allostatic load was associated with increased mortality, and decreased physical and cognitive functioning [51]—and that allostatic load explains the multi-system effects of socio-economic status on mortality [52].

## *1.8 ... Your Appreciation of Health, Dis-ease and Disease Changes*

- 'Feeling healthy' and 'being healthy' is the rule, experiencing dis-ease is uncommon, having a disease is rare.
- Physiological network interactions assure homeostasis and the state of health; *excessive* **or** *prolonged low-level* perturbations by internal and external factors will result in homeokinetic adaptation, which may result in either a different state of health—even if associated with a disease, a state of dis-ease or a state of disease without the experience of health.

- Activation and regulation of the *physiological stress response pathways* are the principle mechanisms that maintain, cause and—most of the time—restore health.
- The diagnosis of health, dis-ease and disease is *a clinical one*—biomarker assays at large are supporting, but not confirming, clinical judgement.

## 2 Looking Differently: At *Healthcare Delivery*

Seeing 'health' differently raises questions about the way we provide 'health care'. Some obvious questions include:

- What should be the focus of 'healthcare' delivery?
- What actually should occur in the consultation between a healthcare provider and his patient?
- Can the current composition of healthcare providers actually meet 'health needs'?
- Who are the missing providers necessary required to ensure delivery of 'health care' that can achieve 'health'?

These questions are linked and need to be explored as one rather than on their own. They raise issues that span across the domains of health professional education—what is taught (culture, content and context) and what is shown (culture and praxis)—to healthcare organisation—the prevailing delivery structures around organ- or technology-based silos. A disease-focused culture, a disease-focused praxis and a disease-focused delivery system limits mindsets and perspectives, it fails to appreciate '*the whole*', it limits creativity and lateral thinking and it fails to integrate the '*social determinants of health*' to our care delivery.

### *2.1 Health Care: Is That Really What We Do?*

Historically, doctors always dealt with patients—meaning sufferers—lacking the *experience of health*, regardless of its underlying cause. Medical care relied on strengthening the '*self-healing powers within the patient*'. It was the only thing they could do as the causes of almost all ailments were largely unknown. Sitting with the patient through their illness taught an important lesson, namely, you have to know the person who has the disease.[2]

As already outlined above, only since we became able to *see* the causes of *some suffering* has the focus of care shifted from helping the patient to self-heal—making

[2]It is much ***more important to know*** what sort of a patient has a disease than what sort of a disease a patient has.—William Osler.

the patient the producer of his health and his doctor the co-producer—to one of removing the *visualisable* causes of disease behind his *suffering*—and making the person a passive recipient of 'doctor dictated' interventions.

#### 2.1.1 Shifting of the—Mental—Mind Frame

The frame [53] of 'health care' has shifted to one of 'disease management', and with it:

- The way we think about patients
- The way we interact with patients
- The way we see our role and
- The way we ascribe value to what we do

#### 2.1.2 In Essence Health Professionals Are Disease Managers

We are fixated on disease and operate within empires of disease management.

- We think about patients as 'carriers of diseases' that need to be found and managed
- We interact with patients as 'objects of disease'
- We see ourselves—the health professionals—as the 'fixers of diseases', and
- We value overwhelmingly what we do 'in relation to diseases'—rather than 'health'

#### 2.1.3 Disinterest in the Person with the Disease

What we have forgotten is the essence of being a doctor, our prime commitment to the 'person with the disease'[2] [54–56]. We also have forgotten our ***basic sciences***:

- Firstly, the nature of community epidemiology—most people seeking health care will not have a disease, they are *in dis-ease* [1–3], and
- Secondly, the network physiological basis of regulation and dysregulation being responsible for the maintenance of health and the emergence of disease [13, 39].

### *2.2 Disease Care at Work*

'The production unit of clinical care' is the consultation, and how it is conducted determines its effectiveness and efficiency [57]—undoubtedly, the current focus is on diseases and disease management, rather than the person with his illness experience. The way you talk reflects the way you think and act—the consequences are seen in the way you communicate with your patients, what you do, how you use limited health system resources and what you regard as the measures of success of your interventions.

### 2.2.1 Communication: About Disease

Doctor–patient communication is a strong predictor about consultation and health outcomes [58, 59]. Good communication leads to *shared understandings*, creates *trust* and enhances *decision-making*.

Today, communication is focused on the technical aspects of health care—the psychosocial dimension is usually seen as a 'nice add-on'. Thus, it is not really surprising that since the 1980s the average time at which the *doctor interrupts a patient* telling his complaint has decreased from 23 to 11 s [60], despite our knowledge that a patient on average needs between 90 and 120 s to tell the full story of his dis-ease (i.e. his complaint).

The slow and continuing decline in doctor–patient communication has been compared to the 'fleeting relationship' between a cab driver and his or her passenger [61], and the increasing use of provider and client—rather than doctor and patient—as one of a commercial contractual interaction [62, 63].

### 2.2.2 A Protocol-/Guideline-Driven Approach to Disease Management

Current approaches to patients' complaints reflect a culture of fear of failure and subsequent medicolegal consequences. Societal beliefs and expectations are 'objectively' unrealistic; however, they are not unexpected if seen in context. Success breeds contempt—having succeeded in overcoming the common infectious diseases in the early parts of the twentieth century has emboldened the health professionals to promise cure of all other diseases and do so without fail.

Today, a tacit symbiotic culture reigns health care, based on a self-reinforcing illusion—health professionals have 'designed the perfect way' of managing each disease, and 'disease customers' receive the perfect outcome as promised. However, maintaining this illusion becomes ever more difficult, and reinforces, for providers the vicious cycle of fear of failure and medicolegal threat, and for 'disease customers' the vicious cycle of repeated disappointment and loss of trust in the health professionals.

'Clinical practice guidelines are statements that include recommendations intended to optimize patient care that are informed by a systematic review of evidence and an assessment of the benefits and harms of alternative care options' [64]. Despite this clear statement of intent, clinical practice guidelines have emerged as one of the responses to manage the fear of failure and medicolegal threat [65, 66]. Guidelines are perceived as the 'right and only way' to manage disease—one by one. Again, they provide an illusion of certainty in the *complex vague real world of illness* with and without disease. Guidelines after all are mostly based on the limited evidence arising from clinical trials that at large use *surrogate measures*[3] to *determine the effectiveness* of an intervention under study [67–69]. However, *surrogates* not uncommonly are misleading and/or poor indicators of predicting causes of outcomes [70, 71] in terms of improved *quality of life* and *mortality* [72–74].

Many guidelines are problematic as they are conflicted by—usually undisclosed—conflicts of interest [66]. Guidelines, for whatever they are worth, are written for the 'average patient without any co-morbidity'—and cannot encompass the variability amongst patients—and thus *should only* ever be seen as a *guide*, rather than a cookbook and a medicolegal defence [75]. Unfortunately, in many jurisdictions, guideline adherence is now seen as the yardstick for appropriate practice, to a large extent reinforced by the professions' own indemnity insurers. Many insurers argue on purely economic grounds—it is cheaper for them to settle—often spurious—claims outside court than to defend 'appropriate care' in court.

### 2.2.3 Disease Management Results in Wasting Scarce Resources

Guidelines have been heavily promoted as 'a rational means' to standardise practice [76]. Guidelines entail an inherent assumption, in particular that diseases can be clearly defined, and that there is 'one proven way' to rationally manage each disease and thus be able to achieve a predictable predefined outcome.

There are several fundamental flaws in these assumptions, all of which contribute to the waist of scare healthcare resources. They include:

- ***Diseases are defined by unique criteria***—specific, well-defined aetiology, pathology, clinical picture, and specific treatment. This assumption ignores that diseases 'as entities' are socially constructed, and that they undergo constant redefinition [77–84]. As Rosenberg highlighted, one cannot discuss the *what* of disease without discussing the *when* and the *where*, i.e. the disease is as much a definable biomedical entity as a social and cultural entity at a particular point in time and tradition of thinking[4] (Appendix 1 details the definitional changes to three common diseases: hypertension, diabetes and depression).
- ***Disease behaviour is predictable***—a given treatment will have a specific dose–response relationship. This assumption ignores that diseases show a high degree of variability in terms of 'causative aetiology' as well as a high degree of variability in dose–response outcomes (non-linear behaviour of complex adaptive systems, see examples from cancer, hypertension, diabetes, hip fractures and Alzheimer's disease [85–101]).

---

[3] A surrogate is a laboratory measure or a physical sign that is intended to be used as a substitute for a clinically meaningful endpoint, e.g. reduction in tumour size as a measure of effectiveness of chemotherapy; low cholesterol as a measure of low cardiovascular risk; and rating scales as measures of disease/pain/distress/mood.

[4] Often referred to as *Zeitgeist*.

- ***Disease-specific interventions work***—evidenced by randomised controlled trial outcomes that show a 'statistically significant **relative** benefit' as demonstrated by a "$p$-value $\leq$ *0.05*.[5]" (see examples from cancer, diabetes, hypertension, screening and primary prevention [103–114]).

The focus on disease, rather than *dis-ease*, and the belief that early detection of disease saves lives, had other unintended consequence—the medicalisation of everyday life experiences or disease mongering [81, 115] and the rapid rise in overdiagnoses, i.e. finding 'diseases' that would never cause symptoms or death during a patient's remaining lifetime [107, 116–119]. Not only have these developments resulted in much harm to patients [120, 121], they also have been a great cost-driver [122–124]—at the individual as well as the societal level, generated irreconcilable conflicts of interest [123–127], and a marketing tool for ALL whose tacit primary goal is the increase of their profits. The consequences of medicalisation or disease mongering are seen in the rising prevalence of common conditions like hypertension, hyperlipidaemia, diabetes and depression and their respective drug consumption (Fig. 9 and Appendix 2) as well as 'early cancer diagnosis' and its associated treatments [128–130].

Disease management is believed to improve morbidity and mortality; however, as Tudor Hart already pointed out, disease management is of far lesser importance than the common socio-economic factors impacting health—standards of nutrition, housing, working environment and education, and the presence or absence of war [57]. The focus on disease fails to see the bigger picture—the person with the illness, and his ability to cope with the professionals' expectations and demands to self-manage and achieve their—guideline determined—pre-set goals.

Overall, the 'unintended consequences' of disease management are the fragmentation of care, the loss of the therapeutic relationship, higher rates of complications caused by over-treatment and treatment side effects, and lower quality of '*whole of patient care*' at unsustainably rising healthcare costs. Disease management is the unavoidable outcome of the economic rationalist paradigm—the laudable aim to decrease variability and improve quality turned 'sufferers into consumers' and 'health professionals into managerial assistants'.

## *2.3 Health Workforce Composition*

The workforce composition reflects the disease focus of the prevailing health systems. Figure 10 shows the composition of the Australian health workforce, three quarters of which comprise physicians and nurses.

---

[5]Remember—the $p$-value is a function of sample size, the larger the sample size required to achieve a '$p$-value $\leq$ *0.05*, the more likely it is that the difference is ***pragmatically*** meaningless [102].

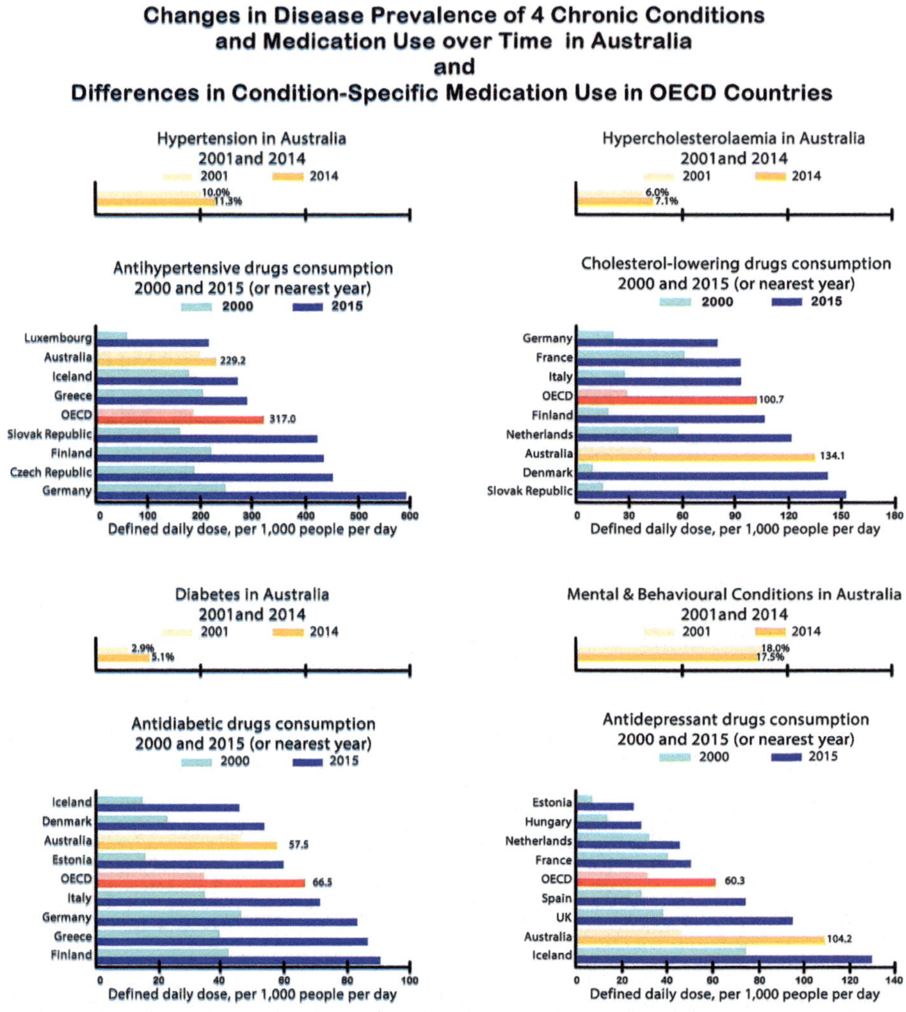


**Fig. 9** Contrasting illness and disease care. Note the wide range of variation in the prescribing rate of medications for hypertension, hypercholesterolaemia, diabetes and depression in selected OECD countries between 2000 and 2015 (Source: OECD (2017), Health at a Glance 2017: OECD Indicators, OECD Publishing, Paris. https://doi.org/10.1787/health_glance-2017-en). The top panels show the prevalence of hypertension, hypercholesterolaemia, diabetes and depression changes between 2001 and 2014—note the decline in Mental & Behavioural Conditions and the marked increase in prescribing of antidepressants (Source: Australian Bureau of Statistics. National Health Survey. Australia 2001: http://www.ausstats.abs.gov.au/Ausstats/subscriber.nsf/0/90A3222FAD5E3563CA256C5D0001FD9D/\protect\T1\textdollarFile/43640_2001.pdf and Australian Bureau of Statistics. National Health Survey. First Results Australia 2014–15: http://www.ausstats.abs.gov.au/Ausstats/subscriber.nsf/0/CDA852A349B4CEE6CA257F150009FC53/\protect\T1\textdollarFile/national%20health%20survey%20first%20results,%202014-15.pdf)

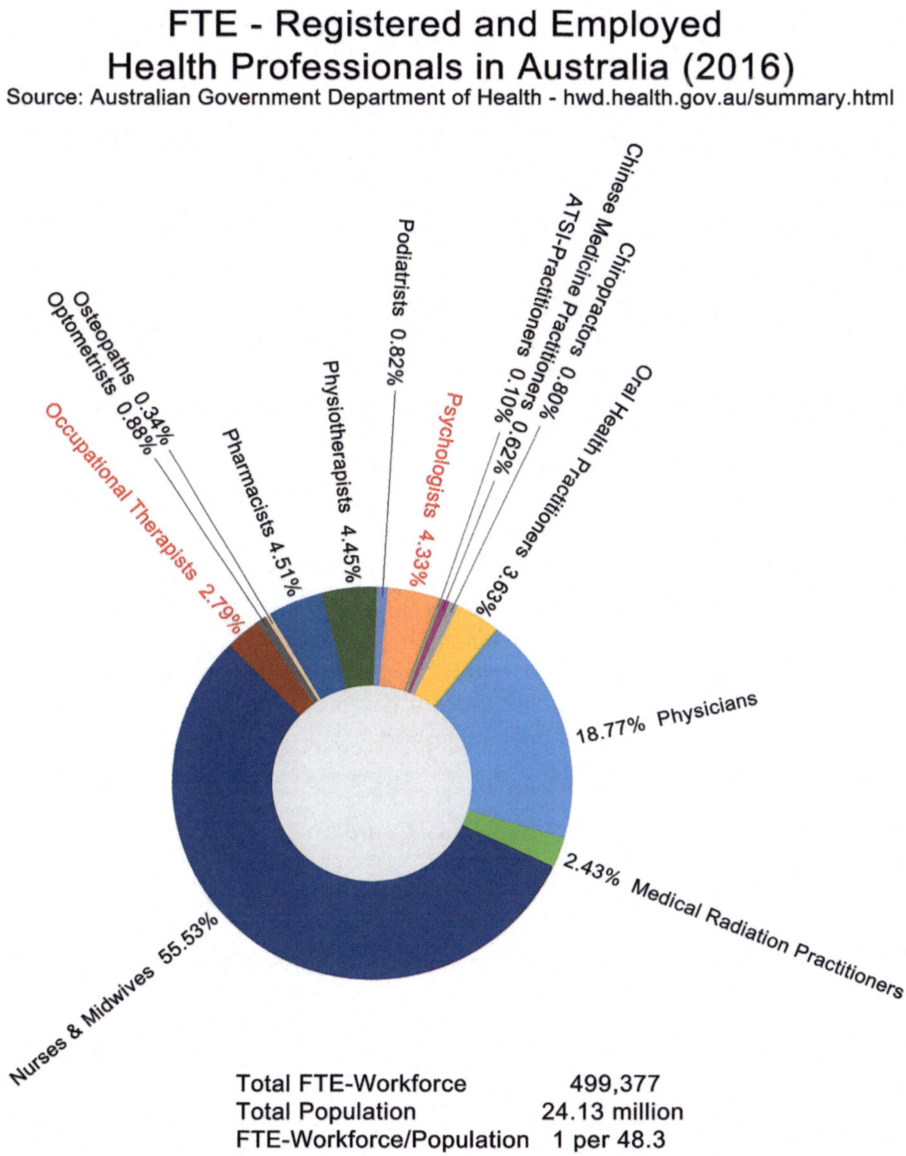


**Fig. 10** Most health professionals' work are focused on disease. The current workforce composition at large consists of health professionals focused on diseases, and thus are clearly better described as *disease managers*. Amongst the workforce, psychologists and occupational therapists (and to some degree physiotherapists) deal with support of people living with disease

The majority of the 102,805 registered medical practitioners work in a disease-focused environment—35% are specialists (134 per 100,000 population), 31.1% specialists-in-training and hospital non-specialists, but only 33.1% are general practitioners (112 per 100,000 population). Of note, of the 35,982 specialists only 655 work in general medicine and 511 in geriatric medicine [131].

The same pattern is evident amongst the 331,804 registered nurses (273,404 registered nurses and 58,000 enrolled nurses)—55.8% of RNs and 45.1% of ENs work in the hospital sector. Only a small number of nurses are working in supportive care services like Aged Care (10% of RNs and 32.7% ENs), Mental Health (6.7% of RNs and 5.5% ENs), Community Health (5% of RNs and 3.1% ENs), Rehabilitation & Disability (2.5% of RNs and 5.7% ENs) and Child & Family Health(1.8% of RNs and 0.4% ENs) [132].

A more patient-oriented health service requires a locally adapted and adaptive health workforce that can manage the needs of its community [133]. This will help to overcome fragmentation of care along disease silos and integration of services across the medical, social and community services [134, 135].

Thus, a largely missing or not counted workforce in the health sector focused on maintaining health and independence, or preventing disease to occur in the first instance include:

- Social workers
- Adolescent health workers
- Social support workers for families with young children
- Support workers for the elderly and the frail
- Workers who create and maintain public infrastructure that enables healthy and independent living like walk and cycle ways, playgrounds and parks, public housing for those in need and public transport

### 2.3.1 Evaluating Outcomes: Which Ones Count?

What matters, and to whom? The focus on disease management demands an evaluation of disease-specific outcomes like diseases cured, disease indicators improved, disease-specific complication rates, impact on disease mortality and disease-specific expenditure impact.

Patients' satisfaction with their management is one of a few outcome measures that involve patient input. However, patient satisfaction is largely an indicator of expectations being met [136], rather than a true indicator of *quality of care* [136–139] or the *impact on patients' ability to cope* or their *experience of well-being* [140].

Overall, outcome measures that matter to patients, other than survival, remain limited [141]. In addition, what outcomes matter to patients and providers in the context of a particular condition vary widely across three key domains—the natural history and treatment effects of the condition; treatment goals and concerns; and treatment options and their effectiveness and impacts (Table 1) [142, 143]. The prevailing disease management focus, unsurprisingly, looks at 'easily measurable' and

**Table 1** Significant differences in priorities between patient and provider priorities (in %) in decision-making for six different conditions

| | | % patients | % providers |
|---|---|---|---|
| Breast cancer [143] | Waiting for 4 weeks to make a treatment decision does not affect survival | 14 | 53 |
| | Keep the breast | 7 | 71 |
| | Do what your doctors think is best | 86 | 14 |
| | Radiation can increase complications and affect cosmetic result of reconstruction | 24 | 60 |
| | Women who do not have reconstruction generally are as satisfied as women who do | 5 | 30 |
| | Avoid using a prosthesis | 33 | 0 |
| | Women with serious health problems may gain less benefit from Chemotherapy/Hormone Therapy | 35 | 5 |
| | Chemotherapy/Hormone Therapy can cause rare, serious side effects (heart problems, cancers, infection and clots) | 24 | 0 |
| | Live as long as possible | 59 | 96 |
| Benign prostatic hyperplasia [144] | Focus on symptoms of BPH | 27 | 61 |
| | Necessity of treatment | 9 | 50 |
| | Avoid surgery | 22 | 68 |
| Herniated disc [144] | Natural history | 48 | 77 |
| | Continuing your usual activities as much as possible will not make a herniated disc worse | 58 | 27 |
| | Avoid taking medication | 39 | 5 |
| | Do what doctor thinks is best | 36 | 9 |
| Spinal stenosis [144] | Natural history | 31 | 59 |
| | Surgery is more likely to help leg pain than back pain | 44 | 73 |
| | Avoid taking medication | 28 | 5 |
| | Do what doctor thinks is best | 46 | 5 |
| Hip osteoarthritis [144] | Do what doctor thinks is best | 84 | 44 |
| Knee osteoarthritis [144] | Quantitative estimates of benefits of total knee replacement | 51 | 88 |
| | Do what doctor thinks is best | 78 | 35 |

'bureaucratically countable[6]' process measures (1181 of 1958 outcome measures in the National Quality Measures Clearinghouse database); while patient-relevant measures of 'functional health' are largely lacking despite the fact that they are those most relevant to patients seeking care [141].

[6]Countable does not equate to *accountable*.

## 2.4 ... *Your Appreciation of the Healthcare Delivery Changes*

- Understanding the person's *health and illness experience* is central to healthcare delivery.
- The aim of the consultation is the improvement of the *person's health experience*, his *ability to cope* and to *keep his independence*, regardless of the underlying nature of his complaints.
- It takes *uninterrupted time* for the patients to convey their concerns. It is time well-spent in the consultation as the *patient's story invariably uncovers* the diagnosis of illness (or *dis-ease*) or disease.
- Health, illness and disease are complex phenomena and thus require adaptive management approaches that consider the interdependency of the patient's biological, social, emotional and cognitive domains.
- Healthcare delivery is driven by the patient's goals rather than his diseases.
- Always consider if earlier diagnosis, latest tests, drugs and interventions, and achieving 'pre-defined' treatment targets is congruent with the patient's needs and goals.
- Assemble the right health, social and support team for your patient and your community.
- The ultimate measure of success in healthcare delivery is the patient's improvement in *self-rated health* (Fig. 11).

# 3 Looking Differently: At the *Healthcare System*

In summary, the health professional mindset is overwhelmingly focused on disease—not health or *dis-ease*—and their work is controlled by guidelines and protocols that have minimal regard to the personal worries and needs of the patients' they are supposed to ***care*** for. Hence, our so-called healthcare systems are in fact nothing more than 'disease management systems' (Fig. 12).

Closer analysis in fact shows that health systems are:

- Fragmented in terms of organisation along disease silos, and
- Controlled by financial interests, be it profit maximisation by private enterprise or cost-control motives by governments and/or insurers [134, 135].

This disease and economics focus has shaped the mindset and the language dominating the 'health system discourse' amongst clinicians, policy-makers and health system managers alike.

Annas—in the mid-1990s—already emphasised how the metaphors of the 'military' and 'market' have pervaded the healthcare system discourse and their consequences to patient care as well as health system organisation and financing (Appendix 3) [144].

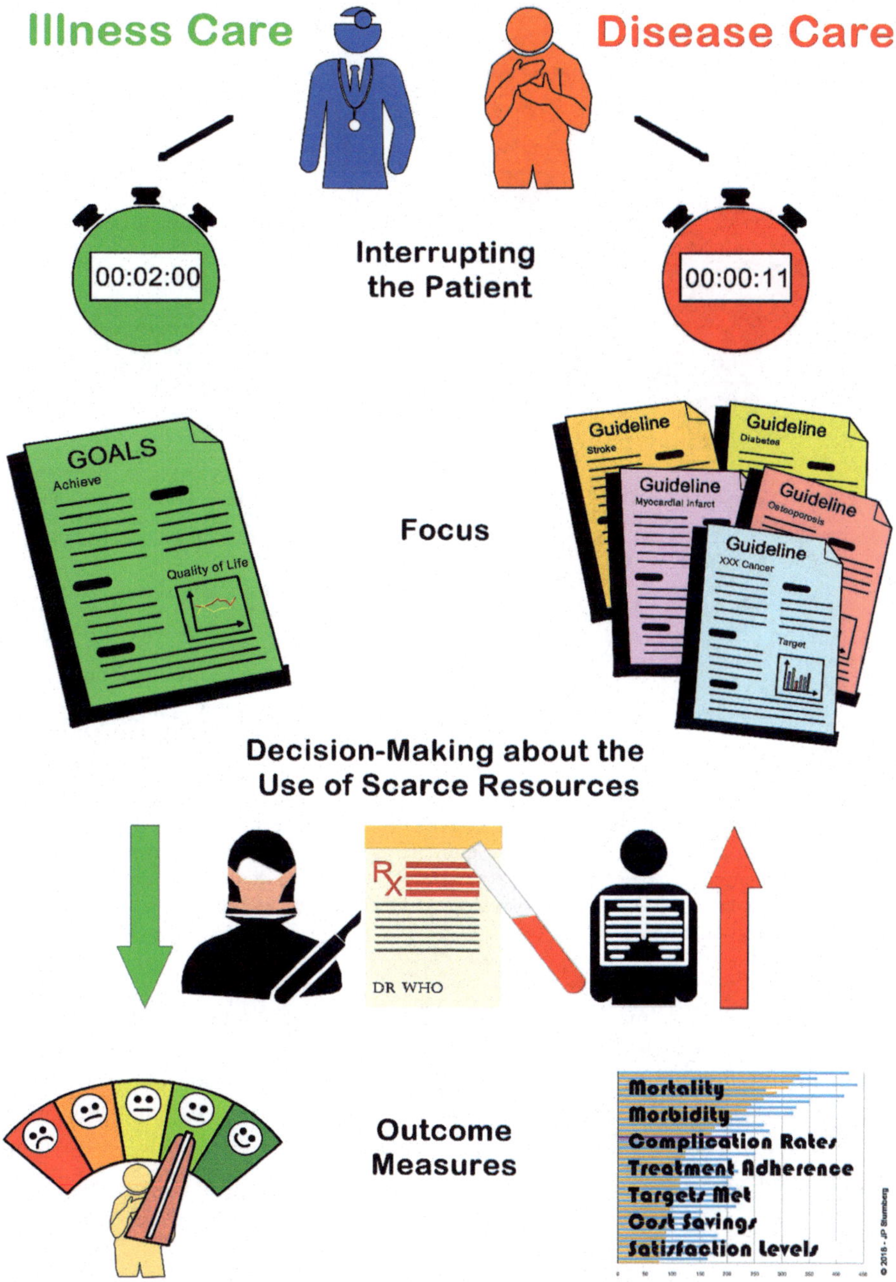


**Fig. 11** Contrasting illness and disease care. *Person-centred* health care has distinctively different approaches to *disease-centred* care—patients can talk *uninterruptedly* to describe their complaints, care elicits and works towards achieving the *patient's goals*, and as a corollary will largely avoid unnecessary and/or harmful interventions. The *person-centred* approach to care measures its success in terms of improving the patient's *self-rated health*. A universal *person-centred* approach to patient care is an important step in ensuring an equitable and sustainable health system

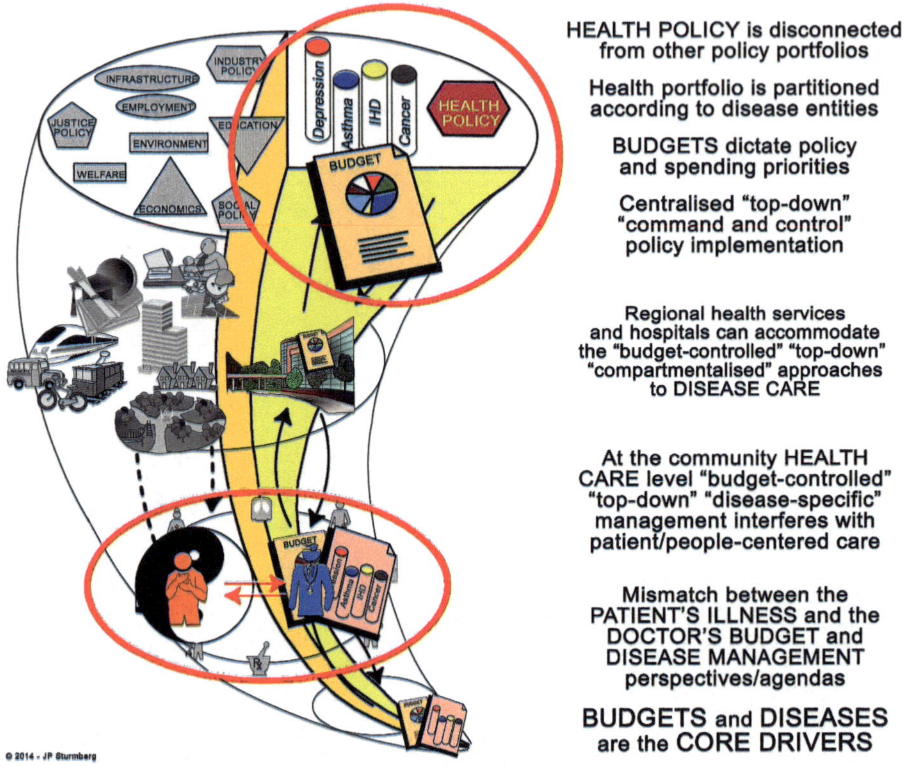


**Fig. 12** The dynamics of the prevailing 'healthcare systems'. Healthcare systems are dysfunctional—their primary focus is on diseases and budgets, permeating through the hierarchy of the system as depicted by the health vortex. Notably, patients and doctors have an agenda of dealing with and managing their concerns; at the policy level, health is disconnected from other policy domains, and health departments themselves are fragmented and silolised according to disease entities and budget item lines

The 'military' and 'market-economic' language clearly support the *status quo*, i.e. they maintain the disease management framework and support vested interest groups that profit from it. These groupings are not limited to the pharmaceutical and device maker industries, but also include health insurers, hospital and other health system organisations, health professionals and 'diseased patient' interest and support groups.

### *3.1 The Disease Focus Diverts Attention and Resources Away from 'Being Healthy' and 'Staying Healthy'*

Health systems are largely focused on the secondary and tertiary level of care delivery which caters for about 4% of the community [1, 2], and only very recently have started to pay more than lip service to primary care—albeit with a focus on disease management—catering for the 16% of the community seeking health care—just a reminder: primary care delivers 80% of all health services.

The greater the disease focus of a health system, as exemplified by the USA, the more expensive it will be—the US health system is nearly twice as expensive as the second most expensive health system (Germany), and about three times more expensive as, e.g. the health systems in the UK, Spain or Sweden. Despite its high spending, the USA has the worst population health status indicators of all OECD countries [145].

The greater disease orientation of health systems has direct negative impacts on morbidity and mortality. More primary care-oriented health systems with a greater number of primary care physicians have better population health outcomes evidenced by lower all-cause mortality, all-cause premature mortality, cause-specific premature mortality from asthma, bronchitis, emphysema and pneumonia, cardiovascular disease and heart disease, stroke, cancer and infant mortality as well as a lower rate of low birth weight infants, an increase in life expectancy and the number of people reporting good, very good or excellent self-rated health [146, 147].

Disease-focused health system fail the equity test, i.e. it affects people in the lower socio-economic strata more—the disease focus perpetuates the *inverse care law*; people with more need have less access to health services and receive less comprehensive care than those with lesser needs from high socio-economic strata [148].

In fact, primary health care with a greater focus on the person and despite its greater complexity [149], largely arising from the multiple morbidities affecting their patients [150], achieve the same disease-specific outcomes at significantly lower cost [151, 152]—disease-oriented specialty care resulted in 41% higher rate of hospitalisation and 12% higher rate of prescribing compared to generalist-oriented care for the same condition.

The benefits of person-focused primary care have been attributed to the development and maintenance of a therapeutic relationship [55, 153] which itself requires a significant level of provider continuity [154] to build the necessary familiarity and trust between the physician and the patient [153, 155, 156]. The benefits of, and thus the justification for, a person-centred therapeutic relationship have been studied extensively and are well-documented in the literature [157–161].

## 3.2 *Reframing Our Metaphors: Achieving Health*

Understanding the *status quo* is a prerequisite to 'reframing' the metaphors [53] necessary to facilitate the redesign of frameworks that allow a different system to emerge—one focused on the person, his health and *dis-ease*, as well as his diseases [162].

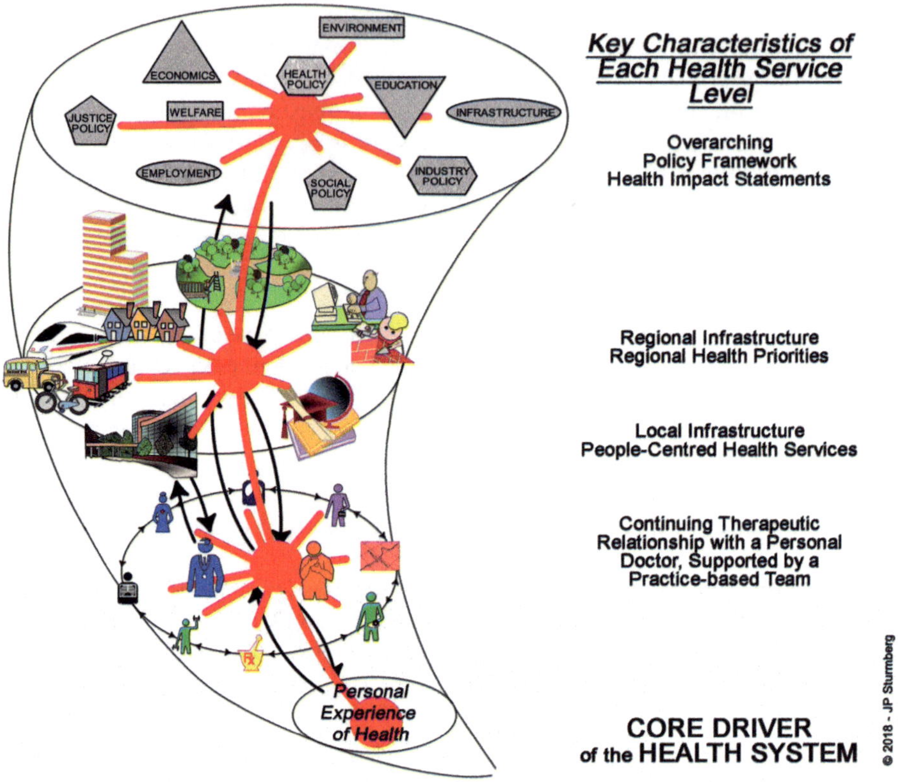


**Fig. 13** The *Health Vortex* as a metaphor for the redesign of a health system focused on health. In a fully integrated health system, all agents at all levels are focused on *the health experience* of the person—the core driver of the system. While various layers within the system have specific work to do, the system only becomes seamlessly integrated if all—despite their different tasks—maintain their focus on the core driver—*the health experience* of the person

A metaphor to achieve a person-centred complex adaptive health system is that of the healthcare vortex (Fig. 13).

- As any complex adaptive social system requires a clearly defined focal point to emerge, a health system focused on the health of people must put the person with his health and dis-ease experiences at its centre [134, 163].
- In addition, it is important to understand the 'causative' relationships across layered human complex adaptive systems—top-down causation imposes *contextual constraints* limiting bottom-up *emergent possibilities* [37, 164].
- The importance of understanding this top-down bottom-up hierarchical relationship explains why it is so important for the policy level to integrate all policy domains in a 'health focus' way—we need to demand from our politicians to provide a 'health impact statement' for *all new policies* to ensure they are health promoting rather than health destroying (Fig. 14).

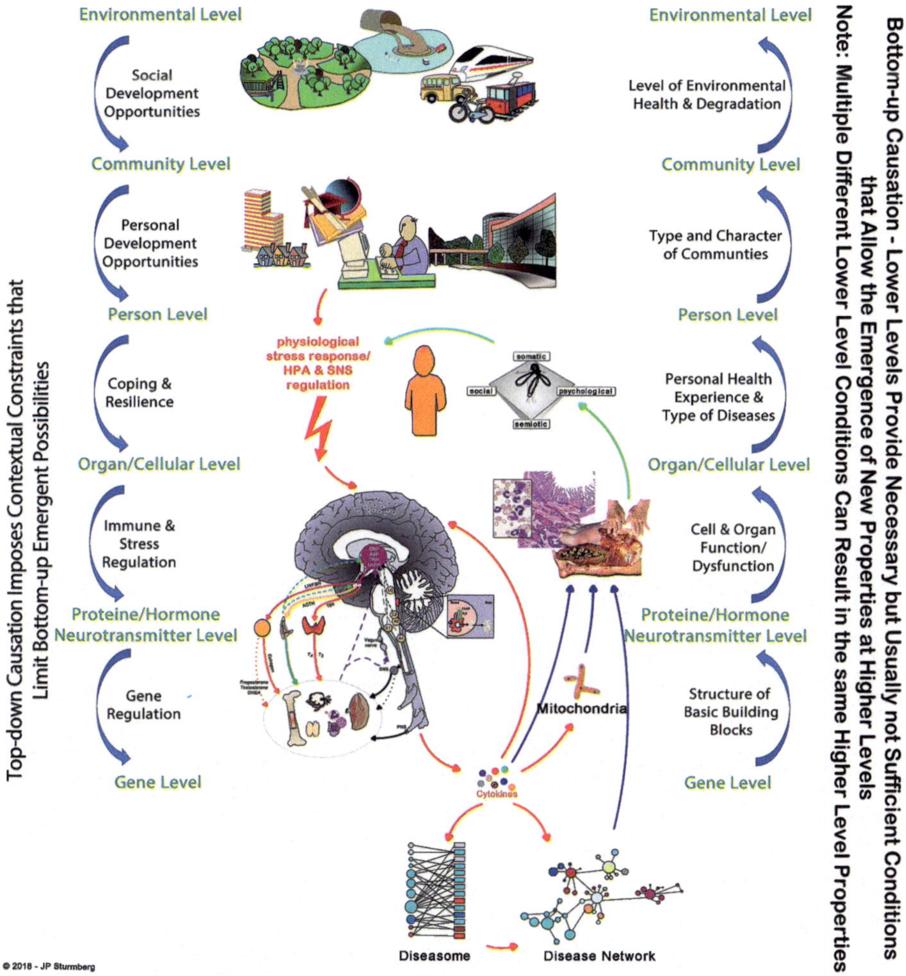


**Fig. 14** Top-down constraints limit bottom-up emergence—implications for health system redesign. Ellis [164] pointed to the top-down bottom-up causational relationship of hierarchical complex adaptive systems. Hierarchical systems, like the health system, are *top-down constraining* its *bottom-up emergent potentials*. In other words, external factors impact the person and—through activation of the physiological stress response and autonomic nervous system regulation—the physiology of organs, cells and genes (left-hand site), limiting the full biological potential of a person, and his abilities to succeed in his environment (right-hand site). Note that different lower level network interactions can result in the same higher level outcome, or what Rothman called the "multiple different combinations of sufficient causes" to achieve the same result [165]

These considerations are a *prerequisite* for *designing* health systems that are effective, equitable and sustainable [162].

## 3.3 ... Your Appreciation of the Healthcare System Changes

- Healthcare systems must embrace the *hierarchical top-down constraining, bottom-up emerging dynamics* between the macro-level policy and the micro-level physiology that effect health at the person level.
- Healthcare systems should have *the needs of the person/patient* at its centre.
- Healthcare systems have to rebuild *trust* that their healthcare professionals act in the *best interest of the patient.*
- Healthcare systems need to be *seamlessly integrated* with other *social services* and all other policy domains.
- Raises the question if healthcare systems should be *common good for-all* or commercial *for-profit* entities.
- Raises the question how best to finance healthcare systems so that they are *person-centred, equitable and sustainable* [162]?

## The Transformative Aspects of This Study

This essay outlines the historical developments of our current health systems. When we were finally able to understand the symptoms in the patients by studying his post-mortem disease findings, followed by seeing the causes of disease under the microscopy or by X-ray, disease had established itself as the focus of the medical enterprise. The successes of dealing with the manifestations of disease had distracted from any question about the 'physiological pathways' resulting in the diseases, and with it the curiosity of pre-emptively working to eliminate those factors that interfered with staying healthy or regaining one's health. Engaging with the fundamentals of health and disease must be the necessary step in redesigning a health system that focuses again on the nature of the healing professionals—it is more important to know the person with the disease.

**Take Home Message**

- The current approach to health care and the organisational structure of the healthcare system must be understood in their historical context—the discovery of the macroscopic and microscopic changes of diseases.
- The experience of disease is emergent with a hierarchical network of macro-level environmental factors to micro-level physiological dys/function.

(continued)

- Stimulation of the physiological stress response—HPA-axis and SNS regulation—controls the immune system dys/function responsible for the maintenance of health as well as the causation of disease.
- Healthcare professionals need to give patients the time they require to uninterruptedly explain their current complaint.
- The key achievement of health care is the improvement of patients' self-rated health. Health system redesign needs to put the patient at the centre of the system.

## Appendix 1: Disease Definitions and Re-definitions

| Hypertension | |
|---|---|
| 1948 | *The blood pressure is* [considered to be] *raised when the systolic pressure is 180 or over, and/or the diastolic pressure is 110 or over, on three consecutive examinations, and in the presence of clinical, radiological and cardiographic evidence of cardiovascular hypertrophy.— Evans W. Hypertension. In: Cardiology. London, England: Paul B. Hoeber, Inc; 1948:204* |
| 1949 | *In a patient with mild benign hypertension*—[defined as a] *blood pressure <200/<100 mm Hg, there is no indication for use of hypotensive drugs. Continued observation is desirable and conservative treatment consisting of reassurance, mild sedatives, and weight reduction is indicated.— Friedberg CK. Diseases of the Heart. Philadelphia, PA: WB Saunders Co; 1949* |
| 1960s | Hypertension = BP > 100+age |
| 1977 | JNC 1— *Moser M. From JNC I to JNC 7-what have we learned? Prog Cardiovasc Dis. 2006;48:303–315*<br>• Diastolic BP >105 mm Hg requires treatment |
| 2003 | JNC 7— *Moser M. From JNC I to JNC 7-what have we learned? Prog Cardiovasc Dis. 2006;48:303–315*<br>• Normal BP 120–129/80–89 |
| 2017 | American College of Cardiology/American Heart Association (ACC/AHA) guidelines—*Whelton PK, Carey RM, Aronow WS, Casey DE, Collins KJ, Dennison Himmelfarb C, DePalma SM, Gidding S, Jamerson KA, Jones DW, MacLaughlin EJ, Muntner P, Ovbiagele B, Smith SC, Spencer CC, Stafford RS, Taler SJ, Thomas RJ, Williams KA, Williamson JD and Wright JT. 2017 ACC/AHA/AAPA/ABC/ACPM/AGS/APhA/ASH/ASPC/NMA/PCNA Guideline for the Prevention, Detection, Evaluation, and Management of High Blood Pressure in Adults. A Report of the American College of Cardiology/American Heart Association Task Force on Clinical Practice Guidelines. Hypertension. 2017;71(6):1269–324*<br>• Hypertension >130/80 mm Hg |

(continued)

| Hypertension | |
|---|---|
| Diabetes mellitus—definition is based on occurrence of diabetic retinopathy | |
| 1979 | National Diabetes Data Group—*Classification and diagnosis of diabetes mellitus and other categories of glucose intolerance. National Diabetes Data Group. Diabetes. 1979 Dec;28(12):1039–57*<br>Based on 77 out of 1213 people developing retinopathy<br>• Fasting plasma glucose (FPG) concentration of $\geq$ 7.8 mmol/L (140 mg/dL), or<br>• 2-h value after 75 g oral glucose of $\geq$ 11.1 mmol/L (200 mg/dL) |
| 1997 | Expert Committee on the Diagnosis and Classification of Diabetes Mellitus—*Report of the Expert Committee on the Diagnosis and Classification of Diabetes Mellitus. Diabetes Care. 1997;20(7):1183–97*<br>Diagnosis of diabetes by linking levels of glycaemia with diabetic retinopathy in populations of Pima Indians (n = 960), Egyptians (n = 1081), and a randomly selected cohort in the Third National Health and Nutrition Examination Survey (NHANES III) (n = 2821)<br>• Fasting plasma glucose (FPG) criterion of $\geq$ 7.0 mmol/L (126 mg/dL) |
| Diabetes mellitus—definition is based on occurrence of diabetic retinopathy | |
| 2010 | American Diabetes Association— *Diagnosis and classification of diabetes mellitus. American Diabetes Association. Diabetes Care. 2010;33(Suppl 1):S62–9*<br>• $HbA_{1c}$ levels $\geq$ 6.5% |
| Depression—disease or syndrome | |
| 1920s–1970s | Textbook definitions of endogenous and reactive depression:<br>• Endogenous depression (severe disorder with delusions and hallucinations)<br>• Reactive depression (milder disorder without delusions and hallucinations; often with the connotation of a vulnerable personality, in the context of life stresses, features of diurnal variation with morning worsening, delayed insomnia with early morning wakening and greater somatic disturbances, such as loss of appetite and weight, and psychomotor retardation or agitation |
| 2013 | DSM-V major depression<br>(**A**) Five (or more) of the following symptoms have been present during the same 2-week period and represent a change from previous functioning; at least one of the symptoms is either (1) depressed mood or (2) loss of interest or pleasure<br>Note: Do not include symptoms that are clearly attributable to another medical condition<br>1. Depressed mood most of the day, nearly every day, as indicated by either subjective report (e.g., feels sad, empty and hopeless) or observation made by others (e.g. appears tearful). (Note: In children and adolescents, can be irritable mood) |

(continued)

| Depression—disease or syndrome | |
|---|---|
| | 2. Markedly diminished interest or pleasure in all, or almost all, activities most of the day, nearly every day (as indicated by either subjective account or observation)<br>3. Significant weight loss when not dieting or weight gain (e.g., a change of more than 5% of body weight in a month), or decrease or increase in appetite nearly every day. (Note: In children, consider failure to make expected weight gain)<br>4. Insomnia or hypersomnia nearly every day<br>5. Psychomotor agitation or retardation nearly every day observable by others, not merely subjective feelings of restlessness or being slowed down)<br>6. Fatigue or loss of energy nearly every day<br>7. Feelings of worthlessness or excessive or inappropriate guilt (which may be delusional) nearly every day (not merely self-reproach or guilt about being sick)<br>8. Diminished ability to think or concentrate, or indecisiveness, nearly every day (either by subjective account or as observed by others)<br>9. Recurrent thoughts of death (not just fear of dying), recurrent suicidal ideation without a specific plan, or a suicide attempt or a specific plan for committing suicide<br><br>(**B**) The symptoms cause clinically significant distress or impairment in social, occupational or other important areas of functioning<br>(**C**) The episode is not attributable to the physiological effects of a substance or to another medical condition<br>Note: Criteria A–C represent a major depressive episode<br>Note: Responses to a significant loss (e.g., bereavement, financial ruin, losses from a natural disaster, a serious medical illness or disability) may include the feelings of intense sadness, rumination about the loss, insomnia, poor appetite and weight loss noted in Criterion A, which may resemble a depressive episode<br>Although such symptoms may be understandable or considered appropriate to the loss, the presence of a major depressive episode in addition to the normal response to a significant loss should also be carefully considered. This decision inevitably requires the exercise of clinical judgment based on the individual's history and the cultural norms for the expression of distress in the contest of loss<br>(**D**) The occurrence of the major depressive episode is not better explained by schizoaffective disorder, schizophrenia, schizophreniform disorder, delusional disorder or other specified and unspecified schizophrenia spectrum and other psychotic disorders<br>(**E**) There has never been a manic episode or a hypomanic episode. Note: This exclusion does not apply if all of the manic-like or hypomanic like episodes are substance-induced or are attributable to the physiological effects of another medical condition |

(continued)

| DSM-V adjustment disorder | |
|---|---|
| | • Emotional or behavioural symptoms develop in response to an identifiable stressor or stressors within 3 months of the onset of the stressor(s) plus either or both of (1) marked distress that is out of proportion to the severity or intensity of the stressor, even when external context and cultural factors that might influence symptom severity and presentation are taken into account and/or (2) significant impairment in social, occupational or other areas of functioning<br>• The stress-related disturbance does not meet criteria for another mental disorder and is not merely an exacerbation of a pre-existing mental disorder<br>• The symptoms do not represent normal bereavement<br>• After the termination of the stressor (or its consequences), the symptoms persist for no longer than an additional 6 months |

## Appendix 2: Prevalence of Long-Term Conditions in the Australian National Health Survey

| | 2001[a] | 2014[b] |
|---|---|---|
| Arthritis | | 15.3% (3.5 million people) |
| Asthma | 12% (2.2 million people) | 10.8% (2.5 million people) |
| Cancer | 1.6% (311,300 people) | 1.6% (370,100 people) |
| High cholesterol | 6.0% (1.1 million people) | 7.1% (1.6 million people) |
| Diabetes | 2.9% (554,200 people) | 5.1% (1.2 million people) |
| Heart disease | | 5.2% (1.2 million people) |
| Hypertension | 10% (1.8 million people) | 11.3% (2.6 million people) |
| Kidney disease | | 0.9% (203,400 people) |
| Mental and behavioural conditions | 18% (3.3 million people) | 17.5% (4.0 million people) |
| Osteoporosis | | 3.5% (801,800 people) |

[a] Australian Bureau of Statistics. National Health Survey. Australia 2001. http://www.ausstats.abs.gov.au/Ausstats/subscriber.nsf/0/90A3222FAD5E3563CA256C5D0001FD9D/\protect\T1\textdollarFile/43640_2001.pdf

[b] Australian Bureau of Statistics. National Health Survey. First Results Australia 2014–15. http://www.ausstats.abs.gov.au/Ausstats/subscriber.nsf/0/CDA852A349B4CEE6CA257F150009FC53/\protect\T1\textdollarFile/national%20health%20survey%20first%20results,%202014-15.pdf

## Appendix 3: Annas' Analysis of the Consequences of the Military and Market Metaphors on Health Care [144]

| Military metaphor | Consequences |
|---|---|
| • Medicine is a *battle* against death<br>• We are almost constantly engaged in wars on various diseases, such as cancer and AIDS<br>• Diseases attack the body, patients fight the disease and doctors *intervene* or counterattack<br>• Doctors are mostly specialists and backed by allied health professionals all of whom are trained to be *aggressive, fight* these *invading* diseases with weapons designed to *knock them out*<br>• Doctors give orders in the *trenches* and on the front lines, using their *armamentaria* in search of breakthroughs<br>• Treatments are conventional or heroic, and the brave patients soldier on<br>• We engage in triage in the emergency department, *invasive procedures* in the operating theatre, and even defensive medicine when a legal enemy is suspected<br>• Health plans and hospitals *market products* to *consumers*, who *purchase them on the basis of price*<br>• Medical care is a business that necessarily involves *marketing* through advertising and competition amongst suppliers who are *primarily motivated by profit*<br>• Health care becomes *managed care*<br>• *Mergers and acquisitions* become core activities | • Ignore *costs*<br>• Strengthens the belief that all problems can be solved with more *sophisticated technology* and scientific advances, prompting hospitals and doctors to engage in medical arms races<br>• War analogies lead to acceptance as inevitable that organisations are *hierarchical* and largely dominated by men<br>• The patient's body becomes a *battlefield*, thus appropriate to have *short-term, single-minded tactical goals*<br>• Concentrates on the physical, sees control as central and encourages the expenditure of massive resources to *achieve dominance*<br>• We failed to assert that medicine, like war, *should be financed and controlled only by the government*<br>• The metaphor has also become mythic. As a historian of war, John Keegan, correctly argues, modern warfare has become so horrible that 'it is scarcely possible anywhere in the world today to raise a body of reasoned support for the opinion that war is a justifiable activity'<br>• Emphasis is placed on:<br>  – *Efficiency*<br>  – *Profit maximisation*<br>  – *Customer satisfaction*<br>  – *The ability to pay*<br>  – *Planning*<br>  – *Entrepreneurship*<br>  – *Competitive models*<br>• The ideology of medicine is displaced by the *ideology of the marketplace*<br>• Trust is replaced by *caveat emptor* |

(continued)

| Market metaphor | Consequences |
|---|---|
| • *Chains* are developed, *vertical integration* is pursued and antitrust worries proliferate<br>• *Consumer choice* becomes the central theme of the market metaphor<br>• In the language of insurance, consumers become 'covered lives' or even 'money-generating biological structures'<br>• Economists become *health-financing gurus*<br>• The role of doctors is radically altered as they are *instructed by managers* that they can no longer be patient advocates (but instead must advocate for the entire group of covered lives in the health plan)<br>• The goal of medicine becomes a *healthy bottom line* instead of a healthy population | • There is *no place for the poor and uninsured* in the market metaphor<br>• *Business ethics* supplant medical ethics as the practice of medicine becomes corporate<br>• *Non-profit medical organisations may tend to be corrupted* by adopting the values of their for-profit competitors<br>• A *management degree* becomes at least as important as a medical degree<br>• *Public institutions*, which by definition cannot compete in the for-profit arena, *risk demise, second-class status or simply privatisation*<br>• *Patients, as consumers*, are to make decisions that are governed by *corporate entities*<br>• The market metaphor *conceals the inherent imperfections of the market* and *ignores the public nature of many aspects of medicine*<br>• *It ignores the inability of the market* to distribute goods and services whose supply and demand are unrelated to price<br>• The metaphor *pretends that there is such a thing as a free market in health insurance plans* and that purchasers can and should be content with their choices when unexpected injuries or illnesses strike them or their family members<br>• The reality is that American markets are:<br>– Highly regulated,<br>– Major industries enjoy large public subsidies,<br>– Industrial organisations tend towards oligopoly and<br>– Require strong laws that protect consumers and offer them recourse through product-liability suits to prevent profits from being too ruthlessly pursued |

Compiled from Annas: reframing the debate on healthcare reform by replacing our metaphors; *italics* emphasise pertinent concepts from the paper. Taken from: Sturmberg et al. [135]

## References

1. White K, Williams F, Greenberg B. The ecology of medical care. N Engl J Med. 1961;265(18):885–92.
2. Green L, Fryer G, Yawn B, Lanier D, Dovey S. The ecology of medical care revisited. N Engl J Med. 2001;344(26):2021–5.
3. Johansen ME, Kircher SM, Huerta TR. Reexamining the ecology of medical care. N Engl J Med. 2016;374(5):495–6.
4. Braun RN. Die gezielte Diagnostik in der Praxis. Stuttgart: Schattauer; 1957.
5. Fink W, Kipatov V, Konitzer M. Diagnoses by general practitioners: accuracy and reliability. Int J Forecasting. 2009;25(4):784–93.
6. Britt H, Miller G, Henderson J, Charles J, Valenti L, Harrison C, Bayram C, Zhang C, Pollack A, O'Halloran J, Pan Y. General practice activity in Australia 2011–12. Sydney: 2012 Contract No.: General Practice Series No. 31.
7. Sturmberg JP. Health: a personal complex-adaptive state. In: Sturmberg JP, Martin CM, editors. Handbook of systems and complexity in health. New York: Springer; 2013. p. 231–42.
8. Sturmberg JP. The personal nature of health. J Eval Clin Pract. 2009;15(4):766–9.
9. Sturmberg JP. Person-centeredness - a paradigm shift for health care? From disease as a "structural problem" to health, illness and disease as the "emergent outcomes of complex adaptive physiological network function". In: Loughlin M, editor. Person Centred Care: the new Professionalism. Understanding the Philosopy. 2019: (Forthcoming)
10. Mackenbach JP. Carl von Linne, Thomas McKeown, and the inadequacy of disease classifications. Eur J Pub Health. 2004;14(3):225.
11. Macklem PT, Seely A. Towards a definition of life. Perspect Biol Med. 2010;53(3):330–40.
12. Que C-L, Kenyon CM, Olivenstein R, Macklem PT, Maksym GN. Homeokinesis and short-term variability of human airway caliber. J Appl Physiol. 2001;91(3):1131–41.
13. Sturmberg JP, Bennett JM, Picard M, Seely AJE. The trajectory of life. Decreasing physiological network complexity through changing fractal patterns. Front Physiol. 2015;6:169.
14. Goh K-I, Cusick ME, Valle D, Childs B, Vidal M, Barabási A-L. The human disease network. Proc Natl Acad Sci. 2007;104(21):8685–90.
15. Heng HH. Heterogeneity-mediated cellular adaptation and its trade-off: searching for the general principles of diseases. J Eval Clin Pract. 2017;23(1):233–7.
16. Tracey KJ. Physiology and immunology of the cholinergic antiinflammatory pathway. J Clin Invest. 2007;117(2):289–96.
17. Glaser R, Kiecolt-Glaser JK. Stress-induced immune dysfunction: implications for health. Nat. Rev. Immunol. 2005;5:243–51.
18. Cole SW. Social regulation of human gene expression: mechanisms and implications for public health. Am J Public Health. 2013;103(S1):S84–S92.
19. Wallace DC. A mitochondrial bioenergetic etiology of disease. J Clin Invest. 2013;123(4):1405–12.
20. Picard M, Juster R-P, McEwen BS. Mitochondrial allostatic load puts the 'gluc' back in glucocorticoids. Nat Rev Endocrinol. 2014;10(5):303–10.
21. Kaur H, Carvalho J, Looso M, Singh P, Chennupati R, Preussner J, Günther S, Albarrán-Jurez J, Tischner D, Classen S, Offermanns S, Wettschureck N. Single-cell profiling reveals heterogeneity and functional patterning of GPCR expression in the vascular system. Nat. Commun. 2017;8:15700.
22. Luo C, Keown CL, Kurihara L, Zhou J, He Y, Li J, Castanon R, Lucero J, Nery JR, Sandoval JP, Bui B, Sejnowski TJ, Harkins TT, Mukamel EA, Behrens MM, Ecker JR. Single-cell methylomes identify neuronal subtypes and regulatory elements in mammalian cortex. Science. 2017;357(6351):600–4.
23. Heng HH. Debating cancer: the paradox in cancer research. Singapore: World Scientific Publishing; 2016.

24. Karatoreos IN, McEwen BS. Annual research review: the neurobiology and physiology of resilience and adaptation across the life course. J Child Psychol Psychiatry. 2013;54(4):337–47.
25. Lazarus RS, Folkman S. Stress, appraisal, and coping. New York: Springer; 1984.
26. Antonovsky A. Health, stress and coping. San Francisco: Jossey-Bass; 1979.
27. Antonovsky A. Complexity, conflict, chaos, coherence, coercion and civility. Soc Sci Med. 1993;37(8):969–74.
28. Rohleder NP. Stimulation of systemic low-grade inflammation by psychosocial stress. Psychosom Med. 2014;76(3):181–9.
29. Wolf JM, Rohleder N, Bierhaus A, Nawroth PP, Kirschbaum C. Determinants of the NF-$\kappa$B response to acute psychosocial stress in humans. Brain Behav Immun. 2009;23(6):742–9.
30. Bierhaus A, Wolf J, Andrassy M, Rohleder N, Humpert PM, Petrov D, Ferstl R, von Eynatten M, Wendt T, Rudofsky G, Joswig M, Morcos M, Schwaninger M, McEwen B, Kirschbaum C, Nawroth PP. A mechanism converting psychosocial stress into mononuclear cell activation. Proc Natl Acad Sci U S A. 2003;100(4):1920–5.
31. Rohleder N, Marin TJ, Ma R, Miller GE. Biologic cost of caring for a cancer patient: dysregulation of pro- and anti-inflammatory signaling pathways. J Clin Oncol. 2009;27(18):2909–15.
32. Cohen S, Janicki-Deverts D, Doyle WJ, Miller GE, Frank E, Rabin BS, Turner RB. Chronic stress, glucocorticoid receptor resistance, inflammation, and disease risk. Proc Natl Acad Sci U S A. 2012;109(16):5995–9.
33. Picard M, McEwen BS. Psychological stress and mitochondria: a conceptual framework. Psychosom Med. 2018;80(2):126–40.
34. Picard M, McEwen BS. Mitochondria impact brain function and cognition. Proc Natl Acad Sci. 2014;111(1):7–8.
35. Naik E, Dixit VM. Mitochondrial reactive oxygen species drive proinflammatory cytokine production. J Exp Med. 2011;208(3):417–20
36. Barabási A-L. Network medicine - from obesity to the "diseasome". N Engl J Med. 2007;357(4):404–7.
37. Sturmberg JP, Bennett JM, Martin CM, Picard M. 'Multimorbidity' as the manifestation of network disturbances. J Eval Clin Pract. 2017;23(1):199–208.
38. Sturmberg JP, Picard M, Aron DC, Bennett JM, Bircher J, deHaven MJ, Gijzel SMW, Heng HH, Marcum JA, Martin CM, Miles A, Peterson CL, Rohleder N, Walker C, Rikkert MGMO, Melis RJF. Health and disease - how network physiology integrates the social and biological determinants of health. A framework for debate. Front Med. 2019;6:59.
39. Bennett JM, Reeves G, Billman G, Sturmberg JP. Inflammation, the body's only efficient way to respond to injuries: implications for clinical care of chronic diseases. Front Med. 2018;(5):316
40. Sterling P, Eyer J. Allostasis: a new paradigm to explain arousal pathology. In: Fisher S, Reason J, editors. Handbook of life stress, cognition and health. New York: Wiley; 1988. p. 629–49.
41. McEwen BS. Stress, adaptation, and disease: allostasis and allostatic load. Ann N Y Acad Sci. 1998;840(1):33–44.
42. McEwen B. Protective and damaging effects of stress mediators: central role of the brain. Dialogues Clin Neurosci. 2006;8(4):367–81.
43. McEwen B. Protective and damaging effects of stress mediators: central role of the brain. Dialogues Clin Neurosci. 2006;8(4):367–81.
44. Edes AN, Crews DE. Allostatic load and biological anthropology. Am J Phys Anthropol. 2017;162(S63):e23146.
45. Juster R-P, McEwen BS, Lupien SJ. Allostatic load biomarkers of chronic stress and impact on health and cognition. Neurosci Biobehav Rev. 2010;35(1):2–16.
46. Read S, Grundy E. Allostatic load - a challenge to measure multisystem physiological dysregulation. National Centre for Research Methods Working Paper 04/12; 2012. http://eprints.ncrm.ac.uk/2879/1/NCRM_workingpaper_0412.pdf.

47. Loucks EB, Juster RP, Pruessner JC. Neuroendocrine biomarkers, allostatic load, and the challenge of measurement: a commentary on Gersten. Soc Sci Med. 2008;66(3):525–30.
48. Robertson T, Beveridge G, Bromley C. Allostatic load as a predictor of all-cause and cause-specific mortality in the general population: evidence from the Scottish health survey. PLos One. 2017;12(8):e0183297.
49. Wiley JFP, Gruenewald TLP, Karlamangla ASMDP, Seeman TEP. Modeling multisystem physiological dysregulation. Psychosom Med. 2016;78(3):290–301.
50. Arbeev KG, Ukraintseva SV, Bagley O, Zhbannikov IY, Cohen AA, Kulminski AM, Yashin AI. "Physiological dysregulation" as a promising measure of robustness and resilience in studies of aging and a new indicator of preclinical disease. J Gerontol A Biol Sci Med Sci. 2018. https://doi.org/10.1093/gerona/gly136.
51. Seeman TE, McEwen BS, Rowe JW, Singer BH. Allostatic load as a marker of cumulative biological risk: MacArthur studies of successful aging. Proc Natl Acad Sci. 2001;98(8): 4770–5.
52. Seeman TE, Crimmins E, Huang M-H, Singer B, Bucur A, Gruenewald T, Berkman LF, Reuben DB. Cumulative biological risk and socio-economic differences in mortality: MacArthur studies of successful aging. Soc Sci Med. 2004;58(10):1985–97.
53. Lakoff G, Johnsen M. Metaphors we live by. London: The University of Chicago Press; 2003.
54. Pellegrino E, Thomasma D. A philosophical basis of medical practice. Towards a philosophy and ethic of the healing professions. Oxford: Oxford University Press; 1981.
55. McWhinney IR. An acquaintance with particulars .... Fam Med. 1989;21(4):296–8.
56. McWhinney IR. Being a GP - what it means. WONCA 2000. 2000 05-07-2000. p. 4.
57. Hart JT. Expectations of health care: promoted, managed or shared? Health Expect. 1998;1(1):3–13.
58. Stewart MA. Effective physician-patient communication and health outcomes: a review. Can Med Assoc J. 1995;152(9):1423–33.
59. Matusitz J, Spear J. Effective doctor-patient communication: an updated examination. Social Work in Public Health. 2014;29(3):252–66.
60. Singh Ospina N, Phillips KA, Rodriguez-Gutierrez R, Castaneda-Guarderas A, Gionfriddo MR, Branda ME, Montori VM. Eliciting the patient's agenda - secondary analysis of recorded clinical encounters. J Gen Intern Med. 2019;34:36–40.
61. Davis F. The cabdriver and his fare: facets of a fleeting relationship. Am J Sociol. 1959;65(2):158–65.
62. McKinlay JB, Marceau LD. The end of the golden age of doctoring. Int J Health Serv. 2002;32(2):379–416.
63. Osorio JH. Evolution and changes in the physician-patient relationship. Colomb Méd. 2011;42:400–5.
64. Graham R, Mancher M, Wolman DM, Greenfield S, Steinberg E, for Committee on Standards for Developing Trustworthy Clinical Practice Guidelines. Board on health care services. In: Institute of Medicine, editors. Clinical practice guidelines we can trust. Washington: The National Academics Press; 2011. Available at http://nap.edu/13058.
65. Samanta A, Mello MM, Foster C, Tingle J, Samanta J. The role of clinical guidelines in medical negligence litigation: a shift from the BOLAM standard? Med Law Rev. 2006;14(3):321–66.
66. Lenzer J. Why we can't trust clinical guidelines. Br Med J. 2013;346:f3830.
67. Fleming T, DeMets D. Surrogate end points in clinical trials: are we being misled? Ann Intern Med. 1996;125:605–13.
68. Institute of Medicine. Evaluation of biomarkers and surrogate endpoints in chronic disease. Washington: The National Academies Press (Institute of Medicine); 2010.
69. Moynihan R. Surrogates under scrutiny: fallible correlations, fatal consequences. Br Med J. 2011;343:d5160.
70. Fleming TR, Powers JH. Biomarkers and surrogate endpoints in clinical trials. Stat Med. 2012;31(25):2973–84.
71. Weintraub WS, Lüscher TF, Pocock S. The perils of surrogate endpoints. Eur Heart J. 2015;36(33):2212–8.

72. Krumholz HM, Lee TH. Redefining quality - implications of recent clinical trials. N Engl J Med. 2008;358(24):2537–9.
73. Kemp R, Prasad V. Surrogate endpoints in oncology: when are they acceptable for regulatory and clinical decisions, and are they currently overused? BMC Med. 2017;15(1):134.
74. Yudkin JS, Lipska KJ, Montori VM. The idolatry of the surrogate. Br Med J. 2011;343:d7995.
75. Mercuri M, Sherbino J, Sedran RJ, Frank J, Gafni A, Norman GP. When guidelines don't guide: the effect of patient context on management decisions based on clinical practice guidelines. Acad Med. 2015;90(2):191–6.
76. Weisz G, Cambrosio A, Keating P, Knaapen L, Schlich T, Tournay VJ. The emergence of clinical practice guidelines. Milbank Q. 2007;85(4):691–727.
77. Rosenberg CE. Disease in history: frames and framers. Milbank Q. 1989;67(Suppl 1):1–15.
78. Brown P. Naming and framing: the social construction of diagnosis and illness. J Health Soc Behav. 1995;35(Extra Issue):34–52.
79. Aronowitz RA. When do symptoms become a disease? Ann Intern Med. 2001;134(9(pt 2)):803–308.
80. Rosenberg CE. The tyranny of diagnosis: specific entities and individual experience. Milbank Q. 2002;80(2):237–60.
81. Moynihan R, Heath I, Henry D. Selling sickness: the pharmaceutical industry and disease mongering. Br Med J. 2002;324:886–91.
82. Rosenberg CE. What is disease? In memory of Owsei Temkin. Bull Hist Med. 2003;77(3):491–505.
83. Sturmberg JP, Martin CM. Diagnosis - the limiting focus of taxonomy. J Eval Clin Pract. 2016;22(1):103–11.
84. Manrai AK, Patel CJ, Ioannidis JA. In the era of precision medicine and big data, who is normal? JAMA. 2018;319(19):1981–2.
85. Wood LD, Parsons DW, Jones S, Lin J, Sjoblom T, Leary RJ, Shen D, Boca SM, Barber T, Ptak J, Silliman N, Szabo S, Dezso Z, Ustyanksky V, Nikolskaya T, Nikolsky Y, Karchin R, Wilson PA, Kaminker JS, Zhang Z, Croshaw R, Willis J, Dawson D, Shipitsin M, Willson JKV, Sukumar S, Polyak K, Park BH, Pethiyagoda CL, Pant PVK, Ballinger DG, Sparks AB, Hartigan J, Smith DR, Suh E, Papadopoulos N, Buckhaults P, Markowitz SD, Parmigiani G, Kinzler KW, Velculescu VE, Vogelstein B. The genomic landscapes of human breast and colorectal cancers. Science. 2007;318(5853):1108–13.
86. Heng HHQ. Cancer genome sequencing: the challenges ahead. Bioessays. 2007;29(8): 783–94.
87. Faber R, Baumert M, Stepan H, Wessel N, Voss A, Walther T. Baroreflex sensitivity, heart rate, and blood pressure variability in hypertensive pregnancy disorders. J Hum Hypertens. 2004;18:707.
88. Mussalo H, Vanninen E, Ikäheimo R, Laitinen T, Hartikainen J. Short-term blood pressure variability in renovascular hypertension and in severe and mild essential hypertension. Clin Sci. 2003;105(5):609–14.
89. Kario K. Blood pressure variability in hypertension. A possible cardiovascular risk factor. Am J Hypertens. 2004;17(11):1075–6.
90. Rothwell PM. Limitations of the usual blood-pressure hypothesis and importance of variability, instability, and episodic hypertension. Lancet. 2010;375(9718):938–48.
91. Mehlum MH, Liestøl K, Kjeldsen SE, Julius S, Hua TA, Rothwell PM, Mancia G, Parati G, Weber MA, Berge E. Blood pressure variability and risk of cardiovascular events and death in patients with hypertension and different baseline risks. Eur Heart J. 2018;39(24):2243–51.
92. Jun JE, Jin S-M, Baek J, Oh S, Hur KY, Lee M-S, Lee M-K, Kim JH. The association between glycemic variability and diabetic cardiovascular autonomic neuropathy in patients with type 2 diabetes. Cardiovasc Diabetol. 2015;14(1):70.
93. Hirsch IB. Glycemic variability and diabetes complications: does it matter? Of course it does! Diabetes Care. 2015;38(8):1610–4.
94. Kanis JA, Odén A, McCloskey EV, Johansson H, Wahl DA, Cooper C, on behalf of IOF Working Group on Epidemiology and Quality of Life. A systematic review of hip fracture incidence and probability of fracture worldwide. Osteoporos Int. 2012;23(9):2239–56.

95. Aussem A, Caille P, Klemm Z, Gasse M, Anne-MarieSchott, Ducher M. Analysis of risk factors of hip fracture with causal Bayesian networks. In: Proceedings IWBBIO. Granada: Copicentro 2014. p. 1074–85.
96. Russ TC, Gatz M, Pedersen NL, Hannah J, Wyper G, Batty GD, Deary IJ, Starr JM. Geographical variation in dementia: examining the role of environmental factors in Sweden and Scotland. Epidemiology. 2015;26(2):263–70.
97. Caillet P, Klemm S, Ducher M, Aussem A, Schott A-M. Hip fracture in the elderly: a re-analysis of the EPIDOS study with causal Bayesian networks. PLoS One. 2015;10(3):e0120125.
98. Stopford CL, Snowden JS, Thompson JC, Neary D. Variability in cognitive presentation of Alzheimer's disease. Cortex. 2008;44(2):185–95.
99. Tractenberg RE, Pietrzak RH. Intra-individual variability in Alzheimer's disease and cognitive aging: definitions, context, and effect sizes. PLoS One. 2011;6(4):e16973.
100. Tarnanas I, Tsolaki A, Wiederhold M, Wiederhold B, Tsolaki M. Five-year biomarker progression variability for Alzheimer's disease dementia prediction: can a complex instrumental activities of daily living marker fill in the gaps? Alzheimers Dement Diagn Assessment Dis Monit. 2015;1(4):521–32.
101. Zolochevska O, Bjorklund N, Woltjer R, Wiktorowicz J, Taglialatela G. Postsynaptic proteome of non-demented individuals with Alzheimer's disease neuropathology. J Alzheimers Dis. 2018. https://doi.org/10.3233/JAD-180179.
102. Sturmberg J, Topolski S. For every complex problem, there is an answer that is clear, simple and wrong. J Eval Clin Pract. 2014;20(5):1017–25.
103. Mittra I. The disconnection between tumor response and survival. Nat Clin Pract Oncol. 2007;4(4):203.
104. Leyvraz S, Pampallona S, Martinelli G, Ploner F, Perey L, Aversa S, Peters S, Brunsvig P, Montes A, Lange A, Yilmaz U, Rosti G, On behalf of the Solid Tumors Working Party of the European Group for B and Marrow T. A threefold dose intensity treatment with ifosfamide, carboplatin, and etoposide for patients with small cell lung cancer: a randomized trial. J Natl Cancer Inst. 2008;100(8):533–41.
105. The Action to Control Cardiovascular Risk in Diabetes Study Group. Effects of intensive glucose lowering in type 2 diabetes. N Engl J Med. 2008;358(24):2545–59.
106. Hemmingsen B, Lund SS, Gluud C, Vaag A, Almdal T, Hemmingsen C, Wetterslev J. Intensive glycaemic control for patients with type 2 diabetes: systematic review with meta-analysis and trial sequential analysis of randomised clinical trials. Br Med J. 2011;343:d6898.
107. Simmons RK, Echouffo-Tcheugui JB, Sharp SJ, Sargeant LA, Williams KM, Prevost AT, Kinmonth AL, Wareham NJ, Griffin SJ. Screening for type 2 diabetes and population mortality over 10 years (ADDITION-Cambridge): a cluster-randomised controlled trial. Lancet. 2012;380(9855):1741–8.
108. Sim JJ, Shi J, Kovesdy CP, Kalantar-Zadeh K, Jacobsen SJ. Impact of achieved blood pressures on mortality risk and end-stage renal disease among a large, diverse hypertension population. J Am Coll Cardiol. 2014;64(6):588–97.
109. Musini V, Gueyffier F, Puil L, Salzwedel D, Wright J. Pharmacotherapy for hypertension in adults aged 18 to 59 years. Cochrane Database Syst Rev. 2017;8:CD008276.
110. Gorricho J, Garjón J, Celaya M, Muruzába lL, Malón M, Montoya R, López A. Blood pressure targets for the treatment of people with hypertension and cardiovascular disease. Cochrane Database Syst Rev. 2017;10:CD010315.
111. Ioannidis JA. Diagnosis and treatment of hypertension in the 2017 ACC/AHA guidelines and in the real world. JAMA. 2018;319:115–116.
112. Han BH, Sutin D, Williamson JD, Davis BR, Piller LB, Pervin H, Pressel SL, Blaum CS, on behalf of the ALLHAT Collaborative Research Group. Effect of statin treatment vs usual care on primary cardiovascular prevention among older adults: the ALLHAT-LLT randomized clinical trial. JAMA Intern Med. 2017;177:955–965.
113. Garrison S, Kolber M, Korownyk C, McCracken R, Heran B, Allan G. Blood pressure targets for hypertension in older adults. Cochrane Database Syst Rev. 2017;8:CD011575.

114. Sturmberg J. Hype and tension in hypertension. Debating the latest hypertension guidelines. Eur J Pers Cent Healthc. 2018;6(1):128–37.
115. Heath I. Combating disease mongering: daunting but nonetheless essential. PLoS Med. 2006;3(4):e146. Available at www.plosmedicine.org.
116. Black W. Advances in radiology and the real versus apparent effects of early diagnosis. Eur J Radiol. 1998;27(2):116.
117. Welch HG, Black WC. Overdiagnosis in cancer. J Natl Cancer Inst. 2010;102(9):605–13.
118. Moynihan R, Doust J, Henry D. Preventing overdiagnosis: how to stop harming the healthy. Br Med J. 2012;344:19–23.
119. Yver M. Surgical pathology in cancer diagnosis: implications for quaternary prevention. Rev Bras Med Fam Comunidade. 2015;10(35):7.
120. Moynihan R, Nickel B, Hersch J, Beller E, Doust J, Compton S, Barratt A, Bero L, McCaffery K. Public opinions about overdiagnosis: a national community survey. PLoS One. 2015;10(5):e0125165.
121. Welch HG, Fisher ES. Income and cancer overdiagnosis - when too much care is harmful. N Engl J Med. 2017;376(23):2208–9.
122. Herndon MB, Schwartz LM, Woloshin S, Welch HG. Implications of expanding disease definitions: the case of osteoporosis. Health Aff (Millwood). 2007;26(6):1702–11.
123. Moynihan R, Doran E, Henry D. Disease mongering is now part of the global health debate. PLoS Med. 2008;5:e106.
124. Drugwatch. Disease mongering and drug marketing. 2018. https://www.drugwatch.com/news/2012/01/22/disease-mongering-and-drug-marketing/.
125. Wolinsky H. Disease mongering and drug marketing. EMBO Rep. 2005;6(7):612–4.
126. Brezis M. Big pharma and health care: unsolvable conflict of interests between private enterprise and public health. Isr J Psychiatry Relat Sci. 2008;45(2):83–9.
127. Prasad V, Cifu A, Ioannidis JPA. Reversals of established medical practices. evidence to abandon ship. JAMA. 2012;307(1):37–8.
128. Prasad V. Powering cancer screening for overall mortality. ecancermedicalscience. 2013;7:ed27. https://ecancer.org/journal/editorial/27-powering-cancer-screening-for-overall-mortality.php.
129. Prasad V, Lenzer J, Newman DH. Why cancer screening has never been shown to "save lives"—and what we can do about it. Br Med J. 2016;352:h6080.
130. Jacklyn G, Bell K, Hayen A. Assessing the efficacy of cancer screening. Public Health Res Pract. 2017;27(3):e2731727.
131. AIHW. Medical practitioners workforce 2015. 2016. https://www.aihw.gov.au/reports/workforce/medical-practitioners-workforce-2015/contents/how-many-medical-practitioners-are-there.
132. Health Workforce Australia. Australia's future health workforce - nurses detailed. Canberra: Department of Health; 2014.
133. Sturmberg JP, M O'Halloran D, McDonnell G, M Martin C. General practice work and workforce. Aust J Gen Pract. 2018;47:507–13.
134. Sturmberg JP, O'Halloran DM, Martin CM. People at the centre of complex adaptive health systems reform. Med J Aust. 2010;193(8):474–8.
135. Sturmberg JP, O'Halloran DM, Martin CM. Health care reform - the need for a complex adaptive systems approach. In: Sturmberg JP, Martin CM, editors. Handbook of systems and complexity in health. New York: Springer; 2013. p. 827–53.
136. Adler KG. Does high patient satisfaction mean high quality of care? Fam Pract Manag. 2016;23(3):4.
137. Kupfer JM, Bond EU. Patient satisfaction and patient-centered care: necessary but not equal. JAMA. 2012;308(2):139–40.
138. Enguidanos ER, Coletti CM, Honigman L, Mazzeo A, Pinson TB, Reed K, Wiler JL. Patient satisfaction surveys and quality of care: an information paper. Ann Emerg Med. 2014;64(4):351–7.

139. Dunsch F, Evans DK, Macis M, Wang Q. Bias in patient satisfaction surveys: a threat to measuring healthcare quality. BMJ Global Health. 2018;3(2):e000694.
140. Howie J, Heaney D, Maxwell M, Walker J. A comparison of a Patient Enablement Instrument (PEI) against two established satisfaction scales as an outcome measure of primary care. Fam Pract. 1998;15:165–71.
141. Porter ME, Larsson S, Lee TH. Standardizing patient outcomes measurement. N Engl J Med. 2016;374(6):504–6.
142. Sepucha KR, Levin CA, Uzogara EE, Barry MJ, O'Connor AM, Mulley AG. Developing instruments to measure the quality of decisions: early results for a set of symptom-driven decisions. Patient Educ Couns. 2008;73(3):504–10.
143. Lee CN, Dominik R, Levin CA, Barry MJ, Cosenza C, O'Connor AM, Mulley Jr AG, Sepucha KR. Development of instruments to measure the quality of breast cancer treatment decisions. Health Expect. 2010;13(3):258–72.
144. Annas GJ. Reframing the debate on health care reform by replacing our metaphors. N Engl J Med. 1995;332(11):745–8.
145. Starfield B. Is US health really the best in the world? JAMA. 2000;284(4):483–5.
146. Macinko J, Starfield B, Shi L. The contribution of primary care systems to health outcomes within Organization for Economic Cooperation and Development (OECD) countries, 1970–1998. Health Serv Res. 2003;38(3):831–65.
147. Macinko J, Starfield B, Shi L. Quantifying the health benefits of primary care physician supply in the United States. Int J Health Serv. 2007;37(1):111–26.
148. Hart J. The inverse care law. Lancet. 1971;I:405–12.
149. Katerndahl DA, Wood R, Jaen CR. A method for estimating relative complexity of ambulatory care. Ann Fam Med. 2010;8(4):341–7.
150. Fortin M, Dionne J, Pinho G, Gignac J, Almirall J, Lapointe L. Randomized controlled trials: do they have external validity for patients with multiple comorbidities? Ann Fam Med. 2006;4(2):104–8.
151. Greenfield S, Kaplan S, Kahn R, Ninomiya J, Griffith J. Profiling care provided by different groups of physicians: effects of patient case-mix (Bias) and physician-level clustering on quality assessment results. Ann Intern Med. 2002;136:111–21.
152. Greenfield S, Rogers W, Mangotich M, Carney M, Tarlov A. Outcomes of patients with hypertension and non-insulin-dependent diabetes mellitus treated by different systems and specialties. JAMA. 1995;274(18):1436–44.
153. Scott JG. Complexities of the consultation. In: Sturmberg JP, Martin CM, editors. Handbook of systems and complexity in health. New York: Springer; 2013. p. 257–77.
154. Hjortdahl P. Continuity of care: general practitioners' knowledge about, and sense of responsibility toward their patients. Fam Pract. 1992;9(1):3–8.
155. Fugelli P. Trust - in general practice. Br J Gen Pract. 2001;51(468):575–9.
156. Freeman G, Olesen F, Hjortdahl P. Continuity of care: an essential element of modern general practice? Fam Pract. 2003;20(6):623–7.
157. Hjortdahl P. The influence of general practitioners' knowledge about their patients on the clinical decision-making process. Scand J Prim Health Care. 1992;10:290–4.
158. Sturmberg JP, Schattner P. Personal doctoring. Its impact on continuity of care as measured by the comprehensiveness of care score. Aust Fam Physician. 2001;30(5):513–8.
159. Saultz JW, Lochner J. Interpersonal continuity of care and care outcomes: a critical review. Ann Fam Med. 2005;3(2):159–66.
160. Guthrie B, Saultz JW, Freeman GK, Haggerty JL. Continuity of care matters. Br Med J. 2008;337(aug07_1):a867.
161. Sweeney K, Gray D. Patients who do not receive continuity of care from their general practitioner - are they a vulnerable group? Br J Gen Pract. 1995;45:133–5.
162. Sturmberg JP. Health system redesign. How to make health care person-centered, equitable, and sustainable. Cham: Springer; 2017.

163. Sturmberg JP, Martin CM. The dynamics of health care reform - learning from a complex adaptive systems theoretical perspective. Nonlinear Dynam Psych Life Sci. 2010;14(4): 525–40.
164. Ellis GFR. Top-down causation and emergence: some comments on mechanisms. Interface Focus. 2012;2(1):126–40.
165. Rothman KJ. Causes. Am J Epidemiol. 1976;104(6):587–92.

# Fail Small, Fail Often: An Outsider's View of Physiologic Complexity

**Bruce J. West**

## 1 Introduction

Human beings distrust statistics, in large part, because they are uncomfortable with uncertainty and are suspicious of unpredictable variability. This was not always the case, however. Primitive man was sensitive to variability in the environment, because change could be dangerous. This mechanism actually found its way into our physiological makeup through macroevolution, so that humans could adapt to small predictable changes, whereas intermittent changes would trigger defensive responses. We note the vestige of this mechanism in our ability to fall asleep in a motel room despite the traffic noise outside the window, or how quickly we no longer hear the murmurings of a large dinner party when we begin to chat with our neighbor, and are no longer conscious of the aroma of cheese in the deli shortly after entering. This mechanism has been given the name habituation, and is how our nervous system adapts to sensory variability.

Scientists, who quantify everything, in order to get at a measure of the underlying regularity, developed the first mathematical theory of empirical unpredictability at the turn of the nineteenth century. Gauss in Europe and Adrian in America, simultaneously, constructed a mathematics to explain why two ostensibly identical experiments never produced the same results. They independently reasoned that all the data from an ensemble of such experiments could be best represented by a numerical average. The scatter in data around the average they determined to be best characterized by the standard deviation of the data, which provides a measure of how well the average characterizes the experimental data. These two quantities, the average and standard deviation, were shown to completely determine

B. J. West (✉)
Information Science Directorate, Army Research Office, Research Triangle Park, NC, USA
e-mail: bruce.j.west.civ@mail.mil

 
J. P. Sturmberg (ed.), *Embracing Complexity in Health*,
https://doi.org/10.1007/978-3-030-10940-0_2

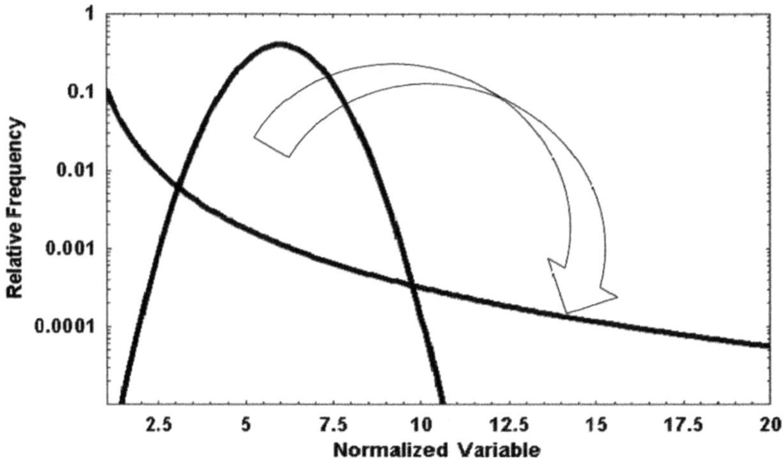


**Fig. 1** The parabolic solid curve is a normal distribution, whereas the other curve is an inverse power-law Pareto distribution. The arrow depicts a control process discussed in the text

the properties of the measurements in terms of a bell-shaped ensemble distribution function centered on the average and a width given by the standard deviation. This is the normal distribution depicted in Fig. 1 on log-linear graph paper by the bell-shaped parabolic curve.

The bell-shaped distribution was given the unfortunate name, the law of frequency of error (LFE). It is unfortunate because that name solidified the interpretation that the average is the correct value for the quantity being measured and therefore deviations from the average must be errors. This was, in fact, the original interpretation and was consistent with clock-work view of the universe given by Newton's laws of motion in physics, but it led to misinterpretations of the more complex phenomena in medicine, as we shall see.

The LFE guided the development of manufacturing processes during the Machine Age of the nineteenth century. The center of the LFE became the engineer's design specification for the widget being manufactured, and the LFE's width became the accepted tolerance. The necessity for having the specifications for a widget to be within a certain range of tolerance reinforced the notion that the width of the distribution should be as narrow as possible, in order to reduce the variability in the product's dimensions coming off the assembly line. The controlled sameness of everything we buy in Western society, from the cars we drive, to the tools we use, to the clothes we wear, all reinforce the notion that variability is bad and should be suppressed. This weaned the typical Westerner from the limited comfort they had historically enjoyed with uncertainty. It also fostered the mistaken belief that variability was the enemy.

While complexity in the physical sciences was being understood using simple feedback loops and the statistical methods of the LFE, these ideas were also finding their way into the social and biological science, as well as medicine. It is not clear exactly when the mechanical view of how the human body works began to permeate society, but in medicine the concept reached maturity with Claude Bernard's introduction of homeostasis [1] in the second half of the nineteenth century. The concept was popularized a half-century later by Walter Cannon [2] and became the guiding principle of medicine.

One reason for its adoption was the overwhelming evidence that body temperature, heart rate, breathing rate, stride interval, and so on all have well-defined average values. The interpretation of LFE is that the average value is characteristic of the physiologic process being measured and what is needed is a feedback loop to stabilize the system. Homeostasis, the result of eons of macroevolution, provides the mechanism to explain how the appropriate subnetwork, within the body, controls both internal fluctuations and external disruptions to maintain the average level of temperature, heart rate, and so on.

## 2 Complex Is Typical Not Normal

We have briefly presented a pleasing picture of how physiological networks behave. Unfortunately, it is less fact than it is fiction. The sad truth is that neither the cardiovascular system, nor the respiratory system, nor the motor control system, nor any other physiological system for which there is data that behaves in this way. The tightly knitted argument, centered on the LFE, began to unravel in the decade of the 1990s, with the research of Peng et al. [3] on the statistics of heart rate variability (HRV). They determined that the time interval between successive heartbeats fluctuates, and the statistical distribution of those interval fluctuations looks nothing like the LFE.

It was determined that the physiologic time series data scale and such scaling entails important physiologic advantages associated with the adaptability of response [4, 5]. The work of Peng et al. [3] was the first of many studies on the scale-invariant properties of HRV time series, the output of an integrative control system, see West [6] for subsequent review of this area. HRV time series fluctuate in a complex, erratic manner in healthy individuals, even those at rest. The same manner of fluctuation was also observed in stride rate variability (SRV) [7, 8] and in breath rate variability (BRV) [9, 10].

The spectrum of the interbeat increment time series data scales as an inverse power law (IPL) in frequency:

$$S(f) \propto \frac{1}{f^{2H-1}}, \tag{1}$$

and using a Tauberian theorem, the mean-square level of the interbeat fluctuations increases in time as $t^{2H}$. The spectrum is a consequence of the correlations in events, say heartbeats, in which different dynamics can occur at different timescales in the physiologic time series. Costa et al. [11] demonstrate a high level of chaos in cardiac dynamics along with a high degree of entropy in normal HRV time series and suggest that this fractal behavior regulates HRV [12].

The IPL index replaces the average as the metric for a complex system. It is the IPL index that quantifies the imbalance in physiology of the reliance that one scale within a network has on another, so that no one scale dominates the network dynamics. What is truly being measured is the complexity in the underlying phenomenon and mathematically this is the fractal dimension. The ultimate conclusion reached, after looking at a variety of physiologic phenomena, is that the traditional notion of disease as the loss of regularity must be replaced with the idea that disease is the loss of complexity, where here that complexity is measured by the variability in the process [13]. This is discussed nonmathematically in *Where Medicine Went Wrong* [14], and mathematically in a number of other places, for example [15].

## 3 But Why Multifractal?

Living matter is significantly more complex than inanimate matter and consequently we do not have fundamental laws and principles to govern living phenomena equivalent to those in physics. Some may object to this harsh characterization, but there are no equivalents to Newton's force law, Maxwell's equations, and Boltzmann's principle in physiology. Biophysics was, in fact, invented to seek out and establish the existence of such *Laws of Life* and relate them to known physical laws, so that both the animate and inanimate aspects of living matter can be better understood. However, the aim here is much more modest than identifying such fundamental biophysical principles. The aim is to present a strategy for understanding a diverse set of physiological data in terms of an underlying complexity and to introduce a data processing method that reveals a hidden symmetry in the data that can be exploited to gain insight into how the body might gain control over complex physiological processes.

If you have not already guessed, the complexity we explore herein is multifractality in physiologic time series. For our purposes, we introduce the notion of scaling, such that if $X(t)$ defines an observable $X$, say HRV, SRV, BRV, or cerebral blood flow (CBF), at a time $t$, and if we change the resolution of timescale by a factor $\lambda$, we obtain the scaling relation:

$$X(\lambda t) = \lambda^H X(t) \tag{2}$$

where $H$ is a scaling index. Mandelbrot [16] introduced $H$ to honor the civil engineer Hurst who first used Eq. (2) to quantify the scaling behavior of hydrostatic data sets and he (Mandelbrot) used it to define the fractal dimension of data with fractal statistics, in which case this equation is interpreted in terms of a probability density function (PDF).

The most well-known scaling PDF is the normal distribution of Gauss, in which case $H = 1/2$ for Brownian motion. More generally, the scaling index falls in the range $0 \leq H \leq 1$ and we then have fractional Brownian motion (fBm) for which the PDF can be written in scaled form:

$$P(x,t) = \frac{1}{t^H} F\left(\frac{x}{t^H}\right). \tag{3}$$

In the case of fBm, the fractal dimension is a constant and the process is said to be monofractal. Using this PDF, one can show that the scaling of the average value of the observable is given by:

$$\langle X; \lambda t\rangle = \int x P(x, \lambda t) dx = \lambda^H \langle X; t\rangle, \tag{4}$$

which is of the same form as Eq. (2), but scaling is expressed in terms of the average value and not the dynamical variable.

A monofractal time series is characterized by a single fractal dimension. In general, time series have a local Hölder exponent $h$ that varies over the course of the trajectory defined by the time series and is related to the fractal dimension by $D = 2 - h$. Note that for an infinitely long time series, the exponent $h$ and the Hurst exponent $H$ are identical; however, for a time series of finite length they need not be the same. We stress that the fractal dimension and the Hölder exponent are local quantities, whereas the Hurst exponent is a global quantity; consequently, the relation $D = 2 - H$ is only true for an infinitely long time series. The function $f(h)$, called the multifractal or singularity spectrum, describes how the distribution of local (fractal) exponents contributes to such time series [17].

One way multifractality manifests itself is through the statistical fluctuations of the IPL index. A relatively simple way to model this is through a random walk process in which the time series data are used to generate a diffusion process, such as the multifractal random walk [18]. Formally, we can write the solution to any such process as [17]:

$$\Delta X(t) = X(t) - X(0) = \int_0^t K_\alpha(t - t')\xi\left(t'\right) dt' \tag{5}$$

where $\xi(t)$ is a fBm statistical process, which scales as $\lambda^H$. The memory kernel $K_\alpha(t)$ contains all the dynamics of the physiologic system being considered. We assume that both the random forcing function $\xi(t)$ and the memory kernel $K_\alpha(t)$ scale, allowing us to write

$$\Delta X(\lambda t) = \lambda^{H+\alpha} \Delta X(t). \tag{6}$$

This scaling of the memory kernel with parameter $\alpha$ implies that the underlying dynamics requires a new mathematical infrastructure for its understanding and that infrastructure is given by the fractional calculus [19]. Here, the parameter $\alpha$ is the order of the fractional derivative in the interval $0 \leq \alpha \leq 1$. Moreover, the multifractal nature of the time series is entailed by the fractional derivative being a random variable.

Different physiological processes are described by different PDFs for the fractional derivatives. Consider a fractional derivative to be a random variable with normal statistics. This model yields a singularity spectrum, or spectrum of Hölder exponents that is quadratic in the exponent and the width of the spectrum is determined by the standard deviation of the normal distribution $\sigma$ [20]:

$$f(h) = f(H) - \frac{(h - H)^2}{4\sigma}. \tag{7}$$

Here, $H$ is the Hurst exponent (asymptotic value for the scaling exponent) and $h$ is the exponent from the time series.

### 3.1 Some Results

Ten CBF time series for ten normal subjects were averaged and gave rise to the spectrum of exponents shown in Fig. 2a where it is clear that the model spectrum, the curve generated by Eq. (7), fits the data, given by the dots, quite well. A group of 13 subjects that suffer from migraine headaches yield the narrowed spectrum depicted in Fig. 2b by the dots and fitted using Eq. (7). The loss in multifractality between the two groups is evident from the reduced width of the multifractal spectrum.

A similar reduction in the multifractality spectrum was obtained for HRV time series after a heart attack [3], as well as, for other physiologic time series, reviewed in West [6, 14]. This change in the width of the singularity spectrum represents a loss in the normal variability of the physiologic process and is diagnostic of a pathology.

## 4 Control of Variability

How does the body control the level of variability in physiologic systems? In Fig. 3, a qualitative sketch of the data denotes the PDFs for heartbeat interval variability (HRV) $I(t)$, from a study [21] of a collection of 670 post-AMI patients using 24-h Holter monitor data sets. This figure schematically depicts the statistical distributions for those from this collection who suffered a cardiac death, those who died by noncardiac causes, and those who survived. Notice that not one of the three empirical PDFs has Gaussian statistics, which in terms of the standardized variable would coincide with the dashed curve. The empirical PDFs all have non-Gaussian forms, with the survivors and those succumbing to noncardiac death nearly coinciding.

On the other hand, the PDF for the variability statistics of the cardiac death patients is very different from those who survive, even though there is a great deal of overlap in the central regions of the PDFs. The difference between the survivor and the cardiac fatality curves suggests that cardiac-induced death can be modeled

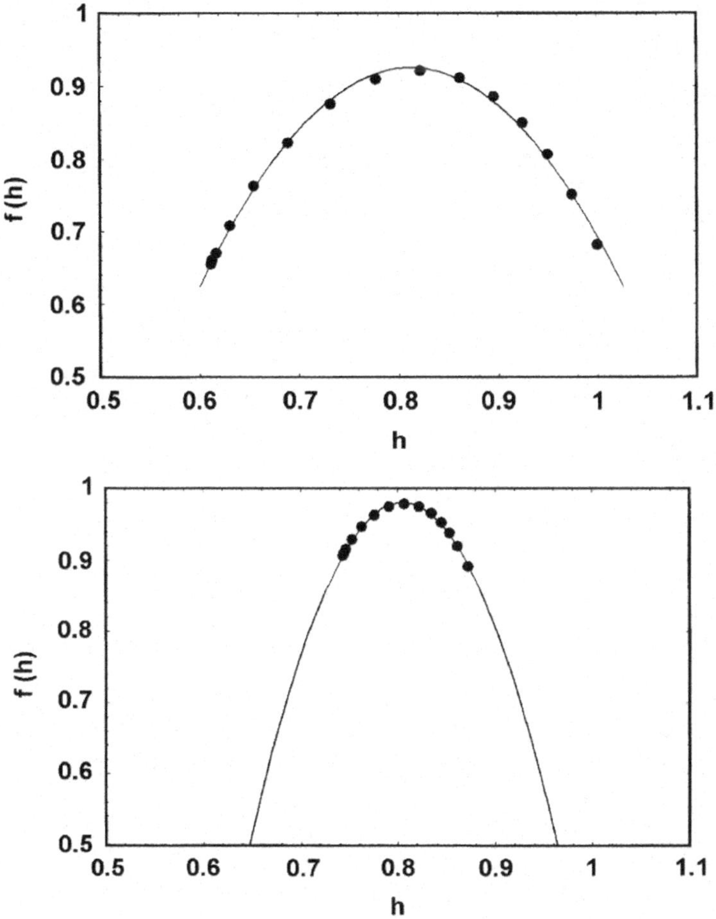


**Fig. 2** Top, (**a**): Depicted is the averaged singularity spectrum $f(h)$ of the healthy subjects (filled circles). The spectrum is the average of ten measurements of five subjects. Bottom, (**b**): Depicted is the averaged singularity spectrum of the migraineurs (filled circles) calculated in the same way as the data in Top. The spectrum is the average of 14 measurements of 8 subjects. The solid curves are the best least-squares fit of the parameters in Eq. (7) to the singularity spectrum. Adapted from [20] with permission

by a Lévy PDF, whereas those who survive, or suffer noncardiac deaths, might be modeled by a truncated or tempered Lévy PDF. The first identification of HRV with Lévy statistics was made a quarter century ago by Peng et al. [3].

Here, we hypothesize the existence of a cardiac mechanism in the sinoatrial node that produces a tempered Lévy PDF for survivors and more generally for healthy individuals. This hypothesized mechanism is the complement to the kind of filter we have been discussing. It suppresses the largest changes in inter-beat intervals, those being in the tails of the Lévy PDF, which persist in the cardiac fatality group.

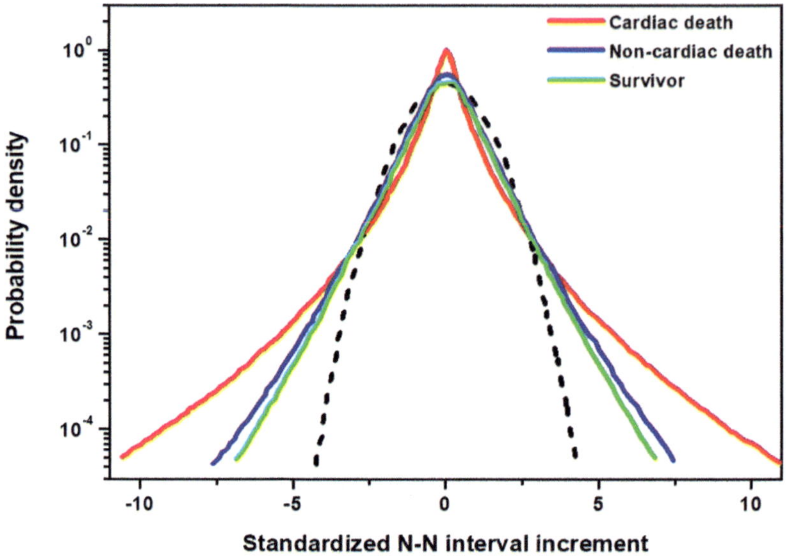


**Fig. 3** The HRV distributions are indicated schematically from 24-h RR interval time series for a group having suffered acute myocardial infarction. The patients are separated into those who suffer cardiac death, another with noncardiac death, and third consisting of survivors (adapted from [21])

The pathophysiology of the HRV PDF being Lévy stable, therefore, results from the suppression of this physiological control process; a process selected for by macroevolution to suppress extreme changes in inter-beat intervals.

For those of you who are mathematically inclined, we can apply the filtering idea to the data shown in Fig. 3. Consider the dynamic model for the inter-beat time intervals in the form of a filtered diffusion process:

$$\frac{dI(t)}{dt} = F(I) + \xi(t) \tag{8}$$

where $F(I)$ is a deterministic driver and $\xi(t)$ is a stochastic driver. The deterministic driver is determined by the dynamics of the sinoatrial node and the random driver by the autonomic signal and can be made functionally specific by what is known about HRV time series.

The HRV time series is the result of competing neuroautonomic inputs. The competition between these two branches of the involuntary nervous system is the mechanism assumed to provide the erratic variability recorded in healthy subjects [4, 13] and therefore determines the statistics of the stochastic driver. We assume that resulting from the competition the statistics are Lévy stable with index $0 < \alpha \leq 2$.

The form of the deterministic driver emerges from the intrinsic dynamic properties of the sinoatrial node pacemaker cells. These properties are modeled herein using the recent observation that biological systems are poised at criticality [22], which can in principle produce the cooperative oscillations, as well as erratic variability, observed in rhythmic heartbeat time series. However, the fluctuations arising from such chaotic dynamics can reasonably be assumed to be overwhelmed by the Lévy statistics of the autonomic input and therefore ignored here. The deterministic force is therefore modeled by the cooperative behavior of the pacemaker cells.

A generic version of this equation has been analyzed [23]. In general, the feedback term is a polynomial, but we restrict the analysis to the largest-order term, since this is the term that dominates the control process and write $F(I) \approx -\lambda_{2n} I^{2n+1}$, where $\lambda_{2n} > 0$ and $n$ is an integer. Note the index is restricted to even order to ensure that higher-order terms to not change the symmetry of the control process from that of a linear feedback term. Note further that the sinoatrial node is comprised of a complex network of interacting pacemaker cells, each with its own internal clock, which acts within the collective to coordinate the heartbeat rhythm. A number of mathematical models have been devised that manifest such collective behavior, providing insight into critical phase transitions in nonphysical networks. One such model is the DMM [17], which near criticality reduces to the $n = 0$ linear and $n = 1$ quartic terms. At criticality, the coefficient of the linear term goes to zero.

Without presenting the details, we assert that the PDF that solves the fractional equation of evolution for the probability density in the steady state has the form [24]:

$$P_{ss}(I) = \frac{N_\mu}{I^\mu} \ ; \mu = \alpha + 2n + 1. \tag{9}$$

It is well known that for an IPL index $\mu \geq 3$, the second moment $\langle I^2 \rangle$ is finite, implying that the central limit theorem holds asymptotically. Consequently, since $\alpha < 2$ for Lévy statistics then it must be $n \geq 1$ in order for the statistics of $I(t)$ to have a finite second moment asymptotically and the steady-state PDF to asymptotically transition from Lévy stable to Gaussian. This transition explains the results obtained by Kiyono et al. [25, 26], without the need to exponentially temper the Lévy driver, relying solely on the sinoatrial dynamics to temper the extreme fluctuations resulting from the competition between the two branches of the involuntary nervous system.

## 5 Discussion and Conclusions

It is often the case in presenting mathematical arguments in support of a clinical interpretation that the latter is lost in the torturous details of the former. So, let us recap the most important aspects of the formal discussion.

The level of complexity in physiologic time series is a balance between regularity and variability, not just variability alone. Thus, the truncated Lévy PDF has this balance built-in with extreme variability at short time intervals, but suppressed variability at very long time intervals. In keeping with this new perspective, homeostasis, which focuses on the long time control of a physiologic process, and inverse power laws that focus on unfettered variability, each have only part of the answer. It has been hypothesized that disease is associated with the loss of complexity [13]. This hypothesis has been repeatedly tested successfully, using HRV data, see [17] for a more detailed discussion.

We hypothesized a collective network mechanism that produces a truncated Lévy PDF for those who survive, not unlike the "kicks" away from the extreme excursions postulated a quarter century ago by Peng et al. [3] to explain the anticorrelation of HRV data. This mechanism would suppress the largest extrema, but they persist in the cardiac death group and therefore this control mechanism, or at least contributions from $n \geq 1$, is not present in this group. The pathology of the HRV distribution being Lévy stable would then be the result of losing the physiological control process, that is, a process not to inhibit events in chronological time but to suppress the size of the interbeat interval.

Scale invariance, the property relating time series across multiple scales, has provided a new perspective on physiological phenomena and their underlying control systems. We have reviewed the change of physiologic time series from the engineering view of "signal plus noise," to fractals in time and finally to multifractals. In the exemplar we discussed, the healthy human brain is perfused by the laminar flow of blood through the cerebral vessels providing brain tissue with substrates, such as oxygen and glucose. It turns out that the CBF is relatively stable between narrow bounds despite substantial variations in systemic pressure. This phenomenon is known as *cerebral autoregulation*, and analogues to this autoregulation occur in all the other physiologic time series mentioned.

Mimicking autoregulation by externally suppressing the natural variability of a physiologic system may seem like the appropriate call, since it reduces the frequency of illness and therefore prolongs the intervals of health and well-being. However, a system "designed" to address adversity when no adversity is encountered over long periods of time becomes less robust, that is, more fragile over time. Thus, such artificial smoothing of natural variability is precisely the wrong thing to do.

## The Transformative Aspects of This Study

Robust health is not being free of all illness, since such a strategy would paradoxically increase the probability that when a risk does occur, the failure would be catastrophic. This is a consequence of the coupling across scales in complex phenomena, and reducing variability on short timescales for scaling phenomena only guarantees a devastatingly large-scale variation when it does occur. This particular perspective was developed in a political context by Taleb and Blyth [27], in which the subtitle of their paper says it all: *How Suppressing Volatility Makes the World Less Predictable and More Dangerous.* The point is that it is not the straw that breaks the camel's back, it is the entire history of load carried by the camel plus the final straw. It is a mistake to assign causation to the fluctuation that finally produces catastrophic system failure. The true cause of large-scale failure is a property of the overall system behavior and not the last event before failure.

The probability of a catastrophic failure arising due to a large-scale fluctuation is exponentially small for the diffusive process. However, by smoothing away the small failures that occur quite often, the probability of a catastrophic failure occurring is of the Pareto form. The result of filtering is to transform a robust system that has frequent nonlife-threatening-failures into one that is fragile and dominated by a few possible events, those being Taleb's Black Swans [28].

**Take Home Message**

- Physiologic complexity is the balance between randomness and regularity, both contributing in equal amounts to the variability necessary for robust health.
- Failure (disease) is a consequence of the loss of physiologic complexity, as defined in 1.
- The mechanism of physiologic autoregulation is maintained by permitting small failures to occur regularly, thereby enabling the regulator to retain a robust status over time.
- Artificially suppressing physiologic randomness (small failures) inhibits one aspect of complexity in autoregulation and paradoxically increases the probability of catastrophic failure (death).

## References


1. Bernard C. Introduction to experimental medicine. New York: Dover Publications; 1865.
2. Cannon WB. The wisdom of the body. New York: W W Norton & Co.; 1932.
3. Peng C-K, Mietus J, Hausdorff JM, Havlin S, Stanley HE, Goldberger AL. Long-range anticorrelations and non-Gaussian behavior of the heartbeat. Phys Rev Lett. 1993;70(9):1343–6.
4. Goldberger AL, West BJ. Fractals in physiology and medicine. Yale J Biol Med. 1987;60(5):421–35 and references therein.
5. Shlesinger MF, West BJ. Asymmetric branching of the mammalian lung. Phys Rev Lett. 1991;67:2106.
6. West BJ. Fractal physiology and chaos in medicine, 2nd ed. New Jersey: World Scientific; 2013.
7. Hausdorff JF, Peng CK, Ladin Z, Ladin JY, Wei JY, Goldberger AL. Is walking a random walk? Evidence for long-range correlations in stride interval of human gait. J Appl Physiol. 1995;78(1):349–58.
8. Griffin L, West DJ, West BJ. Random stride intervals with memory. J Biol Phys. 2000;26(3):185–202.

9. Peng CK, Meus J, Li Y, Lee C, Hausdorff JM, Stanley HE, Goldberger AL, Lipsitz LA. Quantifying fractal dynamics of human respiration: age and gender effects. Ann Biomed Eng. 2002;30(5):683–92.
10. West BJ, Griffin LA, Freerick HJ, Moon RE. The independently fractal nature of respiration and heart rate during exercise under normobaric and hyperbaric conditions. Respir Physiol Neurobiol. 2005;145(2–3):219–33.
11. Costa MD, Peng CK, Goldberger AL. Multiscale analysis of heart rate dynamics: entropy and time irreversibility measures. Cardiovasc Eng. 2008;8(2):88–93.
12. Yaniv Y, Lyaskov AE, Lakatta EG. The fractal-like complexity of heart rate variability beyond neurotransmitters and autonomic receptors: signaling intrinsic to sinoatrial node pacemaker cells. Cardiovasc Pharm Open Access. 2013;2:111.
13. Goldberger AL, Rigney DR, West BJ. Chaos and fractals in human physiology. Sci Am. 1990;262(2):42–9.
14. West BJ. Where medicine west wrong. Singapore: World Scientific; 2006.
15. Bassigthwaighte JB, Liebowitch LS, West BJ. Fractal physiology. Oxford: Oxford University Press; 1994.
16. Mandelbrot BB. Fractals, form, chance and dimension. San Francisco: W.H. Freeman & Co; 1977.
17. West BJ. A mathematics for medicine: the network effect. Front Physiol. 2014;5:456.
18. Bacry E, Delour J, Muzy JF. Multifractal random walk. Phys Rev E. 2001;64(2):026103.
19. West BJ. Fractional calculus view of complexity: tomorrow's science. Boca Raton: CRC Press; 2016.
20. West BJ, Latka M, Glaubic-Latka M, Latka D. Multifractality of cerebral blood flow. Physica A. 2003;318(3–4):453–60.
21. Hayano J, Kiyono K, Struzik ZR, Yamamoto Y, Watanabe E, Stein PK, Watkins LL, Blumenthal JA, Carney RM. Increased non-Gaussianity of heart rate variability predicts cardiac mortality after an acute myocardial infarction. Front Physiol. 2011;2:65.
22. Mora T, Bialek W. Are biological systems poised at criticality? J Stat Phys. 2011;144(2):268–302.
23. Chechkin AV, Gonchar YY, Klafter J, Metzler R. Natural cutoff in Lévy caused by dissipative nonlinearity. Phys Rev E. 2005;72(1 Pt 1):010101.
24. West BJ, Turalska M. Hypothetical control of HRV (under review).
25. Kiyono K, Struzik ZR, Aoyagi N, Sakata S, Hayano J, Yamamoto Y. Critical scale invariance in a healthy human heart rate. Phys Rev Lett. 2004;93(17):178103.
26. Kiyono K, Struzik ZR, Aoyagi N, Yamamoto Y. Multiscale probability density function analysis: non-Gaussian and scale-invariant fluctuations of healthy human heart rate. IEEE Trans Biomed Eng. 2006;53(1):95–102.
27. Taleb NN, Blyth M. The black swan of Cairo: how suppressing volatility makes the world less predictable and more dangerous. Foreign Aff. 2011;90(3):33–9.
28. Taleb NN. The black swan: the impact of the highly improbable. New York: Random House; 2007.

# Part II
# Physiology

# A Puzzling Question: How Can Different Phenotypes Possibly Have Indistinguishable Disease Symptoms?

**Tilo Winkler**

Organisms live in environments that may change at any time. If the internal structure and function of organisms would be fully exposed to all of these changes, it could have a substantial negative impact on their survival as individuals and potentially as a species. The ability of single and multicellular organisms to create and maintain an internal milieu results in homeostasis and provides more stable conditions for the internal processes of the organism. Homeostasis is the result of autoregulation. However, the mechanisms of homeostasis are not fully understood. In fact, our knowledge about the mechanisms of homeostasis are typically approximations that may describe the autoregulation within a narrow range of the normal state but not within the larger context of the organism's development and its overall function. Also, diseases are very likely to involve interactions among the mechanisms of homeostasis but are rarely understood in the larger context of systems biology.

A deeper understanding of diseases and their relationship to health requires an approach beyond the statistical significance of linear correlations. Peter Macklem had actively argued for such an approach [1, 2], and published an excellent review article titled "Emergent phenomena and the secrets of life" [3]. Revisiting his article inspired a review of the literature and further analysis of the origins of emergent behaviors that are the foundations of life and of evolution.

T. Winkler (✉)
Department of Anesthesia, Critical Care and Pain Medicine, Massachusetts General Hospital, and Harvard Medical School, Boston, MA, USA
e-mail: twinkler@mgh.harvard.edu

 
J. P. Sturmberg (ed.), *Embracing Complexity in Health*,
https://doi.org/10.1007/978-3-030-10940-0_3

# 1 Basic Mechanisms Allowing the Emergence of Life

Deeper understanding of health and disease requires insights into the basic building blocks that are the foundation for structure and function of organisms. What were the physical constraints for the development of life on earth? The structure of organisms requires obviously some stable arrangement of molecules. Such stable arrangements exist in the physical world in the form of crystals where molecules are confined to their position within a three-dimensional grid. Their thermal movement is very small and there is no rearrangement among neighboring molecules in crystal. However, that stability is a problem for the function of organisms because it does not allow any rearrangements among molecules in response to a stimulus. Freedom in the molecular arrangements exists in the physical world in the form of liquids. The thermal movement of molecules in liquids is higher than in crystals, and neighboring molecules are free to move along each other, which allows functional responses but no stable structures. Since living organisms require both structural stability and functional rearrangements, it seems as if these two physical states lead to a confinement of life at the very edge of chaos in the transition between the frozen world of crystals and the chaotic world of liquids (Fig. 1).

Crystals or liquids consist of many individual elements. But, this is largely irrelevant if the behavior of the individual elements is virtually the same, if all interactions hold the elements tightly together as in crystals or all allow the free flow of elements as in liquids. In this case, the behavior of the whole system is characterized by the average behavior of the individual interactions among its elements.

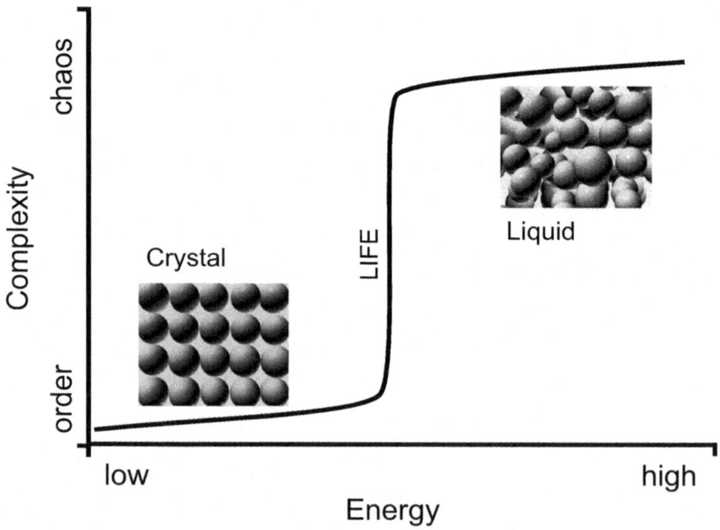


**Fig. 1** Schematic of the relationship between energy and the level of complexity. In crystals, particles are locked in a frozen state that is highly ordered. In contrast, the behavior of particles in liquids is very chaotic and unsuitable for a persistent structure or information storage

A fundamental change occurs, however, when changes in conditions lead to unstable interactions among the elements, and positive feedback mechanisms amplify small fluctuations. In this case, the constructionist approach that extrapolates from single elements to the whole system behavior breaks down [4], and emergent behaviors arise that are "more than the sum of the elements."

## *1.1 The Role of the Chemical Bond*

The first emergent phenomenon that is relevant for the evolution of life is the chemical bond between two atoms. Unlike the three-dimensional fixation in a crystal, chemical bonds lock the atoms in their distance in one dimension. That results in complete freedom for the orientation of the bond. In case of multiple bonds like in a water molecule, the relative position of the bonds may assume a somewhat confined state, which has in the water molecule a *v*-shape, but without fixing the atoms otherwise.

Peptide bonds link consecutive amino acid monomers in long chains resulting in peptides or proteins. The Nobel laureate Erwin Schrödinger described such chains as quasicrystals, and they are truly crystal-like in one dimension meaning that the atoms in peptides are stable in their sequence [5]. But, there is a second feature that is fundamental for life, and that is the high degrees of freedom in the links between the elements of the chain allowing the emergence of protein folding and highly complex protein structures that can interact with other proteins. In the context of how life is possible between the world of crystals and liquids, proteins are clusters of atoms in a relative solid state that float a protein soup behaving like a liquid.

## *1.2 Phase Separation*

Phase separation, like between solid and liquid states, is a key concept of emergent behavior, and has long been assumed to be involved in many biological processes. But, experimental results provided only recently direct evidence that this is true. One extraordinary example of phase separation in cells is observed in T cell signaling [6, 7]. In a very elegant paper, the authors demonstrated in a model system of the cell membrane using only 12 components that a stimulus can trigger the emergence of a dotted pattern separating different components, and that another stimulus can resolve the pattern. This process is linked to T cell receptor signaling that triggers a signaling cascade and leads to actin polymerization.

Similar emergent behaviors have also been observed in the physical world. For example, a temperature difference between two sides of a liquid layer leads to heat transfer by the random movement of molecules in the liquid, called Brownian motion. Higher temperature differences increase the movement of the molecules resulting in a higher heat transfer. But, there is a critical point for the heat transfer at which a positive feedback mechanism leads to self-organization among the molecules triggering a phase separation in the movement of the molecules and the emergence of convection cells, called Rayleigh–Benard cells. Demonstrations of the spontaneous emergence of the Rayleigh–Benard cells are truly fascinating [8]. Another extraordinary visual display of an emergent phenomenon is the Belousov–Zhabotinsky reaction where an autocatalytic reaction leads to local waves in color patterns [9] clearly demonstrating how local feedback can lead to strong spatial discrimination between different states.

The previous examples of emergent phenomena at different length scales illustrate that the principle is essential for life. It plays also an important role in the self-organized development of individuals from a single egg cell to a complex organism. It is obvious that describing an egg cell with average values would not yield any insight into interactions among elements of the egg cell that lead to phase separation and increasing differentiation during the development of the organism. Similarly, genetic determinism should fail if it is assuming that genes completely program an organism, and that interactions among elements of the system or with the environment of the organism are irrelevant.

## 2 Emergent Processes in Disease

In disease, most of the mechanisms that are relevant for the homeostasis of a healthy organism may be perfectly normal but could nevertheless contribute to the disease state. In asthma for example, an asthma attack causes severe difficulties in breathing, and experiments with isolated airways or tissue strips of airway smooth muscle have shown that airway smooth muscle constricts in response to a stimulus. However, studies have not yielded any consistent difference in the properties of airway smooth muscle between patients with asthma and healthy subjects. This shows that patients with asthma may not have different airway smooth muscles compared to healthy subjects although they are clearly affected by the constriction of airways during asthma attacks.

### *2.1 Patterns of Ventilation Defects in Asthma*

Imaging studies of the lung during airway constriction have led to the remarkable discovery of an emergent behavior in asthma: regions with very low or no ventilation, also referred to as ventilation defects (VDefs), in positron emission tomography images of ventilation suggesting regional clustering of severe airway narrowing or complete airway closure (Fig. 2), and a mathematical model showing that the emergence of these VDefs could be explained by self-organized clustering of airway constriction [10]. This emergent behavior is the result of interactions among airways and occurs only after airways reached a critical point of airway

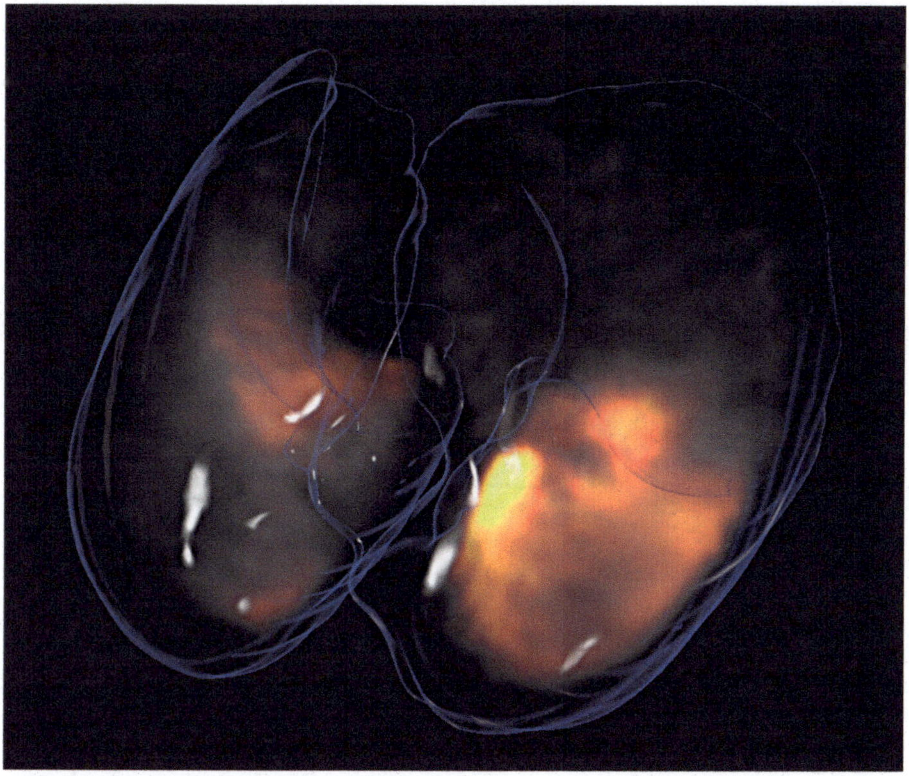

**Fig. 2** Gas trapped in the lungs during an asthma attack. The regional concentration of the gas shows that severe airway narrowing or closure during an asthma attack is highly clustered in some regions of the lungs while regions remain relatively well-ventilated. The gas concentration in the lungs is visualized with a color scale that is fully transparent for low values and shows increasing concentrations in red, yellow, and white for the highest. The lungs are visualized like glass with a blue glow. The three-dimensional rendering is based on imaging data from a study using positron emission tomography and computer tomography (PET-CT) to investigate the effects of asthma attacks on regional ventilation

narrowing. In principle, it is a phase separation in airway behavior resulting in a separation between VDefs and well-ventilated regions. The basic mechanism of the feedback loop causing VDefs can be explained on a single bifurcation of the airway tree: assuming that a perturbation leads to a slightly lower airflow in one of the two daughter airways resulting in lower expansion of the parenchyma surrounding the airway, the lower parenchymal forces would allow increased constriction of its airway smooth muscle, narrowing its lumen, increasing its resistance, and further decreasing the airflow, which triggers a vicious cycle of constriction in this airway. The redistribution of airflow to the other daughter airway increases the tidal expansion of the parenchyma surrounding this airway, which increases the forces pulling on the airway wall counteracting the smooth muscle and that leads to some degree of dilation [11] (Fig. 3).

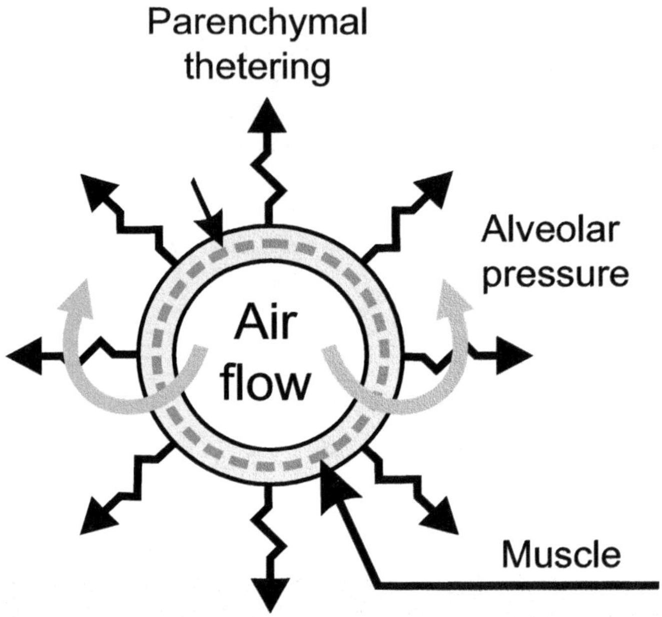


**Fig. 3** Schematic of the single airway model that describes the dynamic behavior during airway constriction. The forces of the airway smooth muscle pull the wall inwards, while all other forces including the parenchymal tethering, the increase in parenchymal tethering from the airflow filling the lung parenchyma, and the pressure difference across the airway wall pull outwards. The key feature of that model is that a critical level of airway narrowing leads to airway instability and closure. Adopted from [12]

Are VDefs associated with asthma symptoms? No study has investigated the direct relationship between asthma symptoms and the emergence of VDefs yet. However, the theoretical model suggests that the critical point of the transition from homogeneous and stable airway diameters to instability and VDefs is affected by a variety of different factors including, for example, the wall thickness of the airways, lung volume, and degree of airway smooth muscle stimulation [11]. Assuming that asthma symptoms are indicators of changes in some of these factors then VDefs should emerge at a lower level of smooth muscle stimulation, which is thought to correspond to an increased sensitivity in tests of airway hyperresponsiveness.

## 2.2 *Asthma Phenotypes*

Identification of different asthma phenotypes (Fig. 4) has been a focus of recent research to improve treatment. The current evidence suggests that there are different underlying causes for asthma. For example, many patients with asthma are allergic, and an allergic response inside the airways of these patients is associated with their

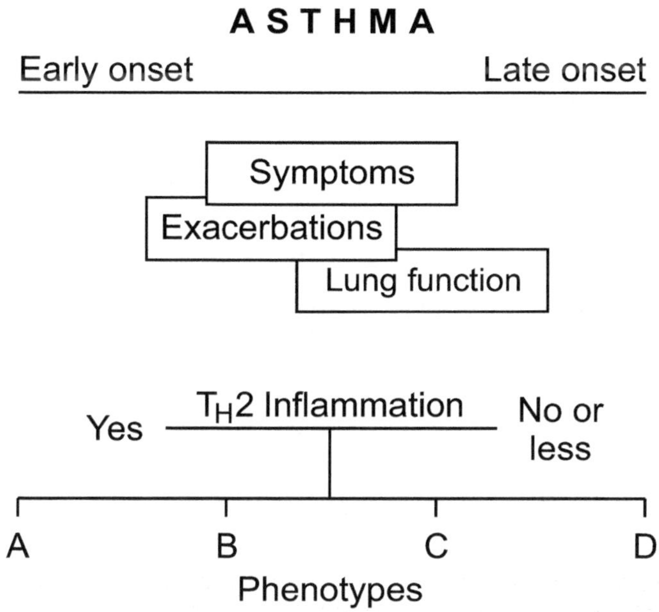


**Fig. 4** Schematic representation of asthma. Schematic representation of asthma with its key clinical features of severity (symptoms, exacerbations, and lung function), TH2 immunity (inflammatory characteristics), and their division into not fully characterized phenotypes. Adopted from [13]

asthma. Choosing treatments that target specifically the allergic response in this phenotype of asthma is expected to improve the efficiency of the treatment and reduce the burden of asthma for these patients. But, the allergic response cannot explain why other patients without allergies have asthma.

## 3 One Symptom: Different Mechanisms?

A puzzling question is: why do clinical symptoms of asthma not allow us to differentiate the different phenotypes? It is possible that the underlying mechanisms of different phenotypes do propagate into clinical symptoms, and that the symptoms are simply too unspecific to allow a clear differentiation. However, the examples of emergent behaviors show that interactions among the different elements of a larger system such as the organism are highly relevant and may prevent a direct propagation from underlying mechanisms to clinical symptoms. This is similar to the failure of the constructionist hypothesis [4], where extrapolation from the behavior of an element to the behavior of the whole system fails when interactions among elements result in emergent behaviors.

Implications for emergent behaviors in diseases with different underlying mechanisms constituting phenotypes may be:

1. That treatment of the actual cause rather than the symptom can restore the healthy state of homeostasis, which would be the optimal outcome; or
2. That the disease may originate from different underlying mechanisms but perturbations of the healthy state have led to manifestations of changes at a different level such that both the mechanism related to the phenotype and the subsequent change elsewhere require treatment.

In the case of asthma, it seems that the mechanisms of different phenotypes may all have in common that they increase the thickness of the airway wall, increase the stimulation of force of airway smooth muscle, or affect both. Such changes would result in increased risk for the emergence of VDefs, and the severe constriction of airways within VDefs could cause secondary airway injury and amplify asthma symptoms. Under these conditions, treating the underlying mechanism related to the phenotype only may not restore the healthy state of homeostasis if the secondary injury persists.

## 4 Conclusions

In summary, understanding emergent behaviors is essential for our understanding of the development of life, the development from an egg to a complex organism, and for a deeper understanding of the origins of diseases. For complex behaviors that underlie major changes in the behavior of a system, it is essential to take the whole system and interactions among its elements into account. Emergent behaviors may explain why different phenotypes with specific underlying mechanisms of the disease may not have different clinical symptoms. The implications for treatment are that targeting of the phenotype's specific disease mechanism is relevant but may not be sufficient to cure the patient. In other words, focusing on a single mechanism of a phenotype may fail to address the overall emergent behaviors in the disease process, or as Peter Macklem had argued: "To focus on the moves of the individual pieces without understanding the strategy misses the point." [1].

## The Transformative Aspects of this Study

Emergent phenomena are a key principle for development and evolution of life, which can only exist at the edge of chaos where phase transitions of elements of the system and interactions among the elements create an infinite world of possibilities with stable structures in crystal-like states and liquid-like transitions between different states. In disease, different underlying causes related to disease states could potentially lead to different clinical symptoms. But in the human body, different underlying causes interact with other processes like the interactions among the elements of a complex system, and such interactions may trigger an emergent behavior that is the same for different underlying causes so that the clinical symptoms may—in the end—be identical.

**Take Home Message**

- Emergent phenomena are the biggest secrets of life.
- Transitions between crystal and liquid states provide both stability and flexibility.
- If different underlying causes of a disease would radiate like an evolutionary tree, then the disease should show different symptoms for the different causes.
- In a complex system like the human body, different underlying causes of a disease may interact with other processes triggering an emergent behavior that leads to the identical disease symptoms.

## References


1. Macklem PT. Con: greater funding of cell and molecular biology has not delivered what was promised to respiratory medicine. Am J Respir Crit Care Med. 2004;169(4):438–9.
2. Macklem PT. Is cell and molecular biology divorcing from clinical practice? Am J Respir Crit Care Med. 2003;167(9):1164–5.
3. Macklem PT. Emergent phenomena and the secrets of life. J Appl Physiol. 2008;104(6):1844–6.
4. Anderson PW. More is different. Science. 1972;177(4047):393–6.
5. Schrödinger E. What is life? The physical aspect of the living cell. Cambridge/New York: University Press/The Macmillan Co.; 1946.
6. Dustin ML, Muller J. Liquidity in immune cell signaling. Science. 2016;352(6285):516–7.
7. Su X, Ditlev JA, Hui E, Xing W, Banjade S, Okrut J, et al. Phase separation of signaling molecules promotes T cell receptor signal transduction. Science. 2016;352(6285):595–9.
8. Anwar T. Benard-Marangoni instability [Internet]. Available from: https://www.youtube.com/watch?v=v2vMXmuC818. Cited 29 May 2018.
9. nater06. Belousov-Zhabotinsky reaction [Internet]. Available from: https://www.youtube.com/watch?v=IBa4kgXI4Cg. Cited 29 May 2018.
10. Venegas JG, Winkler T, Musch G, Vidal Melo MF, Layfield D, Tgavalekos N, et al. Self-organized patchiness in asthma as a prelude to catastrophic shifts. Nature. 2005;434(7034):777–82.
11. Winkler T, Suki B. Emergent structure function relations in emphysema and asthma. Crit Rev Biomed Eng. 2011;39(4):263–80.
12. Anafi RC, Wilson TA. Airway stability and heterogeneity in the constricted lung. J Appl Physiol. 2001;91(3):1185–92.
13. Wenzel SE. Asthma phenotypes: the evolution from clinical to molecular approaches. Nat Med. 2012;18(5):716–25.

# Complexity Sciences Dramatically Improve Biomarker Research and Use

**James Caldwell Palmer**

*"Panta rhei" Everything flows.*
Lucretius [1]

*Most of an organism most of the time is developing from one pattern to another not from homogeneity into a pattern.*
Alan Turing [2]

## 1 Introduction

### *1.1 How Average Can Be "Below-Average"—An Analog to Remember*

Consider you are departing Denver International Airport, as I have done many times, plane lifting, turning west toward massive mountains, up to 14,000 feet high. The pilot announces a new altimeter has been installed that provides the average altitude over the previous 10 min of flight. It is easier to use than the last altimeter and much cheaper. The challenge is that average altitude could mean a below-average flight for you—or perhaps the last!

Like average altitudes, average readings of vital signs in medicine may not be adequate but are easy to calculate. Point measures or thresholds are often used in medical practice—beats per minute (bradycardia or not), current temperature (febrile or not), and 750 Hounsfield units (emphysema or not). Average is easy to

J. C. Palmer (✉)
DMan, Denver, CO, USA



J. P. Sturmberg (ed.), *Embracing Complexity in Health*,
https://doi.org/10.1007/978-3-030-10940-0_4

calculate. Point measures can be done once. But, the scientific method does not endorse doing what is easiest—it calls for using the right measures and tools of inquiry appropriate to the subject of study.

The core clinical practice and applied research topic of this chapter asserts that complexity sciences and mathematics can significantly improve the finding and application of biomarkers that improve patient care. This will be demonstrated throughout this chapter focusing on the rather ancient standard four vital signs—heart rate, respiratory rate, blood pressure, and temperature.

## *1.2 Why Is It That Complexity Sciences and Mathematics Do Particularly Well in Pursuing Biomarkers?*

Complexity sciences provide explanations of particular types of change. Complexity sciences add value by improving insights into previously unrecognized or unanalyzed dynamic patterns and pattern dynamics. These patterns can be emerging and self-organizing, being thermal disequilibrium or nonthermal disequilibrium based—with relevance to a myriad of medical topics—and their biological, bioenergetics, physics, and chemical foundations.

The corollary theoretical proposition of this paper is that human interactions are characterized by qualities and capacities for interaction with the continuous dynamic variability of the exigencies of existence. Humans exist as patterns of interactions with self, others, and environments—built and natural. Humans experience wellness and illness not just in the sense of resisting change, but in the sense of resilience or endurance to change. Embodied self-aware humans engage and interact fully with change in such ways as to proactively leverage and shape change to fit the fundamental requisites of the human organism—to survive, replicate, and thrive.

Complexity sciences support the core proposition that: ***Continuous dynamic variability of human interactions provides the primary sources of continuous sustained viability.***

The various complexity sciences have provided useful insights for improved clinical care. Heart rate variability dynamics (HRVD)—as R–R interval fractal patterns—can provide early detection of neonate ICU infection/sepsis. Blood pressure variability (BPV) can serve as an indicator for risk of stroke and the efficacy of different hypertension drug classes [3–5]. Complexity analytics of temperature curve complexity were predictive of survival or mortality [6].

## 1.3 Vital Signs as Biomarkers

To locate our topic in clinical practice and research, we will use examples involving the long-used standard vital signs—pulse, respiratory rate, blood pressure, and temperature—as biomarkers.[1]

The following definition of biomarkers by Snell and Newbold [7] is used in this chapter:

> …any measurement that predicts a patient's disease state (a diagnostic or prognostic marker) or response to treatment (a clinical endpoint or surrogate for such a measure) can be called a biomarker.

Biomarkers are not just physical samples, nor just measures of direct effect—as shown in this chapter changes in variability of function can indicate physiological alteration, and change in variability of structure can identify anatomical alteration. Responding to changes in the "biomarker" HRVD in the context of a febrile patient is about combating imminent sepsis, rather than the direct change of "the measure" HRVD.

## 1.4 Mathematics of Complexity Sciences

Complexity sciences are now multiple research fields of particular concepts and methods, measures, and analytics. These include: Complex Responsive Processes [8], Coordination Dynamics [9], and Complex Dissipative Systems [10]. Others include Chaos [11], Complex Adaptive Systems Type I (agents and rules do not change) and Type II (agents and rules can change, innovating what can be done), Synergetics [9, 12], Criticality [13], and Statistical Mechanics (e.g., the Tsallis generalization of Boltzmann–Gibbs applied with wavelet and Tsallis entropy analysis).

Fractal analysis, for example, detrended fluctuation analysis (DFA) and mathematical information entropies (MSE, SampEn, and Tsallis entropy) have become key contributors over the last 30 years to understanding heart rate variability as a diagnostic and prognostic biomarker.

Fractal analysis is derived from fractal geometry [14] and can be used to analyze time series data (like HRVD, and temperature variability) or structures (branching lung structures, vasculatures, and blood clots). Fractals are temporal–spatial scaling symmetries that are adept at quantifying patterns within seemingly biological irregularities across the human phenotype (healthy heart rate variations or vasculature patterns).

Mathematical information entropies, simply stated, look at complexity as probabilities of patterns of expected/unexpected patterns in numerical runs in data.

[1] Arterial pulse has been measured over 2000 years in Asia and Europe.

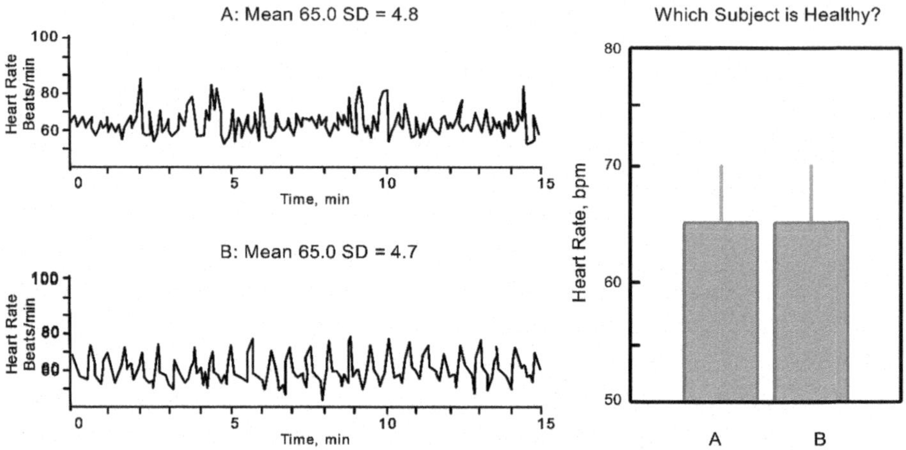


**Fig. 1** BP mean and SD does not distinguish a healthy from a diseased heart. Mean and standard deviation of heartbeats per minute may not differentiate between health (**A**): mean 65.0 SD = 4.8 and disease (**B**): mean 65.0 SD = 4.7. From variability and complexity, Goldberger and DaCosta, www.physionet.org

Generally, a higher entropy numerical calculation indicates a greater degree of complexity, whereas a lower one indicates a greater degree of order. Humans exist in continual critical transitions, in Turing's terms they are "*becoming new patterns*" [15]—a dynamic balancing between patterns as "*too orderly*" or "*too disorderly*."

## 2 Vital Signs Variability

This section will look at pragmatic examples of nonlinear, dynamic complexity sciences analysis of vital signs variability—heart rate, respiratory rate, blood pressure, and temperature variability.

### *2.1 Heart Rate Variability*

Heart rate variability dynamics (HRVD) refers to the continuously variable patterning of size and frequency of R–R intervals, typically measured in milliseconds. This provides very different information as a dynamic biomarker than often used "average variability," "standard deviation," or other summary statistics (Fig. 1). *Averaging removes and obscures information.* An important example highlighting the advantage of dynamic analysis of HRVD is the earlier detection and diagnosis of infection and/or sepsis. Time is particularly vital for effective treatment of infection and especially sepsis.

#### 2.1.1 HRVD for Neonate Infection and Sepsis, Clinical Use, and Significance

A heart rate characteristics (HRC) biomarker is in daily clinical use in over 30 neonatal ICUs across the USA and in Europe [16]. Combined with other patient risk data, it helps provide up to a 24-h added window of diagnostic and prognostic warning of imminent infection/sepsis. Mortality reductions around 20% have been achieved [17]. The index measures heart rate dynamics with SampEn, Standard Deviation, and Sample Asymmetry (transient accelerations—transient decelerations). Clinical use was preceded by a multiyear NIH-sponsored RCT with 3000 infants at nine ICUs [17].

In contrast to information from HRVD about infection/sepsis, the systemic inflammatory response criteria (SIRS) have included heart rate of 90 or greater, along with respiratory rate of $\geq$20 breaths/min or $PaCO_2 \leq 32$ mm Hg. In the latest, 3rd Sepsis Guidelines, heart rate and respiratory rate have been dropped as not being of significant contribution. However, these measures were not replaced by their variability counterparts—indeed, it appears that this has never been considered.

#### 2.1.2 HRV Dynamics Potential for Increased Prognostic Window of Infection/Sepsis in Ambulatory Bone Marrow Transplant (BMT) Recipients

The compelling HRV dynamics tracings below show HRV dynamics of ambulatory BMT recipients at high risk for sepsis—14 had an infection/sepsis, and three who remained healthy. The HRVD of those who developed infection/sepsis declined and became more orderly (in red)—calculated using a discrete wavelet transformation (other analytics including DFA confirmed results)—and showed a 35-h prognostic window before the clinical onset of infection. These findings illustrate the strikingly large window for earlier treatment that HRVD might afford to diagnosing and treating infection and/or sepsis—and the attendant implications for outcomes (Fig. 2).

### 2.2 *Blood Pressure Variability*

Common practice of blood pressure monitoring almost exclusively focuses on mean—generally interpreted as "true"—blood pressure. However, Peter Rothwell's and colleagues' research on blood pressure variability over the last decade [3–5] has shown that BPV is a better prognostic indicator of stroke risk. Their work also showed differential effects of antihypertensive drug classes on BPV, concluding that:

> The opposite effects of calcium-channel blockers [reduction] and $\beta$ blockers [increase] on variability of blood pressure account for the disparity in observed effects increase on risk of stroke and expected effects based on mean blood pressure. To prevent stroke

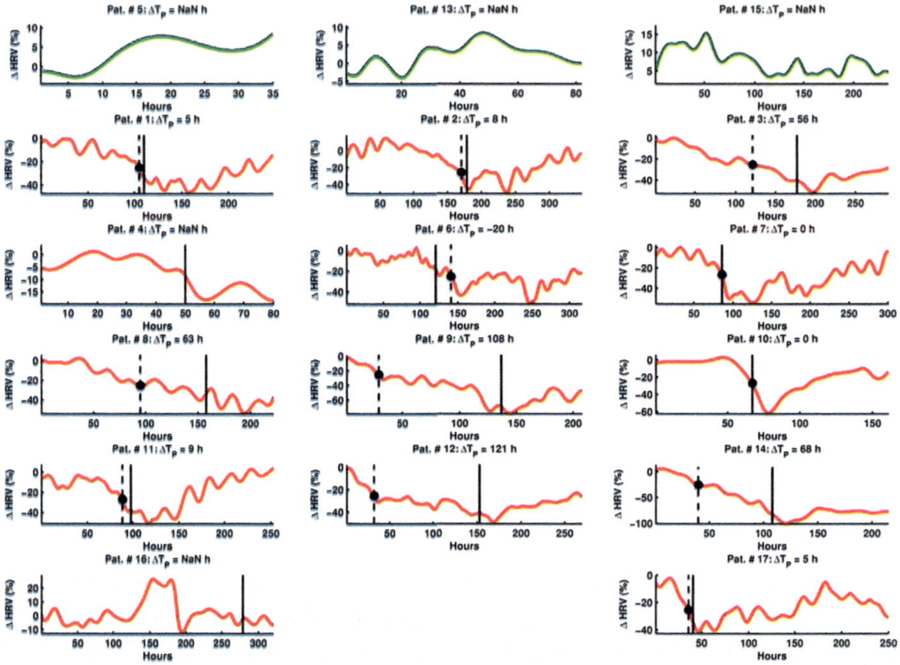


**Fig. 2** Heart rate variability (HRV) in patients with sepsis. Solid black line indicates treatment administered, taken as point of sepsis diagnosis in these high-risk, immunocompromised patients of sepsis. Dotted black line indicates that HRV has dropped 25% below baseline (reproduced from Ahmad et al. Continuous Multi-Parameter Heart Rate Variability Analysis Heralds Onset of Sepsis in Adults, PLoS ONE. 2009;4(8):e6642. (Creative Commons Attribution License))

> most effectively, blood-pressure-lowering drugs should reduce mean blood pressure without increasing variability; ideally they should reduce both [4].

These findings have implications for the design of "flexipills" (i.e., compounding several drugs in one tablet) for the treatment of hypertension and the prevention of strokes. As O'Brien [18] a member of the Rothwell group explains, such combinations give physician the ability to achieve two treatment objectives—lowering mean blood pressure levels ***and*** reducing BPV.

> Blood pressure variability (BPV), which predicts cardiovascular outcome, especially stroke, should be considered as a target for treatment. The recent introduction of variable doses of combination drugs in "flexipills" ...provides a means of not only lowering BP, but of also reducing BPV by using medication with contrasting modes of action. Recently, amlodipine/perindopril has been show to significantly reduce total and cardiovascular mortality, compared with atenolol/diuretic.

These findings show that **average can be a below-average** in terms of one measure relating to a desired outcome—obsessional attention to mean blood pressure ignores the role of BP variability.

> Peter Rothwell argues that the management of hypertension has been clouded by the fact that physicians and scientists have been distracted from consideration of variability by giving obsessional attention to mean blood pressure (BP). The hypertension guidelines, which insist on reduction of BP per se and remove BP variability from consideration, may have done science a disservice by obscuring the influence of BP makes a very valuable contribution to outcome, it does not always account fully for the benefit of therapeutic intervention, which might also be due in part, to a reduction in BPV [19, p. 25].

Shifting or broadening the perspective to include variability of a vital sign, like blood pressure, has implications for clinical practice. As O'Brien [19] observed:

> ...the sternest historical indictment from future generations will be directed at our insistence on permitting isolated BP measurements to dictate diagnostic and management policies of hypertension in the light of an abundance of evidence... How many patients have been subjected to unnecessary or inappropriate therapy and continue to be so mismanaged at the time of writing.

O'Brien cites predecessors to current BPV studies, particularly the landmark publication in 1904 of Theodore Janeway's work and the later work during the 1960s by Pickering's Oxford group. Their research showed marked elevation in BP during doctor visits—the "white-coat effect"—resulting in much unnecessary prescribing, overtreatment, and patient harm.

The introduction of ambulatory blood pressure monitoring in the 1960s provides multiple measures taking into account temporal and contextual conditions, providing a reasonable idea of BPV. Rothwell's team [3, 4] limited their analysis to summary statistical methods, and future work on BP variability will use more advanced analytics as this applied research advances. More important than issues of measurement is the general acceptance of the importance of variability for clinical care.

## 2.3 *Temperature Curve Variability*

Use of the clinical thermometer gained routine use in the 1800s with innovative reduction of thermometer length from a foot to about 5 in. and time to take a reading from twenty minutes to five [20]. Expected human temperature, discerned in the history of temperature taking, is generally viewed as the set-point of, or range around, 98.6 °F or about 37 °C.

Varela [21] noted the challenge arising from temperature averages—"*Measuring body temperature is one of the oldest clinical tools available. Nevertheless, after hundreds of years of experience with this tool, its diagnostic and prognostic value remains limited.*" Papaioannou [22] pointed out the paradox that temperature is in fact a "*continuous quantitative variable,* [but] *its measurement has been considered* [only as a dichotomous] *snapshot of a process, indicating* ... [a] *febrile or afebrile* [state]."

The works by Varela, Papaioannou, and others illustrate the "nonlinear dynamic turn," in which researchers across sciences are turning away from averages, set-points, and linear approximations arising from complex adaptive data-sets. Temperature Curve Complexity analysis mines the data between temperature measures to improve diagnostic and prognostic insights. Varela and colleagues [23] showed that temperature curve complexity[2] in critically ill patients suffering multiple organ failure has high clinical utility:

- An inverse correlation between the clinical status and ApEn temperature curve complexity
- Reduced mean and minimum ApEn complexity indicating high likelihood of fetal outcome
- An increase in 0.1 units in minimum or mean ApEn increased the odds of surviving 15.4 and 18.5-folds, respectively

Papaioannou [22] confirmed Varela et al.'s. [23] earlier findings showing that

> …complexity analysis of temperature signals can assess inherent thermoregulatory dynamics during systemic inflammation and has increased discriminating value in patients with infectious versus non-infectious conditions, probably associated with severity of illness.

and that:

> …the analysis of a continuously monitored temperature curve in critically ill patients using sophisticated techniques from signal processing theory, such as wavelets and multiscale entropy, was able to discriminate patients with systemic inflammatory response syndrome (SIRS), sepsis and septic shock with an accuracy of 80% [25].

### 2.3.1 Temperature Curve Variability in Preterm Infants

Preterm infants are at increased risk of morbidity and mortality due to poor control of their body temperature. Temperature curve complexity dynamics, expressed as scaling exponent $\alpha$ ($T_\alpha$) calculated from DFA of a temperature time series, showed a negative association with gestational age and a positive association with the need for ventilatory support. $T_\alpha$ provides an assessment of an infant's autonomic maturity and disease severity. These findings point to possible added diagnostic and prognostic insights, and improve decision-making when to transfer a neonate from the incubator to an open cot which currently is more trial and error based on weight [26].

## *2.4 A Multiple Variability Biomarker Index for Sepsis*

These findings suggest that it might be possible to create a multiple variability biomarker index for sepsis status and morbidity and mortality risk incorporating HRC/HRV, BPV, and temperature curve variability.

---

[2]Measured as ApEn (approximate entropy) [24].

# 3 The Fractal Nature of Structure and Function

The fractal nature of structure and function allows for the most energy efficient vital organ function. This section briefly describes the fractal branching structure of the airways on respiratory physiology.

## *3.1 The Fractal Nature of the Branching Airways*

As a measure fractal dimension (DF) quantifies how the branching structures of airways make more use out of the available chest cavity than an equivalent Euclidean structure could make [27]. Calculating DF can distinguish healthy from diseased lungs [28] (Fig. 3).

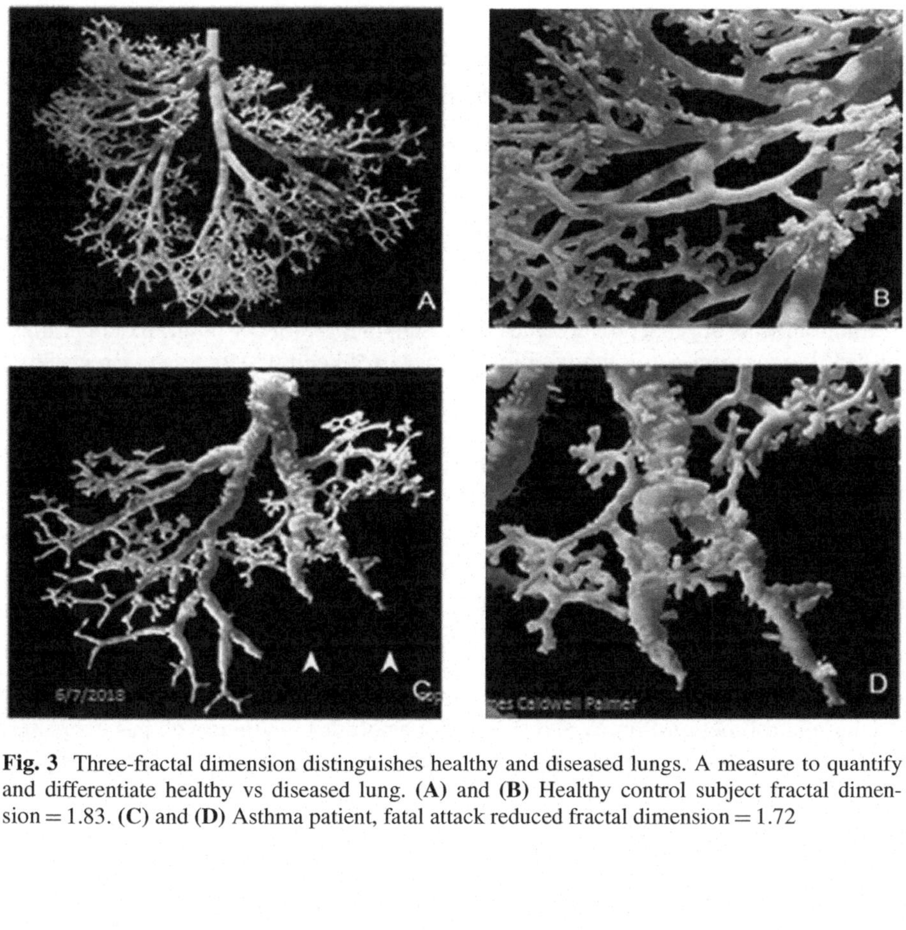


**Fig. 3** Three-fractal dimension distinguishes healthy and diseased lungs. A measure to quantify and differentiate healthy vs diseased lung. **(A)** and **(B)** Healthy control subject fractal dimension = 1.83. **(C)** and **(D)** Asthma patient, fatal attack reduced fractal dimension = 1.72

The advantage of the fractal lung structure seems to be at least two-folds, given the volume used: the surface exchange area is increased and transport costs are reduced. Other branching structures, such as the retinal vasculature, also tap into this advantage.

## *3.2 Respiratory Rate Variability*

Papaioannou and colleagues [29] used several complexity analytics to study difficulties of weaning from mechanical ventilation. DFA, SampEn, fractal dimension (here applied to time series), and largest Lyapunov exponent (measures phase space divergence in three-dimensional space of system states). They concluded that "*…complexity analysis of respiratory signals can assess inherent breathing pattern dynamics and has increased prognostic impact upon weaning outcome in surgical patients.*" The team thought advantages of variability analysis included:

- Observing over longer time periods
- Different perspective—why and how much values deviate from the mean
- Continuous real-time information for any weaning process point

They did not assume stationary time series behavior.

### 3.2.1 Biologically Variable Artificial Ventilation

Biologically Variable Artificial Ventilation describes the use of noisy mechanical ventilation. This approach overcomes the disadvantages of set-point, fixed parameter ventilation, mimicking the breathing patterns of healthy people. As Brewster et al. [30] pointed out:

> Most ventilators monotonously deliver the same sized breaths, like clockwork; however, healthy people do not breathe this way. This has led to the development of a biologically variable ventilator—one that incorporates noise.

They applied a static compliance function [31] with insights from Jensen's inequality about nonlinear averaging [32] to determine the best way to add "noise" to vary ventilation rate and tidal volume.

The benefit of adding "noise" leads to "*higher mean volume (at the same mean pressure) or lower mean pressure (at the same mean volume)* …[resulting in] *enhanced gas exchange or less stress on the lungs.* [31]" The fractal nature of structure and function improves respiratory performance—increased gas exchange area at reduced respiratory effort—and improves post-anesthetic outcomes (Fig. 4).

**Fig. 4** Graphs illustrating Jensen's inequality. From Denny [32]. **(a)** Linear function average value equals function evaluated at average input. **(b)** Convex function average is greater than function evaluated at average input. **(c)** Concave function average value is less than function evaluated at average input

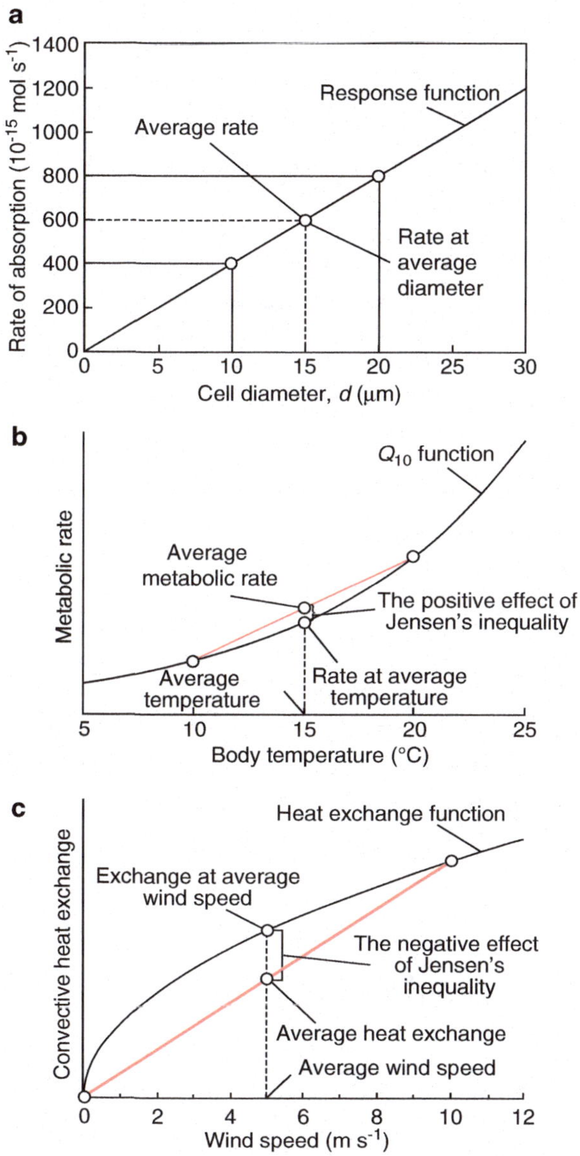


## 4 Jensen's Inequality—or the "Fallacy of the Average"

This section explains in more detail Jensen's inequality proposition used in the work above by Brewster et al. [30] for Biologically Variable Mechanical Ventilation. Jensen's inequality is a durable example (since 1904!) of how to understand difficulties in biology and medical inquiry using (1) averages and summary statistics and (2) assumed bell shape/normal distributions. Denny [32] states:

> Biologists often cope with variation in physiological, environmental and ecological processes by measuring how living systems perform under average conditions. However, performance at average conditions is seldom equal to average performance across a range of conditions. This basic property of non-linear averaging—known as 'Jensen's inequality' or 'the fallacy of the average'—has important implications for all of biology.

Averages are not necessarily helpful to detect, diagnose, or extrapolate information from typically nonlinear biological processes, but more importantly, they may well overlook proper therapeutic choices or suggest incorrect/harmful treatments. This is clearly seen in Brewster et al.'s [30] analysis in relation to mechanical ventilation where fixed parameter "monotonous" mechanical ventilation results in lung injury and is prevented by biologically variable "noise-assisted" ventilation.

Uses of Jensen's inequality occur across research fields and disciplines. It is progressing in ecology and evolutionary studies to better explain, e.g., population dynamics. The evaluation of risks and uncertainty in the "human generated financial asset market" reveals the flaw—or fallacy—of averages; they are below average in usefulness for evaluations of nonlinear functions [33].

Denny [32] concludes:

> Because nature is variable and biological response functions are typically nonlinear, it is dangerous to assume that average performance is equal to the performance under average conditions. Ecological physiologists and evolutionary biologists have heeded this warning in their attempt to predict the effects of the looming shifts in Earth's climate. For example …increased variance in temperature is likely to have greater impact [on species] than the increase in average temperature .

Jensen's inequality provides the mathematical scaffolding for the role complexity sciences are providing for biomarkers and cautions about nonlinear averaging superseding use of averages and linear assumptions.

## 5 Implications

*The future is already here, it's just unevenly distributed.*
William Gibson [34]

Vital signs variability analysis provides major advantages over the use of averages, point measures, and threshold indicators in detecting important diagnostic and prognostic signs. The demonstrated advantages of vital sign variability described herein indicate how the use of averages, point measures, and thresholds may generate missed diagnostic and prognostic insights. These insights raise two important questions:

- What is the cost of missing the early signs of sepsis for the patient's morbidity and mortality arising in the context of constant time pressures on care staff? and
- How can we design better search strategies for variability biomarkers?

Ongoing applied research will find added uses for the integration of dynamic biomarkers. The "Nonlinear Dynamic Turn" is not just a matter of better data analysis compared to mechanistic models [35] but also entails the need to change our fundamental assumptions of the nature of health, wellness, and illness—we need a new theory of disease. The abductive question that comes to mind is:

- If omnipresent variability characterizes human interactions and requires proper analytics—then, what abductive explanation, what theory, describes ontological fundamentals of being human, as having qualities and capacities that enable continuous variability for continuous viability?

Besides of these philosophical questions, we also need pragmatic questions to enhance the future of clinical care like:

- What applied research can develop a biomarker variability index for infection/sepsis? Candidate markers could include [36, 37]:
  - HRVD (infection/sepsis risk, vasopressor independence)
  - Temperature curve variability (survival prospects)
  - Systolic BPV (28 days mortality)
  - Clot structure variability (sepsis coagulopathies)
- How do humans actually embrace and leverage, not just survive, and be resilient to continuous change? How does the embrace of change help generate persistence?
- A thread to follow here is that fractals are "fractal temporal–spatial scaling symmetries" [14]. Mathematical symmetries, in a simple definition, describe actions taken on a particular object that leave that object changed in its essential aspects [9]. For example, the heart as it was at the start of the day resembles the heart as it still is at the end of the day (ceteris paribus). How do fractal symmetries help understand that persistence?

The implications of bio-symmetries of interaction point to the entrained presence (pari passu as to biological not physics symmetries, q.v. Longo & Montévil [38]) of conservation laws (inherent in symmetry mathematics), here in the biological context of energy and momentum. This indicates, importantly, that when an integrated bio-symmetries variability index is altered—episodically like in sepsis, or chronically like in COPD—information may be present to investigate the correlated disruptions of useful energy generation in the body, e.g., the higher resting energy expenditure (REE) seen in various chronic diseases.

**Acknowledgements** The learning by my colleague, David Introcaso, is much appreciated from our conversations with multiple clinicians and researchers over the last few years. Thanks for conversations about HRV and infection/sepsis to Drs. Ryan Arnold, Barnaby Douglas, and Andrew Seely.

## The Transformative Aspects of This Study

- Consolidates evidence-based examples of current or potential advantageous clinical use of particular complexity sciences and mathematics to improve care processes and outcomes.
- Highlights a general mathematical analysis issue of using averages across nonlinear functions by illustrating Jensen's inequality.
- Points to integrative potential and lines of research on the implications of biological mathematical symmetries as characterized by the ubiquitous usefulness of analysis by fractal temporal–spatial scaling symmetries.

**Take Home Message**

- Complexity sciences, applied as *Dynamic Variability Analysis*, already has improved clinical care arising from variability biomarkers.
- More resources should be used to apply complexity sciences to search for and accelerate the clinical use of dynamic biomarkers.
- The "*Nonlinear Turn*" of improved dynamic analytics of process and structure (epistemology) invokes the abductive question: How do we develop a matching processual human ontology—what does it mean to be continuously dynamically variable?

## References

1. Panta rhei. Lucretius. Heraclitus, quote on change. In: Hicks RD, editor. Diogenes Laërtius's lives of eminent philosophers. Boston: Harvard University Press; 1925.
2. Turing AM. The chemical basis of morphogenesis. Philos Trans R Soc. 1952;B237:37–52.
3. Rothwell PM. Limitations of the usual blood-pressure hypothesis and importance of variability, instability, and episodic hypertension. Lancet. 2010;375(9718):938–48.
4. Rothwell PM, Howard SC, Dolan E, O'Brien E, Dobson JE, Dahlöf B, et al.; ASCOT-BPLA and MRC Trial Investigators. Effects of $\beta$ blockers and calcium-channel blockers on within-individual variability in blood pressure and risk. Lancet Neurol. 2010;9(5):469–80.
5. Rothwell PM. Does blood pressure variability modulate cardiovascular risk? Curr Hypertens Rep. 2011;13(3):177–86.
6. Varela M, Churruca J, Gonzalez A, Martin A, Ode J, Galdos P. Temperature curve complexity predicts survival in critically ill patients. Am J Respir Crit Care Med. 2006;174(3):290–8.
7. Snell N, Newbold P. The clinical utility of biomarkers in asthma and COPD. Curr Opin Pharmacol. 2008;8(3):222–35.
8. Stacey R. Complex responsive processes in organizations: learning and knowledge creation. London: Routledge; 2001.
9. Kelso JAS, Engstrøm D. The complementary nature. Cambridge: MIT Press; 2006.
10. Prigogine I, Stengers I. Order out of chaos. Boulder: New Science Library; 1984.
11. Lorentz EN. Deterministic nonperiodic flow. J Atmos Sci. 1963;20(2):130–41.
12. Haken, H. The science of structure: synergetics. New York: Van Nostrand Reinhold; 1984.

13. Bak P. How nature works: the science of self-organized criticality. New York: Copernicus; 1996.
14. Mandelbrot BB. Fractal geometry: what is it and what does it do? Proc R Soc Lond A. 1989;423(1864):3–16.
15. Turing A. The chemical basis of morphogenesis. Philos Trans. 1952;B.237:37–72.
16. Palmer JC, Introcaso D, O'Shea M. Heart Rate Variability: A Diagnostic and Prognostic Biomarkers for Identifying Infection-Associated Sepsis. Available from https://www.healthcarecommunities.org/ResourceCenter.aspx?CategoryID=834659&EntryID=102172
17. Fairchild KD, O'Shea TM. Heart rate characteristics: physiomarkers for detection of late-onset neonatal sepsis. Clin Perinatol. 2010;37(3):581–98.
18. O'Brien E. Stabilizing blood pressure variability: a new therapeutic target in hypertension. Medicographia. 2012;34:1.
19. O'Brien E, Fitzgerald D. The history of blood pressure measurement. J Hum Hypertens. 1994;8(2):73–84.
20. Pearce JMS. A brief history of the clinical thermometer. Q J Med. 2002;95(4):251–2.
21. Varela M, Churruca J, Gonzalez A, Martin A, Ode J, Galdos P. Temperature curve complexity predicts survival in critically ill patients. Am J Respir Crit Care Med. 2006;174(3):290–8.
22. Papaioannou ME, Chouvarda IG, Maglaveras NK, Pneumatikos IA. Temperature variability analysis using wavelets and multiscale entropy in patients with systemic inflammatory response syndrome, sepsis, and septic shock. Critical Care. 2012;16(2):R51.
23. Varela M, Calvo M, Chana M, Gomez-Mestre I, Asensio R, Galdos P. Clinical implications of temperature curve complexity in critically ill patients. Crit Care Med. 2005;33(12):2764–71.
24. Pincus S. Approximate entropy (ApEn) as a complexity measure. Chaos. 1995;5(1):110–7.
25. Papaioannou VE, Chouvarda IG, Maglaveras NK, Baltopoulos GI, Pneumatikos IA. Temperature multiscale entropy analysis: a promising marker for early prediction of mortality in septic patients. Physiol Meas. 2013;34(11):1449–66.
26. Jost K, Pramana I, Delgado-Eckert E, Kumar N, Datta AN, Frey U, et al. Dynamics and complexity of body temperature in preterm infants nursed in incubators. PLOS ONE 2017;12(4):e0176670.
27. West G, Brown JH, Enquist BJ. A general model for the origin of allometric scaling laws in biology. Science. 1997;276(5309):122–6.
28. Boser SR, Park H, Perry SF, Ménache MG, Green FH. Fractal geometry of airway remodeling in human asthma. Am J Respir Crit Care Med. 2005;172(7):817–23.
29. Papaioannou VE, Chouvarda I, Maglaveras N, Dragoumanis C, Pneumatikos I. Changes of heart and respiratory rate dynamics during weaning from mechanical ventilation: a study of physiologic complexity in surgical critically ill patients. J Crit Care. 2011;26(3):262–72.
30. Brewster JF, Graham MR, Mutch W. Convexity, Jensen's inequality and benefits of noisy mechanical ventilation. J R Soc Interface. 2005;2(4):395–6.
31. Venegas JG, Harris RS, Simon BA. A comprehensive equation for the pulmonary pressure-volume curve. J Appl Physiol. 1998;84(1):389–95.
32. Denny M. The fallacy of the average: on the ubiquity, utility and continuing novelty of Jensen's inequality. J Exp Bio. 2017; 220(Pt 2):139–46.
33. Savage S. The flaw of averages: why we underestimate risk in the face of uncertainty. Hoboken: Wiley; 2009.
34. Gibson W. The future is already here – it's just unevenly distributed. NPR Talk of the Nation, 30 November, 1999 show. www.npr.org/templates/story/story.php?storyId=1067220
35. Aerts JM, Haddad WM, An G, Vodovotz Y. From data patterns to mechanistic models in acute critical illness. J Crit Care. 2014;29(4):604–10.
36. Evans PA, Hawkins K, Williams PR. Rheometry for blood coagulation studies. Rheo Rev. 2006:255–91.
37. Brown MR, Curtis DJ, Rees P, Summers HD, Hawkins K, Evans PA, et al. Fractal discrimination of random fractal aggregates and its application in biomarker analysis for blood coagulation. Chaos Solitons Fractals. 2012;45(8):1025–32.
38. Longo, Montévil M. Perspectives on organisms: biological time, symmetries and singularities. Heidelberg: Springer; 2014.

# Analyzing Complex Medical Image Information: Convolution Versus Wavelets in a Neural Net

**Jason H. T. Bates, Elena A. Doty, and C. Matthew Kinsey**

## 1 Introduction

The recent revolution in deep learning applied to image recognition is demonstrating how bio-inspired computer architectures can achieve levels of object classification accuracy that, in some cases, rival the abilities of the human brain [1]. The number of application areas for this new technology is virtually limitless. Perhaps one of the most compelling from a societal perspective is the diagnosis of disease from medical images, something that plays a central role in modern medicine. For example, pathologists diagnose disease by identifying pathologic features in micrographs of human tissue samples, while detection of anatomic abnormalities using a variety of imaging modalities is the domain of the radiologist. Reading a medical image of any kind typically takes a great deal of training because what separates normal from abnormal usually rests on a relatively small number of features that must be parsed out from a background of irrelevancy. This can be extremely difficult even for an expert. The potential benefits of a machine learning tool to assist in these tasks are obvious, especially given that such tools may obviate variances in human capability.

The specific problem we address here is the detection of malignant lung tumors in CT images of the thorax. Lung cancer is the most common form of cancer in western society, and is largely due to smoking exposure [2]. It also has a very poor prognosis unless caught early, usually before symptoms appear. Regular CT screening of high-risk subjects based on the two most prominent risk factors, heavy smoking and advanced age, thus seems an obvious public health strategy. Unfortunately, the vast majority of suspicious lung nodules identified in this way turn out to be benign [3]. This means that most screened individuals who are pulled aside for

J. H. T. Bates (✉) · E. A. Doty · C. M. Kinsey
Larner College of Medicine, University of Vermont, Burlington, VT, USA
e-mail: jason.h.bates@uvm.edu; elena.a.doty.20@dartmouth.edu; matt.kinsey@med.uvm.edu



J. P. Sturmberg (ed.), *Embracing Complexity in Health*,
https://doi.org/10.1007/978-3-030-10940-0_5

further invasive investigation are subjected to rather unpleasant and potentially dangerous procedures that may be unnecessary. Improving the specificity of lung cancer screening is thus a very important public health problem.

Lung nodules are identified as being suspicious largely on the basis of their size [4], yet there is presumably a substantial amount of information contained in the appearance of the surrounding parenchyma as well as in the shape of the nodule itself that pertain to its likelihood of being malignant. For example, the nature of any emphysematous changes surrounding a nodule is known to contain information related to malignancy since emphysema is also a smoking-related disease [5]. Extracting this information seems perfectly suited to deep learning. Indeed, we are certainly not the first to pursue this notion (e.g., [6]), and a web-based competition entitled the "Data Science Bowl 2017" [7] has recently been instigated to stimulate research in this area.

Nevertheless, there are innumerable ways in which a deep learning net can be designed, with limited theory as to how best to do this in any particular situation. Accordingly, current practice tends to be somewhat empirical [1]. For example, a set of convolutional filters are often included at the start of a deep learning net, being inspired by the structure of the visual cortex of the brain [8]. The power of such convolutional nets appears to accrue from their ability to isolate key primitive features in an image (e.g., lines of various orientation together with other simple local structures that can be detected at specific locations throughout an image). When such nets are trained, the filter coefficients must be learned along with all the (usually very numerous) synaptic weights connecting neurons of different layers. Training is thus typically a very time-consuming process. In the present study, we develop a theoretical basis for replacing the trainable filters with pre-specified wavelet filters, and investigate the relative merits of the two approaches on a set of CT images of lung nodules.

## 2 Theoretical Aspects of Convolutional Deep Leaning

We have a set of CT images of the thorax (512 $\times$ 512 pixels each) that we wish to segregate into two mutually exclusive classes corresponding to *cancer* and *benign*. The goal is to assign each image to its correct class on the basis of a set of measured attributes contained within the image. The most immediately accessible attributes are the Hounsfield unit values of each pixel in the image. Radiological diagnosis of lung cancer rests on there being a unique mapping between all possible thoracic CT images and the two diagnostic classes, and that this mapping can be expressed with a useful degree of accuracy by some function only of the Hounsfield unit values. That is, if $\{O_i\}, i = 1, \ldots, m$ is a set of $m$ images, $\{H_j\}_i, j = 1, \ldots, 512 \times 512$ is the set of Hounsfield units associated with the $i$th image (defined, for example, as the linear array created by concatenating each consecutive row of image pixels), and $\{C_k\}, k = 1, 2$ is the set of 2 diagnostic classes, then we seek a function $\Omega$ such that

$$C(O_i) = \Omega(\{H_j\}_i) \tag{1}$$

is a usefully accurate mapping of $\{O_i\}$ on to $\{C_k\}$.

When this problem is solved by a deep learning net, $\Omega$ is comprised of a sequence of operations performed by layers of artificial neurons and ancillary structures. For the purposes of the present development we will suppose that the input data, namely the $H_j$, are first processed through a set of parallel convolutional filters. In the deep learning literature, it is common to see the operations associated with convolution expressed as cross-correlations, but this is immaterial since the weights of the convolutional filters are typically learned as part of the training of the process (so filter direction is of no particular importance). The output of a convolutional filter applied to an image can thus be expressed in tensor notation (i.e., using the summing convention) as

$$A_j = H_i a_{ij} \tag{2}$$

where the $a_{ij}$ are the filter coefficients. In general, there are $n$ different such filters that process the image in parallel, but we will track the path of one of these here.

We assume that this first convolutional layer proceeds directly to the first layer of a multi-layer perceptron such that every one of the outputs from the convolutional layer is passed to each neuron of the first perceptron layer after being scaled by a synaptic weight. That is,

$$B_k = H_i a_{ij} w_{jk} \tag{3}$$

Next, the $B_k$ are processed by the neurons of the first perceptron layer. This means they are subjected to the activation function, $f$, of each neuron which is a saturation-type nonlinearity shifted by a neuron-specific bias $\beta$. The outputs from the neurons are thus

$$C_k = f(H_i a_{ij} w_{jk} - \beta_k) \tag{4}$$

This proceeds through the next neuron layer with weights $u$ and biases $\gamma$ to give

$$D_l = f(f(H_i a_{ij} w_{jk} - \beta_k) u_{kl} - \gamma_l) \tag{5}$$

and so on. Important additional dimension-reducing operations, such as max pooling, take place along the way. These have the effect of reducing the number of values of the indices in the equations that describe operations taking place in the deeper layers of the net until eventually reaching the output layer [1]. The patterns of activity of the output layer correspond in some coded way to the various classes that the input data might possibly belong to.

In order to develop a conceptual picture of what the above operations are achieving, note that a CT image can be represented as an individual point in a $512 \times 512$-dimensional feature space relative to a coordinate system having axes

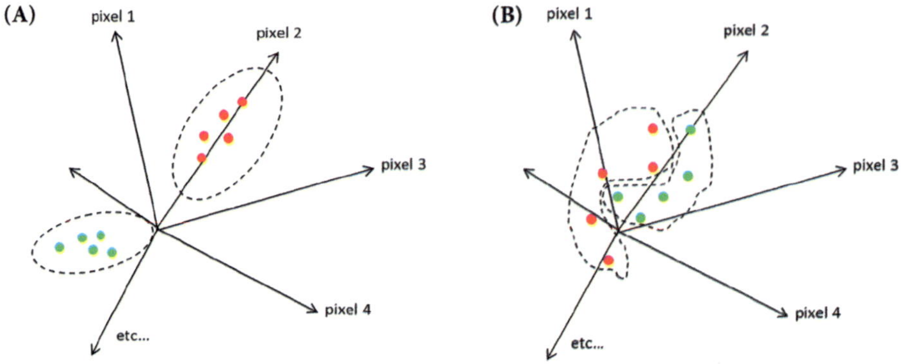


**Fig. 1** A set of images can be represented as a cloud of points in $n$-dimensional feature space, where different image classes (shows as the green and red dots) may be well separated as on the left (**A**), or intermingled as on the right (**B**)

that correspond to the positions of each of the pixels [9]. The coordinates of an image along each of these axes are the $H_j$, so the origin of this coordinate system is the point at which all the $H_j$ are zero. The $H_j$ thus define a vector in feature space corresponding uniquely to a particular image. The vectors corresponding to sets of CT images thus correspond to a cloud of points in feature space. Segregating such a cloud into a sub-set corresponding to *cancer* and a remainder sub-set corresponding to *benign* requires that feature space be partitioned into sub-regions that respectively encompass all possibilities of the two classes. The boundaries of these sub-regions are hyper-surfaces expressible as functions of the coordinate axes. If the classes are well separated, then the classification problem may be straightforward (e.g., Fig. 1a). These functions may be quite complex, however, if the sub-regions exhibit significant overlap within feature space (e.g., Fig. 1b), in which case the classification problem can be very challenging.

A vector corresponding to an image can be expressed in terms of any other coordinate system so long as this other system spans feature space. A straightforward way to construct an alternative coordinate system is to rotate and scale the axes of the original coordinate system. The new system will continue to span feature space so long as none of the new coordinates are collinear, meaning that the new system will continue to have $512 \times 512$ independent axes. Rotation and scaling of coordinates is achieved via linear transformations, expressed in general as

$$H'_k = a_{jk} H_j \tag{6}$$

This is precisely the same kind of operation as performed by a convolutional layer (Eq. (2)) and by a set of synaptic weights (Eq. (3)). It therefore seems reasonable to posit that the classification enhancement properties of a convolutional layer in a deep learning net derive from the way that it re-expresses an image vector in terms of a system of rotated coordinates that are more naturally aligned with the different classes. It presumably also allows some of the coordinates to assume the majority of the classification load while the remainder can be discarded as inconsequential, similar to the retention of only the largest eigenvalues of the covariance matrix in principal component analysis [10]. This is done in a number of different ways corresponding to each of the filters used in the convolutional layer.

Simply realigning the axes in feature space, however, is not enough to completely facilitate a complex classification problem because the vectors corresponding to the different image classes are usually highly intermingled in feature space as defined by the image pixels (i.e., as in Fig. 1b). In order to separate the vectors corresponding to the two classes, *cancer* and *non-cancer*, it is therefore necessary to perform some kind of nonlinear operation that distorts the image space basis vectors in an appropriate way. This is presumably where the highly nonlinear function $f$ becomes crucial. The final operation, $\Omega$, is thus composed of a combination of rotations, scalings, and distortions of the original basis vectors in feature space, with the retention of only those basis vectors that contain significant discriminating information about *cancer* versus *non-cancer*. What started out as highly convoluted boundary in the original feature space separating two mutually invaginating regions becomes transformed into a simpler boundary between two well-separated regions in a feature space of much reduced dimension.

The particular problem we focus on in the present application is how best to perform the initial axis rotations and scalings that are performed by the convolutional layer. In the conventional convolutional net these linear operations are learned as part of the training process, and are done in different ways by each of the convolutional filters in the convolutional layer. Each convolution involves the passage of a relatively small set of filter weights over the entire image, and the output that is fed to the next layer of neurons is a space-frequency analysis of the image. The space component of this analysis is provided by the location of the filter as it moves over the image, while the frequency component is provided by the spatial frequency content of the small patch of image covered by the filter at each location. It is not surprising that these two sets of information are important for identifying complex objects within the image. As a simple example of this concept, consider the 1 large, 2 medium sized, and 6 small circles shown in Fig. 2a. This collection of simple objects of different sizes does not convey anything in particular, yet when the same circles are arranged in a different juxtaposition they are immediately recognizable as a smiley face (Fig. 2b). This recognition is based on the relative sizes of the circles (i.e., their respective spatial frequency contents) and their positions relative to each other. In other words, our recognition of the smiley face is based on a space-frequency analysis of the image.

A convenient general approach to the space-frequency analysis of an image is provided by the wavelet transform [11], which is provided by convolving the image with a set of spatially scaled wavelets of common basic shape. This essentially generates a series of spatial band-pass filters of the image for which the frequency bands are equally spaced logarithmically. The output of the wavelet transform thus converts the original image pixels into a map of the spatial frequency components of the image and where in the image these components are located. In other words,

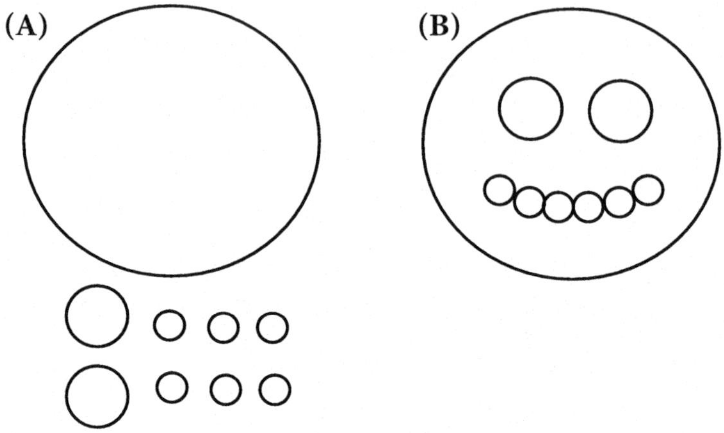


**Fig. 2** The recognizability of an object depends on the sizes of the components of which it is composed as well as the relative spatial locations of those components. The collection of circles shown on the left (**A**) are not recognizable as anything in particular, but when these same circles are arranged differently as on the right (**B**) they are immediately recognizable as a cartoon face

feature space is now expressed in terms of a different set of basis vectors that are arguably better suited to segregating images in terms of the different objects they may contain. Furthermore, pre-specifying the wavelet filters significantly reduces the training burden because the filter weights do not have to be learned, as is typically the case with a convolutional neural network [1].

## 3 Application to Lung Cancer Detection

A set of DICOM CT images of the thorax from the National Lung Screening Trial (NLST) was obtained through a data sharing agreement with the National Cancer Institute (NLST-163). The NLST randomized over 50,000 current or former smokers between the ages of 55 and 74 with at least a 30 pack-year history of smoking to annual screening with either chest X-ray or low-dose CT scan. The CT scans had a reconstructed slice thickness of 2.5 mm and a reconstruction interval of 2.0 mm. We used 10 slices through each of 637 images of lungs with cancerous nodules and 959 images with benign nodules for our study. An example from each group is shown in Fig. 3, demonstrating that there is not an immediately obvious difference between the two groups.

We used the freeware software platform Tensor Flow [12] to construct a multi-layer perceptron (MLP) neural network in which three layers of hidden neurons with 48, 24, and 12 nodes, respectively, connected to two output neurons corresponding respectively to *cancerous* and *benign*. We also constructed two extended versions of the MLP by adding a preceding layer consisting of: (*1*) 64 $3 \times 3$ parallel

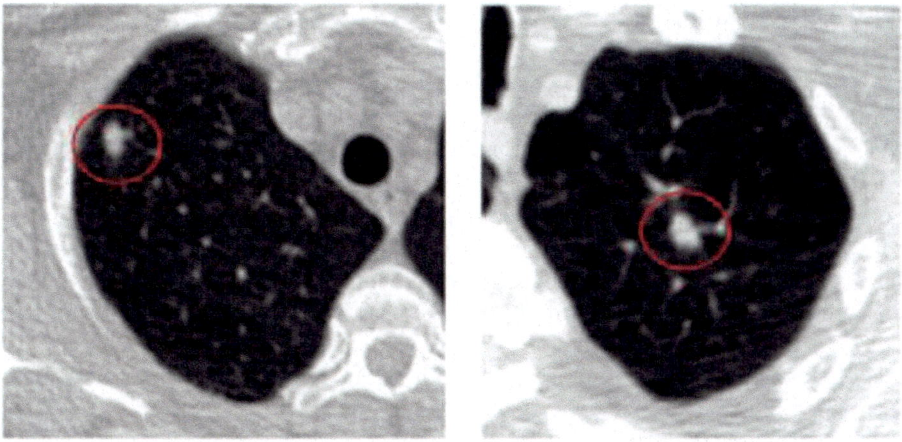

**Fig. 3** An example of a cancerous lung nodule (T1 stage, 11 × 6.5 mm in size, located in the right upper lobe) is shown on the left. On the right is a visually similar benign nodule (11 × 9 mm in size located in the left upper lobe)

convolutional filters with learnable weights (CONV), and (2) 4 wavelet band-pass filters with pre-assigned weights (WAVE). MLP, CONV, and WAVE were each trained on 450 CT images of cancerous lung nodules and 845 images of benign nodules, using batch sizes of 30–100 images run over 30–150 epochs. MLP, CONV, and WAVE were tested on a separate set of 187 cancer and 114 benign images.

CONV and WAVE achieved very similar classification accuracies of $74.3 \pm 1.4\%$ (combined mean). The training times for MLP and WAVE were within a mean of 1.5% of each other, but CONV took an average of 87 times longer to train as a result of its much greater number of free parameters. We thus found little difference in performance between the three approaches, which perhaps suggests that all three nets extracted the maximum discriminatory information about malignancy from the images they were trained on. If so, this underscores the inherent difficulty in detecting lung cancer in CT images of the thorax. On the other hand, the nets correctly classified cancer about 75% of the time, which compares favorably with the performance of expert radiologists, supporting the notion that deep leaning has an important role to play in this arena.

A singular advantage of this approach is that the filter coefficients of the wavelet transform are known a priori and therefore do not have to be learned during training. This presumably saves considerably on both training time and the size of the data set needed for training. Also, the wavelet transform can be performed with different wavelet functions, and we do not yet have a good idea of how to choose the functions that best suit a given problem.

## 4 Implications

Our study suggests that the conventional design of a convolutional deep learning net may be usefully replaced by a design that uses pre-specified wavelet transform filters in place of learned convolutional filters, thereby saving substantially on computational time without undue loss in performance. To place this preliminary conclusion on a solid footing will require larger data sets than the somewhat limited set we employed here, but the results at this stage are promising and performance may be further enhanced with the inclusion of details about smoking history, family cancer history, and relevant co-morbidities such as degree and type of emphysema.

Our study also has implications for the general theory of image recognition and classification. Although much is now known in general terms about how deep learning achieves its spectacular feats of image recognition, many of the precise details about how to optimize deep net performance remain on an empirical footing [1]. Here we view the general classification problem in terms of the manipulation of basis vectors in feature space, something that has a certain natural alignment with the mathematical operations that are performed on information as it percolates through a deep convolution net. As a consequence, we are led to the notion that recognition of objects within an image is based on the sizes of the components of the object (i.e., their spatial frequency content) and the relative juxtaposition of these components (i.e., their spatial locations), as illustrated in Fig. 3. This leads to the notion that transforming an image from a set of pixel intensities to a set of characteristic spatial frequencies and their associated spatial locations would facilitate the subsequent parsing of this information by a multi-layer perception neural net, and the tool most obviously suited to performing a pre-processing step of this nature is the wavelet transform [11].

**Acknowledgement** This study was supported by NIH grants R01 HL-124052 and K23 HL133476.

## The Transformative Aspects of this Study

The work reported herein contributes to the growing body of evidence that deep learning algorithms allow computers to perform feats of image recognition that, until recently, were considered the exclusive purview of the human expert. Indeed, pattern recognition in general has consistently been resistant to recipe-like algorithms based on sequences of logical decisions about apparent features in complex data sets. Neural networks of sufficient structural richness have revolutionized this field by replacing the use of a priori logic with result-based learning, something that has compelling similarity to what apparently transpires in the human brain. The potential impact of deep learning on the practice of medicine is enormous because of the central role that high-resolution imaging has assumed in the diagnosis of many diseases. It is tempting to imagine that computational analysis of medical images may surpass, and thus eventually replace, what is now routinely performed by medical specialists such as radiologists and pathologists. In reality, these techniques will likely be used to complement rather than replace the activities of human experts, allowing the medical professional to focus on the intrinsically human aspects of health care. In any case, there remains much work to be done in determining how the application of deep learning to medical diagnosis can be optimized, and in discovering what is really going on when deep learning nets perform their remarkable feats.

**Take Home Message**

- Improving the specificity of CT screening for malignant lung nodules is an extremely important public health problem, and one that would appear to be an ideal candidate for deep learning.
- Using a deep learning convolutional net with pre-specified wavelet filters on the front end in place of the conventional learned general convolutional filters may substantially reduce learning time.
- Given that the key information in an image relevant to object recognition relates to the relative sizes of the image components and their spatial locations relative to each other, wavelet transformation of an image prior may represent a natural way to parse out this information in a way that makes it easily digestible by a subsequent deep multi-layer perceptron.

## References

1. Goodfellow I, Bengio Y, Courville A. Deep learning. Cambridge: MIT Press; 2016.
2. Siegel RL, Miller KD, Jemal A. Cancer statistics, 2015. CA Cancer J Clin. 2015;65(1):5–29.
3. National Lung Screening Trial Research Team, Aberle DR, Adams AM, Berg CD, Black WC, Clapp JD, Fagerstrom RM, et al. Reduced lung-cancer mortality with low-dose computed tomographic screening. N Engl J Med. 2011;365(5):395–409.
4. Kazerooni EA, Armstrong MR, Amorosa JK, Hernandez D, Liebscher LA, Nath H, et al. ACR CT accreditation program and the lung cancer screening program designation. J Am Coll Radiol. 2015;12(1):38–42.
5. Hohberger LA, Schroeder DR, Bartholmai BJ, Yang P, Wendt CH, Bitterman PB, et al. Correlation of regional emphysema and lung cancer: a lung tissue research consortium-based study. J Thorac Oncol. 2014;9(5):639–45.
6. Hua KL, Hsu CH, Hidayati SC, Cheng WH, Chen YJ. Computer-aided classification of lung nodules on computed tomography images via deep learning technique. Onco Targets Ther. 2015;8:2015–22.
7. Worley P, Prideaux D, Strasser R, Silagy C, Magarey J. Why we should teach undergraduate medical students in rural communities. Med J Aust. 2000;172:615–7.

8. Matsugu M, Mori K, Mitari Y, Kaneda Y. Subject independent facial expression recognition with robust face detection using a convolutional neural network. Neural Netw. 2003; 16(5–6):555–9.
9. Beale R, Jackson T. Neural computing—an introduction. New York: Taylor & Francis; 1990.
10. Jolliffe IT. Principle components analysis. 2nd ed. New York: Springer; 2002.
11. Chui CK. An introduction to wavelets. San Diego: Academic Press; 1992.
12. Sulmasy D. Is medicine a spiritual practice. Acad Med. 1999;74(9):1002–5.

# The Mechanisms of How Genomic Heterogeneity Impacts Bio-Emergent Properties: The Challenges for Precision Medicine

**Henry H. Heng, Guo Liu, Sarah Alemara, Sarah Regan, Zachary Armstrong, and Christine J. Ye**

## 1 Introduction

Bio-systems are typically considered complex adaptive systems. It is now well-accepted that in bio-systems, there are multiple levels of complexity coupled with increased uncertainty. Research areas dealing with complex features of a system can be focused on any level (from molecules to cells, from tissues to organs, and from individuals to populations, all the way up to Earth's biosphere), but the combination of levels can be extremely challenging, not only because "*the whole is greater and different than the sum of its parts*," but also because different laws govern different levels of complexity [1]. While there are valid examples that specific genetic changes of lower-level agents have profound effects on the higher levels of the system (e.g., some gene mutations can be linked to disease phenotype with high certainty), the majority of gene mutations do not. Similarly, higher-level constraints can impact lower-level agents' behavior (e.g., a healthy tissue organization can suppress cancer cells), but cancer will still form from time to time. To fully grasp

H. H. Heng (✉)
Center for Molecular Medicine and Genomics and Department of Pathology, Wayne State University School of Medicine, Detroit, MI, USA
e-mail: hheng@med.wayne.edu

G. Liu · S. Alemara · S. Regan · Z. Armstrong
Center for Molecular Medicine and Genomics, Wayne State University School of Medicine, Detroit, MI, USA
e-mail: gliu@med.wayne.edu; sarah.alemara@wayne.edu; saregan@bu.edu; zarmstrong18@adrian.edu

C. J. Ye
Division of Hematology and Oncology, Department of Internal Medicine, University of Michigan, Ann Arbor, MI, USA
e-mail: jchrisy@med.umich.edu

 
J. P. Sturmberg (ed.), *Embracing Complexity in Health*,
https://doi.org/10.1007/978-3-030-10940-0_6

the idea of such uncertainty, we need to acknowledge the uniqueness of emergent properties of bio-systems.

An emergent property is the key feature for any given complex adaptive system. For various nonliving systems, it is often easier to predict the higher level's emergent properties based on the order or combination of lower-level agents, especially when these agents display homogeneity. For example, it is easier to comprehend that the metal sodium combines with the poisonous gas chlorine, forming the edible compound sodium chloride with a salty taste. In contrast, it is much more challenging to predict emergent properties in biological systems based on a known gene's profile. Although some gene mutations are recognized as cancer causing genes, the relationship between gene mutations and cancer still maintains high uncertainty, as even a pair of identical twins with identical cancer gene mutations can have drastically differing phenotypes [2, 3].

To reduce such uncertainty between the characterization of agents at a lower-level and emergent properties at a higher level, it is anticipated that by using advanced high-throughput -omics technologies, especially with the help of cutting edge computational tools, quantitative profiling at a large-scale level will have high predictability for diseases. Surprisingly, despite the vast amount of data we are dealing with, the only thing we are certain of is that the massive amount of heterogeneity across multiple levels of bio-systems is overwhelming. Furthermore, we are observing an increasing amount of features that display less specificity, challenging our core belief that bio-specificity corresponds to high efficiency at its maximal level. For example, when dealing with DNA–protein interactions, there are many other factors involved in addition to the DNA sequence defined specificity of binding, like the nonspecific "noise." Similarly, a large number of substrates (in the order of thousands) have been identified to various enzymes, suggesting decreasing specificity. Another example is the cancer genome project. This costly project has generated many high-profile publications but has failed to identify common driver mutations (the key initial goal of this project). The most valuable finding was perhaps the high levels of genomic heterogeneity in cancer, as reflected by massive stochastic gene mutations and chromosomal aberrations. Such genomic heterogeneity provides no correlation in accordance to the current framework of the cancer gene mutation theory, where specific common cancer drivers are key. While the result of the cancer genome project was a big shock to many molecular cancer researchers who are sequencing the cancer genome, the results were anticipated by us based on our observations of the patterns of cancer evolution and the fact that cancer represents complex adaptive systems [2, 4, 5].

When faced with such setbacks and even confusion, one must ask: can profiling lower-level agents (gene mutations) explain/predict the emergent properties of cancer (such as overgrowth and invasive phenotypes)? If the answer is no, which factors contribute to this unpredictability? Since increased heterogeneity and nonspecificity are two obvious features of genomic agents following various -omics studies, it is logical to investigate their impact on the predictability of emergent properties. By comparing various types of genomic heterogeneity and their potential contribution to disease phenotypes, we realized that the types of heterogeneity at different levels of a system are responsible for the increased uncertainty in predicting emergent properties based on the genetic profiling of agents. As a result, these analyses shine a new light on the unique features of emergence of bio-complex adaptive systems. Such analysis is crucial to evaluating the significance and limitations of current precision medicine methods, as the rationale of using genomic information to build prospective medicine has ignored the key issue of heterogeneity-mediated emergent properties.

## 2 Heterogeneity Alters Emergent Properties

Emergence can be classified as weak and strong emergence: the stronger the emergence, the more challenging to predict. Unlike nonbiological systems with weak emergence, the task of studying emergence in biological systems is daunting. Due to the fact that the component properties of biological systems are highly state dependent, biological systems belong to very strong emergence types. The reconstruction of emergent properties from lower levels requires a vast amount of information regarding the state dependency of its component properties [6]. Clearly, one of the key component properties (as well as higher levels' system behavior) is bio-heterogeneity.

Indeed high levels of heterogeneity are a key feature for most bio-systems, as heterogeneity should not be considered "noise," but an important adaptive feature [3, 7]. In addition to the fact that there are over 20,000 different genes (agents) in the human genome, and "*more is different*," some unique yet often ignored features of genomic heterogeneity should be considered to understand emergent properties, especially when the status of agents' heterogeneity can change the pattern of emergent properties and its overall predictability. The following are examples that illustrate how genomic heterogeneity alters emergent properties.

### *2.1 Topological Arrangement of Agents (Genes) Changes the Properties of the Genome: Why Chromosomal Coding Rather than Gene Coding is Important for Both Cancer and Speciation*

Current gene-centric molecular genetics has focused on the gene itself and ignored its physical location within the chromosome. Information regarding chromosomal location was used to assist in gene cloning prior to the completion of the human genome sequencing project. For chromosomal translocation studies in cancer, too much emphasis is put on the identification of the fusion genes resulting from the breaking-fusion points, assuming that the function of individual genes outside of the translocation sites will remain unchanged.

In contrast, our studies have revealed that large-scale chromosomal changes are actually the key driving force in cancer evolution, as both translocations and aneuploidy change the genomic topology of all genes [3]. According to the genome theory, the order of genes and regulation elements along and among chromosomes represents a new genomic coding, named chromosomal or karyotype coding, which codes for "*system inheritance*" (to differentiate between the gene-coded "*parts inheritance*" and blueprint). Such information determines the boundaries of the genetic network and defines the platform of gene–gene interactions in 3D nuclei. Recently, increased evidence has supported this new coding system [1, 3, 8–10]. Examples include that karyotype changes can rescue the yeast that loses specific key genes for its essential function, as well as the correlation between karyotype, transcriptome, and various phenotypes. More details can be found from Ye et al. [11].

It makes sense now why chromosomal alterations are a common phenomenon in most cancers. Reorganized genomes produce new systems that represent the most effective ways to system evolution (Fig. 1). Only these fundamentally new systems can break up the normal tissue/immune system constraints and become successful cancers. This is the reason why changing the topological relationships (chromosomal coding) among the same or similar agents (genes) can lead to new emergent properties of cancer. Naturally, the majority of new systems will fail, except for those selected by somatic cell evolution.

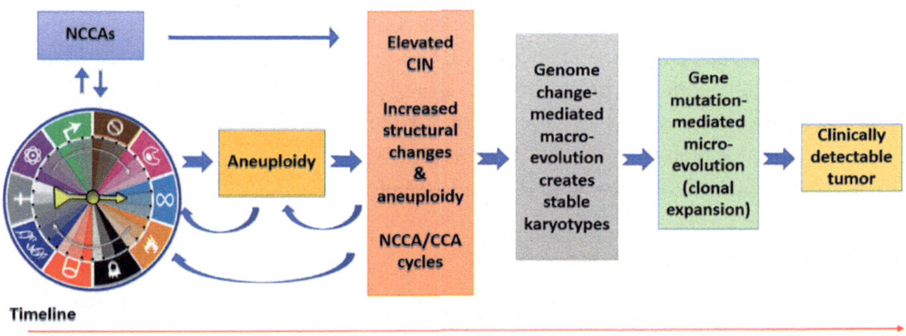


**Fig. 1** Cancer evolution. The proposed timeline illustrates the relationship between various molecular mechanisms (summarized by the hallmarks of cancer), aneuploidy, CIN (often coupled with other karyotype alterations such as structural alterations and polyploidy), macroevolution, microevolution, and the clinically detectable tumor. As NCCAs can be detected from earlier developmental stages, the relationship between various molecular mechanisms and aneuploidy is less clear. It is clear, however, that there is a complex, interactive relationship. Furthermore, elevated CIN is important for triggering macrocellular evolution, followed by microcellular evolution, leading ultimately to the proliferation of the cancer cells with the winning genome. This diagram highlights the complex, dynamic relationship between aneuploidy, CIN, and the two phases (macro and micro) of cancer evolution. Reproduced from Ye et al. [11]. Under Creative Commons Attribution 4.0 International License

Equally important, the same mechanism can be used to explain speciation. It is known that most mammals have similar genes but different karyotypes. Since the main and initial function of sexual reproduction is to preserve the order of genes along chromosomes, changes of gene orders in the germline is the main mechanism of speciation. According to the genome theory, genome reorganization leads to new species, while gene/epigene alterations modify some features of the genome-defined species [3, 12, 13].

Note that there are also nonliving cases of how the topological arrangement of agents can change emergent properties, like the eight allotropes of carbon (including diamond and graphite, for example). Still, bio-heterogeneity is remarkably more complex than these nonliving forms. The amount of heterogeneous states can be too much to comprehend. In addition to the multiple levels of heterogeneity, the large number of agents are different. Unlike the properties of individual carbon atoms, which are identical in bigger or smaller pieces of diamond or graphite, population size clearly changes bio-properties. The system can also change the function of an individual agent, as within a different genome, the same gene plays different functions.

## 2.2 *Quantitative Heterogeneity Leads to Different Emergent Properties*

By tracing genome alteration patterns during cancer evolution using in vitro models, we have unexpectedly demonstrated the importance of the non-clonal chromosome aberrations (NCCAs) in cancer evolution [4]. Not only do the frequencies of NCCAs serve as an index to genome instability, they also provide cell population heterogeneity by supplying different genome systems too. In contrast, the anticipated clonal chromosome aberrations or CCAs are relatively limited, as there is no common CCAs that are shared by the majority of cancer cases in the same type of solid tumors (unlike liquid cancer types (blood cancers) and where recurrent types of CCA is more common). Furthermore, the elevated NCCAs are associated with cancer evolutionary potential, the macrocellular evolutionary transition, and drug resistance [9]. The quantitative nature of NCCAs has drawn our attention. The frequencies of NCCAs seem to correlate with the patient's phenotypes and the treatment response of the cancer [2, 4]. In addition to cancer, the elevated frequencies of NCCAs have also been observed in lymphocytes from individuals with different disease or illness conditions such as Gulf War Illness [9, 14, 15]. Even though genome instability can be linked to many common and complex diseases, as somatic cellular evolution requires genetic components, the specific mechanism of why small portions of NCCAs can lead to different diseases is unknown. We have two hypotheses:

- First, the different genome can generate stress which triggers the succeeding system response. Our data has linked the frequencies of NCCAs to increased ER[1] stress for example [Heng et al., unpublished data].
- Second, the degree of genome heterogeneity itself leads to emergent variable properties at the tissue or organ level, which can be considered an abnormal system response [15].

Interestingly, the heterogeneity of mtDNA[2] (an intracellular mixture of mutant and normal mtDNAs, called heteroplasmy) is well known, and a relatively subtle change in the degree of heteroplasmy can have dramatic impacts on a patient's phenotype displaying different types of diseases [16]. For example, the 3243A>G mutation (mtDNA transfer RNA mutation at nucleotide 3243A>G) disturbs mitochondrial protein synthesis leading to amino acid misincorporation and electron transport chain deficiency. When this mutation is present at 50–90% mtDNA heteroplasmy, it can cause multisystem disease, including the mitochondrial encephalomyopathy, lactic acidosis, and stroke-like episodes (MELAS) syndrome. When the same mutation is at lower heteroplasmy levels, it can contribute to autism and type I and type II diabetes in Eurasians, and at very high levels it can lead to Leigh syndrome (or perinatal lethality) [17]. The phenomenon could be considered a good example of heterogeneity leading to different emergent properties. Surely, when the transcriptome was analyzed for a series of degree of heterogeneity (using mtDNA 3243G mutation as an example, from 0%, 20%, 30%, 50%, 60% 90%, and 100%, within the same nuclear genome background), it showed that the heterogeneity of a single mtDNA point mutation can cause different cellular transcriptional responses. This data set not only explains the mechanism of heteroplasmy but also supports the concept of fuzzy inheritance. Equally important, it also provides evidence of heterogeneity leading to different emergent phenotypes of diseases [13, 15, 17], as the experimental design has set up an excellent model system to illustrate how the quantitative changes of a heterogenic subsystem impacts the emergent properties of a whole system.

In addition, cell density can influence the switching of pathways. For example, the cell density can lead to pathway changes between the e-cadherin-beta catenin (e-cadherin/$\beta$-catenin complex plays an important role in maintaining epithelial integrity) and the TCF (T-cell factor) pathway.

---

[1]Endoplasmic reticulum.

[2]Mitochondrial DNA.

### 2.3 *Selection Pressure Swings the Patterns of Emergent Properties: The Advantages of Average vs. Outliers within Physiological vs. Pathological Conditions*

Current technology of genomic profiling of cancer cells is mainly based on collecting the average data of the cellular population, which unavoidably washes away heterogeneity. Since heterogeneity is inevitably the key feature of cancer, this averaged data no longer truly represents the cancer cell population. To illustrate this point, we have compared single cell growth and its contributions to population growth. The average growth dominates in cell populations with relatively stable genomes (the growth profile among individual cells are similar to average growth), while for highly unstable cancer populations, the main contribution to population growth is often contributed by rapid and massive growth from a few cells (the majority of cells did not contribute to the growth) (Fig. 2). Further syntheses have concluded that unstable cell populations are not reliably characterized by the arithmetic mean, and cancer evolution is the game of outliers [18]. It is thus likely that the emergent properties of the outliers vs. average growth are determined by the overall stability of the cellular population, as well as the level of selection stress. In physiological conditions, for example, selection pressure is lower, and the relatively stable cell populations display homogenous behavior. In pathological conditions however, under high selective pressure, most cells are not able to survive, and only outliers survive and repopulate the new population.

Moreover, during normal development and physiological processes, the karyotypes of most cells are unchanged and the gene/epigene level regulation dominates. In contrast, in the pathological condition, many genomic changes involve

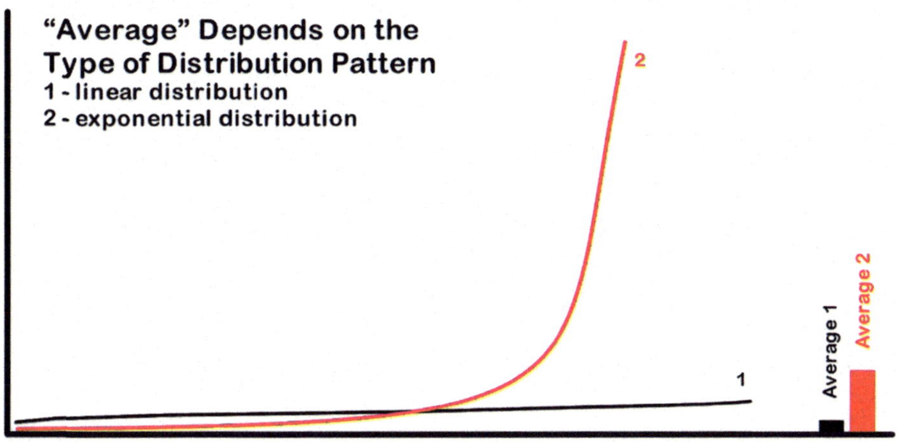


**Fig. 2** Averages can be misleading. Averages do not always reflect the true distribution of a data series. The higher average of the distribution pattern represented in line 2 is caused by the "outliers" at the end of the distribution curve (For original data, see [18])

karyotypes (much more profound changes). Similarly, under low stress, cellular adaptation can be achieved without inducing new genome formation, while under the highest stress (such as high dosage of chemotherapy drugs), only cells with new karyotypes can survive. In a way, cell killing can also trigger the genome chaos-mediated survival strategy [3, 19, 20]. A recent experiment also illustrated that while a moderate suppression of Rad51C reduces HR activity,[3] strong or near complete suppression of this gene paradoxically activates HR activity (15–>50%), possibly by activation of RAD51 independent HR pathways [21].

Clearly, the population emergent patterns are different, even for the same agents under different selection conditions.

## 2.4 The Dynamics of Emergent Properties: Transitional Populations Are Important for Macrocellular Evolution

Genome chaos or karyotype chaos, a rapid and massive genome reorganization, was initially described in the cellular immortalization model [4]. During recent years, this has been confirmed by various cancer genome sequencing projects, although many different names were introduced to describe various subtypes of chaotic genomes including chromothripsis and chromoplexy [20, 22, 23]. Using drug-induced genome chaos as a model, the process of induction, chromosome fragmentation, initial chaotic genome formation, and the selection of stable genomes were studied. Interestingly, most of the initial chaotic genomes were often replaced with simpler and more stable genomes at later stages, despite their crucial importance in serving as transitional karyotypes which pass along features of fuzzy inheritance among cellular generations.

Many initial chaotic genomes are highly dynamic with complex translocations. Some of them display hundreds of chromosomes coupled with new processes of cell division and fusion by which one cell division can generate 20–60 cells (Fig. 3). We hypothesized that the main function of the rapid dividing and fusing is to form a genome package that can survive. These transitional chaotic genomes are essential to passing genetic information to the proceeding stable and fit population. Thus, the same emergent properties can be produced by different agents. Interestingly, the transitional genome chaos can be observed in all major cancer evolution episodes including immortalization, transformation, metastasis, and survival of drug treatment.

Moreover, among many transitional chaotic genomes, we have observed cells with only one giant chromosome. Evident from its size and morphology, this giant chromosome was formed by chromosomal fusion. Due to genome reorganization

[3] Homologous recombination: a type of genetic recombination in which nucleotide sequences are exchanged between two similar or identical molecules of DNA, particularly to repair DNA damage affecting both strands of the double helix.

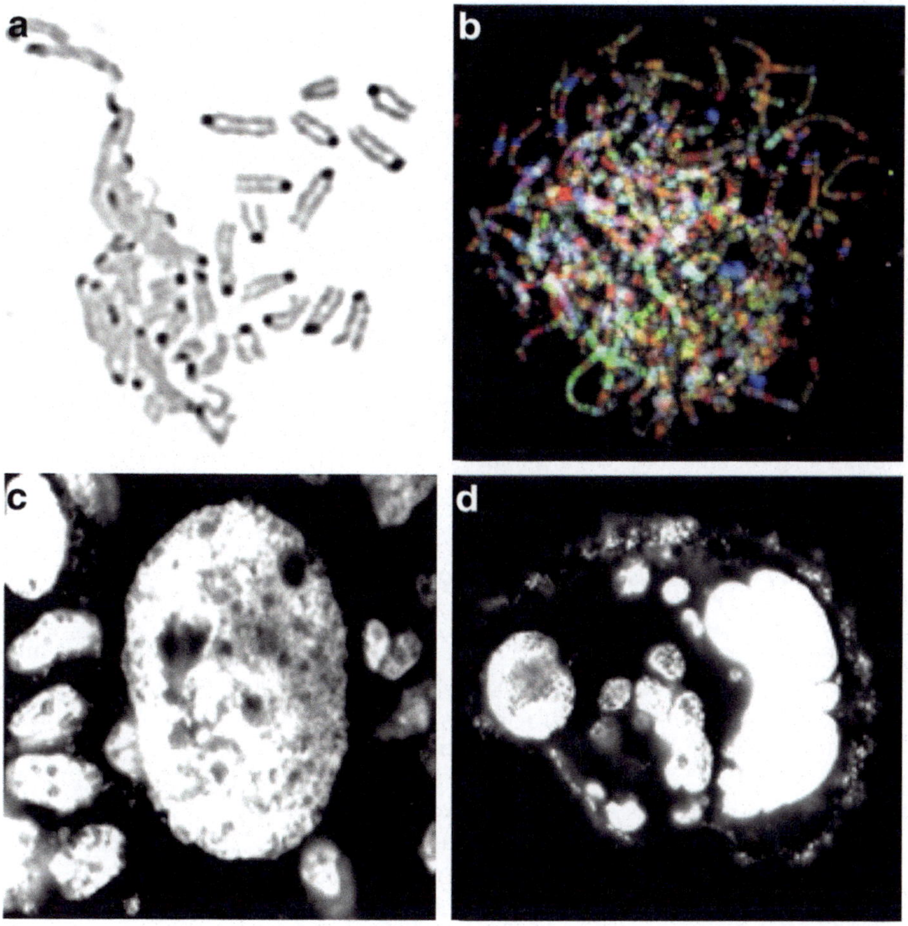


**Fig. 3** Genome chaos. Examples of NCCAs: (**a**) DMF image (reversed DAPI image) detected from mouse cell culture. Left portion shows the decondensed chromosomes tangling together, while some normal condensed chromosomes are nearby. (**b**) SKY image of a chaotic genome detected from a Dox-treated mouse cell. Each normal chromosome should have one unique color. However, for these massively reorganized chromosomes, there are multiple colors detected from each single chromosome, indicating the multiple events of chromosomal shattering and stitching. Note that there are many extremely long chromosomes. (**c**) An image of a giant nucleus (DAPI image) detected from HT-29 cells cultured in situ. Typical normal-sized nuclei are surrounding the giant nucleus. (**d**) An image of a cluster of cells derived from one giant nucleus. Since many of these cells are stochastically generated and display different amounts of DNA, these cells represent NCCAs when they enter into metaphase. Live imaging shows that there are continuous division/fusion events for unstable cancer cells, suggesting a new means of generating fuzzy inheritance. Reproduced from Heng et al. [10]. Under Creative Commons Attribution 4.0 International License

during crisis, the entire genome became one new chromosome. Clearly, this type of giant chromosome is only observed from earlier stages of genome chaos. It is likely that they lost the evolutionary competition, as all robust genomes have much simpler karyotypes. Recently, one giant functional yeast chromosome has been formed by linking 16 individual chromosomes together with CRISPR-Cas9-mediated genome editing technology (another research group also obtained a yeast with only 2 giant chromosomes using similar technology) [24, 25]. Even though this artificial yeast can grow under lab conditions and displayed similar features compared to its parental wild type, the new yeast cell with one giant chromosome displayed incompetence when co-cultured with a wild type and will likely be eliminated if prolonged in culture. This supports our viewpoint regarding the drug-induced giant chromosome formation in our experiments.

Nevertheless, these transitional unstable genomes might represent an important step for the success of system emergence. Despite that they are often invisible, they are essential for the process as a whole.

## 2.5 Emergence Based on Collaborative Agents

Studying cancer drug resistance has revealed an interesting phenomenon: while many clones become stable displaying clonal karyotypes following selection, some surviving clones can keep a highly heterogeneous population for years of culture. When the majority of the cellular population is highly dynamic, the population is stable.

Different explanations can be considered: there are powerful collaborations among these unstable individual cells. It is likely that these highly dynamic cells cannot survive on their own but are able to when collaborating together. If true, then survival can be managed through the emergence of independent unviable agents.

It is also possible that some of these transitional genomes function as collaborative agents necessary for transition (more details can be found in Sect. 3).

There are many examples that support this idea:

Heppner and Miller have pointed out that the heterogeneity from the mixture of sublines is essential for tumorigenicity. Moreover, tumor subpopulation interactions, influencing both growth and drug sensitivity, resulted in treatment responses that were either better or worse than would be expected [26]. Clearly, emergence is different in terms of function and predictability than individual agents.

Recently, using the mouse model, Heppner's observation that interclonal cooperation is essential for tumor maintenance has been confirmed [27].

In our drug resistance experiment, isolated clones were not viable, even though the highly heterogenous population was fine (unpublished observation).

Finally, it has concluded that phenotypic heterogeneity and cell-to-cell differences in stress tolerance are emergent properties when cells cooperate in metabolism [28].

### 2.6 *Multiple Levels of Heterogeneity*

To further complicate the situation, there are multiple levels and multiple stages of heterogeneity involved in most biological processes, which unavoidably contribute to many human diseases. Recently, there have been some important realizations as to why there is an overwhelming amount of genomic heterogeneity in human systems, and why many common and complex diseases are difficult to cure.

***First.*** Heterogeneity is the key feature for most bio-systems with advantages in evolutionary selection. Systems with high levels of heterogeneity display high resilience and robustness, as well as evolvability, even though this means a larger cost for both individuals and populations. Karyotype heterogeneity is especially important for macroevolution [1, 3, 13]. Furthermore, separation of the germline and somatic cell allows somatic heterogeneity to rise to the highest level. As long as the germline displays the same karyotype, the somatic genome can be drastically altered in delivering the adaptive function.

***Second.*** The genomic basis of heterogeneity has been identified as fuzzy inheritance. Different than traditional inheritance, fuzzy inheritance suggests that most genes code for a range of potential phenotypes. From this "fuzzy" range of phenotypes, the respective environment can then allow the best-suited status to be "chosen." Meanwhile, a similar range of potential phenotypes will be passed on to offspring, and again, environments will select the specific phenotype [3, 13, 29]. This new concept points out that the genetic coded message is rather fuzzy, which serves as the basis for inherited heterogeneity or phenotypic plasticity.

***Third.*** Successful cellular adaptation requires increased heterogeneity to deal with dynamic environmental changes. Increased heterogeneity can have big advantages, particularly during development, aging, repair, and regeneration. However, as a trade-off, the altered genomic landscape can contribute to diseases [30]. In a sense, as long as cellular adaptation is needed, variant-mediated diseases will stick around [31].

## 3 The Challenges for Precision Medicine

Precision medicine (or personalized medicine) refers to the personalization of medical treatment to the individual characteristics of each patient. Following a research initiative from the Obama administration, precision medicine has become a popular term [32].

Precision medicine represents one of the biggest promises since the original human genome project (which was completed 15 years ago) as well as the current cancer genome project (that is why the short-term goal of the US government's initiative focuses on precision medicine in cancer research). Despite the fact that precision medicine was designed to combine different approaches including the profiling of people's genes, environments, and lifestyles, and due to the popularity of current various -omics technologies, profiling genomics has become the priority. The rationale seems rather straightforward:

- There is a strong correlation between genotype and phenotype. Since environmental factors are too diverse and hard to control in a human population, accessing genotypic information is more reliable and practical.
- Even though many gene mutations have been identified so far, by sequencing many cancer patients, the list of key driver gene mutations will be identified.
- Sequencing and other efforts will provide precision genomic profiles and molecular causation for each patient, including cancer-specific pathways, which offers the individualized molecular targets for medical benefit.

The massive cancer genome sequencing data is now available. Surprisingly, it challenges the original rationale of the cancer genome project.

- The anticipated *common driver mutations cannot be identified from the majority of cancer patients*. There are actually many more diverse gene mutations that are not shared among patients, and most of the gene mutations identified do not make sense based on current gene mutation theory of cancer.
- There is a *high level of chromosomal changes and epigenetic changes*. The multiple levels of genomic heterogeneity are overwhelming.
- The *genomic landscape is often unique even among different portions of the same tumor*, not to mention the heterogeneity among different patients.
- The *genomic landscape is highly dynamic*. When targeted by tailored molecular treatment, a new genomic landscape will emerge to replace the previous one, with altered targets.

Clearly, only focusing on a snapshot of a gene mutation is not very useful in predicting the trend of cancer evolution. To monitor the overall heterogeneity and system stability, as well as to distinguish the phases of cancer evolution (either micro- or macrocellular phase), is of more significance. For example, multiple studies have illustrated the *power of using genome instability (CIN) to predict clinical outcomes*, which is more reliable than using gene mutation profiles. This raises some important questions for precision medicine:

- Which genomic level should we monitor, and what types of biomarkers (gene mutations, molecular pathways, or instability-mediated system behaviors) should we develop?
- How do we deal with the concept of heterogeneity?
- Knowing the aspect of fuzzy inheritance, should more attention be turned to environmental factors?
- How do we integrate system constraints into disease management?
- And how do we apply molecular medicine in the context of holistic medicine?

Many physicians and researchers have started studying these issues through the lens of complex and adaptive systems prior to the era of precision medicine [5, 33–35]. Since multiple levels of genomic heterogeneity are the key features of many diseases such as cancer, studying how genomic/epigenetic heterogeneity contributes to emergence is of ultimate importance. Our analyses of this issue will directly benefit our understanding of precision medicine in terms of its goals and limitations. Hopefully, knowing the limitations of the characterization of lower-level agents, especially with a high level of heterogeneity involved, precision medicine will adjust its goals and strategies by focusing more on holistic medicine, as monitoring system dynamics and measuring system heterogeneity will not only simplify the process but also provide enhanced benefits for patients.

**Acknowledgement** This chapter is part of a series of studies entitled "*The mechanisms of somatic cell and organismal evolution.*"

## The Transformative Aspects of This Study

While the promise of precision medicine has generated excitement and high expectations, there are challenges for some key assumptions on which the concept is based. Since most common and complex diseases belong to adaptive systems where fuzzy inheritance interacts with the dynamic environment during nonlinear somatic cell evolution, both disease progression and treatment response are less predictable if based only on the precision of gene profiles. Although increasingly voices have expressed their concerns for this neo-reductionist approach (reduction based on big data), few have directly studied the conceptual limitations of precision medicine. In this chapter, we have focused on the relationship between bio-heterogeneity and emergent properties, a subject crucial to understanding why the targeting of lower-level agents (genes and pathways) provides unsatisfactory results at higher levels of this system such as clinical outcomes, which is practically the ultimate goal. Such analyses illustrate that dynamic interactions of heterogeneity in lower-level agents lead to the unpredictability of complex adaptive systems. As a result, stress-induced multiple genomic heterogeneity-mediated evolutionary processes present the greatest challenges for precision medicine.

**Take Home Message**

- Multiple levels of bio-heterogeneity impact emergent properties.
- Heterogeneity is the key factor that complicates the goals of precision medicine.
- Further studies are needed to illustrate the relationship between heterogeneity and emergent system behaviors.

## References


1. Heng HH. The genome-centric concept: resynthesis of evolutionary theory. Bioessays. 2009;31(5):512–25.
2. Heng HH. Cancer genome sequencing: the challenges ahead. Bioessays. 2007:29(8):783–94.
3. Heng HH. Debating cancer: the paradox in cancer research. Hackensack, NJ: World Scientific; 2015.
4. Heng HH, Stevens JB, Liu G, Bremer SW, Ye KJ, Reddy PV, et al. Stochastic cancer progression driven by non-clonal chromosome aberrations. J Cell Physiol. 2006;208(2):461–72.
5. Heng HH. The conflict between complex systems and reductionism. JAMA. 2008;300(13):1580–1.
6. Kolodkin A, Simeonidis E, Westerhoff HV. Computing life: add logos to biology and bios to physics. Prog Biophys Mol Biol. 2014;111(2–3):69–74.
7. Heng HH, Bremer SW, Stevens JB, Horne SD, Liu G, Abdallah BY, et al. Chromosomal instability (CIN): what it is and why it is crucial to cancer evolution. Cancer Metastasis Rev. 2013;32(3–4):325–40.
8. Heng HH, Liu G, Stevens JB, Bremer SW, Ye KJ, Abdallah BY, et al. Decoding the genome beyond sequencing: the new phase of genomic research. Genomics. 2011;98(4):242–52.
9. Heng HH, Liu G, Stevens JB, Abdallah BY, Horne SD, Ye KJ, et al. Karyotype heterogeneity and unclassified chromosomal abnormalities. Cytogenet Genome Res. 2013;139(3):144–57.
10. Heng HH, Regan SM, Liu G, Ye CJ. Why it is crucial to analyze non clonal chromosome aberrations or NCCAs? Mol Cytogenet. 2016;9:15.
11. Ye CJ, Regan S, Liu G, Alemara S, Heng HH. Understanding aneuploidy in cancer through the lens of system inheritance, fuzzy inheritance and emergence of new genome systems. Mol Cytogenet. 2018;11:31.
12. Ye CJ, Liu G, Bremer SW, Heng HH. The dynamics of cancer chromosomes and genomes. Cytogenet. Genome Res. 2007;118(2–4):237–46.
13. Heng HH. Genome chaos: rethinking genetics, evolution, and molecular medicine. Cambridge: Academic Press; 2019.
14. Liu G, Ye CJ, Chowdhury SK, Abdallah BY, Horne SD, Nichols D, et al. Detecting chromosome condensation defects in Gulf war illness patients. Curr Genet. 2018;19(3):200–6.
15. Heng HH, Liu G, Regan S, Ye CJ. Linking Gulf war illness to genome instability, somatic evolution, and complex adaptive systems. In: Sturmberg J, editor. Putting systems and complexity sciences into practice. Cham: Springer; 2018. p. 83–95.
16. Wallace DC, Chalkia D. Mitochondrial DNA genetics and the heteroplasmy conundrum in evolution and disease. Cold Spring Harb Perspect Biol. 2013;5(11):a021220.
17. Picard M, Zhang J, Hancock S, Derbeneva O, Golhar R, Golik P, et al. Progressive increase in mtDNA 3243A>G heteroplasmy causes abrupt transcriptional reprogramming. Proc Natl Acad Sci USA. 2014;111(38):E4033–42.
18. Abdallah BY, Horne SD, Stevens JB, Liu G, Ying AY, Vanderhyden B, et al. Single cell heterogeneity: why unstable genomes are incompatible with average profiles. Cell Cycle 2013;12(23):3640–9.
19. Liu G, Stevens JB, Horne SD, Abdallah BY, Ye KJ, Bremer SW, et al. Genome chaos: survival strategy during crisis. Cell Cycle. 2014;13(4):528–37.
20. Ye CJ, Liu G, Heng HH. Experimental induction of genome chaos. Methods Mol. Biol. 2018;1769:337–52.
21. Pal J, Nanjappa P, Kumar S, Shi J, Buon L, Munshi NC, et al. Impact of RAD51C-mediated homologous recombination on genomic integrity in Barrett's adenocarcinoma cells. J Gastroenterol Hepatol Res. 2017;6(1):2286–95.
22. Stephens PJ, Greenman CD, Fu B, Yang F, Bignell GR, Mudie LJ, et al. Massive genomic rearrangement acquired in a single catastrophic event during cancer development. Cell. 2011;144(1):27–40.

23. Baca SC, Prandi D, Lawrence MS, Mosquera JM, Romanel A, Drier Y, et al. Punctuated evolution of prostate cancer genomes. Cell. 2013;153(3):666–77.
24. Luo J, Sun X, Cormack BP, Boeke JD. Karyotype engineering by chromosome fusion leads to reproductive isolation in yeast. Nature. 2018;560(7718):392–96.
25. Shao Y, Lu N, Wu Z, Cai C, Wang S, Zhang LL, et al. Creating a functional single-chromosome yeast. Nature. 2018;560(7718):331–5.
26. Heppner GH, Miller BE. Therapeutic implications of tumor heterogeneity. Semin Oncol. 1989;16(2):91–105.
27. Cleary AS, Leonard TL, Gestl SA, Gunther EJ. Tumour cell heterogeneity maintained by cooperating subclones in Wnt-driven mammary cancers. Nature. 2014;508(7494):113–7.
28. Campbell K, Vowinckel J, Ralser M. Cell-to-cell heterogeneity emerges as consequence of metabolic cooperation in a synthetic yeast community. Biotechnol J 2016;11(9):1169–78.
29. Heng HH. Heterogeneity-mediated cellular adaptation and its trade-off: searching for the general principles of diseases. J Eval Clin Pract. 2017;23(1):233–7.
30. Horne SD, Chowdhury SK, Heng HH. Stress, genomic adaptation, and the evolutionary trade-off. Front Genet. 2014;5:92.
31. Heng HH, Regan S, Ye CJ. Genotype, environment, and evolutionary mechanism of diseases. Environ Dis. 2016;1(1):14–23.
32. Collins FS, Varmus H. A new initiative on precision medicine. N Engl J Med. 2015;372(9):793–5.
33. Heng HH. Bio-complexity challenging reductionism. In: Sturmberg JS, Martin CM, editors. Handbook of systems and complexity in health. New York: Springer; 2013. p. 193–208.
34. Sturmberg JS, Martin CM, editors. Handbook of systems and complexity in health. New York: Springer; 2013.
35. Sturmberg JP, Bennett JM, Martin CM, Picard M. 'Multimorbidity' as the manifestation of network disturbances. J Eval Clin Pract. 2017;23(1):199–208.

# Part III
# Health Care

# The Health System Quartet: Four Basic Systems—Cure, Care, Heal, and Deal—To Foster the Co-production of Sustained Health

**Jan van der Kamp and Thomas Plochg**

## 1 Introduction

The development of life on Earth was an emergent process, which is called evolution. If evolution is the natural process of development, we ought to ask the question how can we harness emergent properties for healthcare policy and practice. The theory of complex adaptive systems (CAS) provides tools to understand the features of this question.

Millions of years ago life began, developed and sustained itself without human interventions. It is only for the past 200 years, with Semmelweis seen as a founding father, that medical sciences were developed, mainly focusing on pathology and cure. It is curious that almost at the same time Darwin launched the theory of evolution; however, medicine hardly learned anything from it for use in the health sciences, while evolution resulted in the features of growth, maintenance and recovery.

Our observations demand us to think about how to harness the intrinsic features of health, in particular our self-healing capacities, back into the healthcare system. Positive support of biological, mental and behavioural characteristics is rapidly gaining in importance to restore health and to make health systems sustainable.

A better insight in the possible use of the self-healing potential of human beings can facilitate the emergence of a more ecological approach to health and health care. Like the wind and the sun can help us with energy transition, the energy of life and well-being are important sources to sustain health. Utilising resources without using

J. van der Kamp (✉)
Health Systems Innovations, Blaricum, Netherlands
e-mail: kampjan@ziggo.nl

T. Plochg
Netherlands Public Health Federation, Amersfoort, Netherlands
e-mail: t.plochg@nphf.nl



J. P. Sturmberg (ed.), *Embracing Complexity in Health*,
https://doi.org/10.1007/978-3-030-10940-0_7

them up—the principle approach to ecological management—is the basis for an ecological approach to health, and as a consequence, the sustainability of healthcare systems. This idea resonates with the call for the adaptation of systems thinking in public health [1], in medical sciences (e.g. [2, 3]) and in policy making more general [4].

Life, health, evolution, biology, neurology, behaviour, social systems, culture, economy, management, organisation and communication, amongst others, are normally studied trying to isolate cause–response relationships.

When agents in an open system are sensitive to external influences and interact with each other over time, relationships become complex and this is typically the case in matters of health and disease. For instance, Friel et al. [5] showed that the dietary behaviour of neighbourhood residents might depend on local availability of healthy food choices, while the choice of available foods in shops depends on the buying behaviour of the same people. In a complex adaptive system (CAS), the aforementioned interaction (or feedback loop) between agents over time results in agents adopting new properties, i.e. systems become emergent. This way of thinking helps to distinguish between the multidimensional aspects of health, and their single-dimensional representations in disease, which is crucial to advance our understanding of health and disease.

Thereby, the term "complex adaptive system" refers to a system that emerges over time into a coherent form, and adapts and organises itself without any singular entity deliberately managing or controlling it [6]. These complex relationships can be seen at all possible levels and scales: global, national and local policy, the health care system, two or more people dealing with each other, a person dealing with his health (health problem/s), the immune system, homeostasis, the functioning of a cell and more. Systems and scaling in CAS are bottom-up self-organising and self-balancing dynamic processes, adaptive at all scale levels. The adaptivity results in positive developments by creating conditions such as that nourish, challenge and support.

Modelling is a powerful tool to understand the agents and their possible interactions within a CAS. Understanding the current behaviour of a CAS allows one to develop different scenarios by changing agent configurations or interactions and evaluate these changes on the system as a whole. Comparing different scenarios allows one to find patterns of successful system change. It is the means of understanding "emergent practice" [1].

The central thrust of this chapter is that applying CAS understandings to human health, medicine, public health and healthcare systems is needed to better understand the processes of health and disease, and it ultimately will help to improve the functioning of our healthcare systems. Notwithstanding leading health scientists have made the case for CAS in health research (e.g. [2, 3, 7]); however, the consequences of CAS-based health knowledge for the functioning of medicine and health care more generally remain poorly understood. Thinking in terms of CAS will require the rethinking of the cure and care dominated healthcare systems. We will argue that it will be the driver for a so-called heal and deal support system that complements the existing cure and care ones: *the health systems quartet*.

## 2 Human Health as a CAS

Let us look after a human being in another way than usual. One is familiar with the different levels of the human body's structure, such as the molecule level, the cell level, the organ system level, the human as a whole level, and the context in which the person resides, all of which influence his health. Normally, we are looking after horizontal relationships within these levels, like cells in a tissue (e.g. cells of the immune system). Only recently did we start to look after the processes between the different levels—how they are interrelated. Figure 1 provides a simplified schematic overview how human health functions as a whole across different levels. In this model, five horizontal levels are used—molecule, cell, functional system/organ, man and context/environment. These levels are functionally integrated vertically.

The core of the system consists of molecular agents that create the functional systems around the cell and ensure ***homeostasis***. Around the functional system of cells and the man as a whole arises the living system or ***life***. The man living in his context and interrelated systems results in ***well-being***. Homeostasis, life and well-being, together forming the human biotope-a dynamic system. Whereas the component levels behave as adaptive agents, working together they entail the complex adaptive system of health.

Can it be helpful to see a human's health as a CAS to be able to improve his/her health? Recently, a published obesity study showed a relationship between cellular fat content (cell level), exercise, food intake and individual rates of metabolism (function system level), and the microbiome and gene expression (molecule level) on well-being [8, 9]. This study demonstrated that metabolic change occurred within

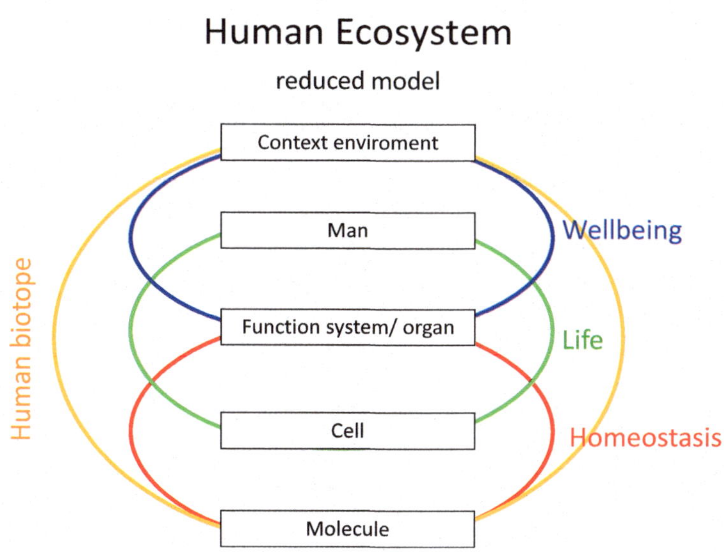


**Fig. 1** The human ecosystem is horizontally and vertically integrated

physically active children resulting in the formation of easily burnable brown fat instead of structural, metabolically inactive white fat. Changes solely focused on one factor without taking account of others, this factor had little impact on overall weight control. The authors concluded that insight from self-organising systems theory can be helpful to solve the obesity problem.

Within this theory, all the different factors and their interrelationships behave like agents and are adaptive. As such, the problem of obesity could be approached as a CAS problem—including all identifiable factors into a system model could identify which ones are dominant, and which ones are easiest to influence to reduce being overweight and to help maintaining a steady normal weight. Then, the objective is no longer the fight against obesity as a risk factor, but to create a system that maintains optimal body weight. It could be that improving self-respect and well-being are the key for the majority of people, whereas the few with a "lazy metabolism" or an "unfavourable gene expression" require more specific treatments. Behaviour in the system "well-being" will play an important role as a conductor of the underlying systems [10]. Let us next have a look at the role of acting and adapting human behaviour and well-being in CAS.

## 2.1 The Evolving Human Role

During the WHO Alma Ata Conference (1978), one of the turning points in health policy was the acknowledgement of the role of human beings in the healthcare system. No longer only an object requiring good practice approaches, attention shifted to their participation in the healthcare system. In the Alma Ata Declaration, this participation mainly concerned the emancipatory role arising from the democratisation of the system—active participation in health care, recognising that health is a human right, and the importance of lay care for health, well-being and system sustainability.

Ten years later during the WHO Adelaide Conference on Healthy Public Policy (Adelaide Recommendations [11]), the Director General Mahler underlined the importance of participation, by mentioning the parable of the chicken and the pig discussing a joint venture to start a ham and egg restaurant. The pig suddenly became aware of a problem and said to the chicken: "for you it is only participation, but for me it will be total involvement". Humans are constantly involved in their health responding to their biological, emotional, cognitive and behavioural experiences [12, 13].

At that time, there was a strong belief that achieving best possible health would be achieved by identifying disease conditions and for the health system to provide necessary services to control or cure them. In that view, people with health problems were mainly seen as victims of their biological systems that had failed them. Health policy makers were left behind—the emancipation movement had caught on and people were willing and able to manage their own lives. Nothing much has changed; in 2018, we still have ethical problems dealing with the tension of policy being responsible to protect human health as much as possible whilst at the same time recognising the importance of individuals having a right to make—albeit at times poor—decisions for themselves. Respecting the human right for health includes both people having the right to be protected as well as being respected in their autonomy. Recognising this duality can help to bridge the gap between both sides with an open mind.

Thirty years ago, human behaviour was mainly seen through medical eyes—one mainly saw what was going wrong. The relationship between behaviour and conditions/diseases became an area of do's and don'ts. This is an impediment to recognising "the human spirit" as a positive resource for health. The change in appreciation can be exemplified in relation to sport—initially, sport was highly suspected to be a potential cause of injuries, but today we recognise the importance of sport as a resource for health even in those with severe and disabling conditions and the frail.

The positive appreciation of human behaviour deserves more attention. Basically, humans are competent to manage their own lives, including their health. Through their essential involvement, they are natural partners; people are no longer only "consumers of healthcare services" but should be regarded more and more as the "*co-producers of their own health*". Self-determined people develop their commitment and skills to become as independent as possible. Not at least this is facilitated by the digitalisation of society as manifested in web-based information, e-health applications and social media. Thereby, empowering people's competence is a major goal.

## 2.2 Competence

It is clear that not everybody is equally competent at managing their own health [14]. And even when they are, it is far from self-evident that people will manage their own health in a societal context that incites them to behave unhealthily. Starting from their existing competence, most people can improve their skills, self-reliance and commitment to look after themselves. However, there are also groups who will need more specific approaches to engage them in their own health care.

Figure 2 depicts the possible combinations of levels/lack of commitment and available skills, the intersection between the two indicating the level of competence for self-care [14]. Strengthening self-care competence will vary for each of the four segments:

1. People, with an ordinary level of skills and commitment (segment 1), can maintain/enhance their competence by both maintaining/increasing their commitment and available skills for self-care.
2. People, committed but with a lack of skills and an inability to develop them, will need an additional (individual) services (segment 2). Many adolescents belong to this group.
3. People with neither the skills nor the commitment to look after their own health (segment 3) will require special individualised help to increase their skills and

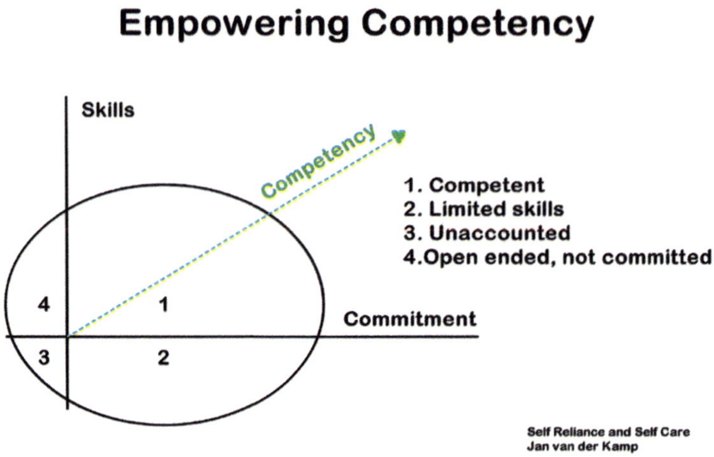


**Fig. 2** Enhancing people's health competence

commitment for self-care. This group often has "multiple—congenital and/or acquired—problems".

4. People, who have the skills but no commitment to look after their own health (segment 4), will require professional help to change their attitudes towards a more appropriate balance between personal and professional healthcare expectations. They exhibit the typical behaviour of "free riding", i.e. they demand that health professionals and society will come to their help and fix their illnesses whenever they occur.

## 3 A New Era in Health Care

If people are considered competent to manage their own health, healthcare services need to adapt accordingly opening up a whole array of innovative health interventions. The traditional way of healthcare professionals to provide cure and care services and patients consuming those services does not fit any more. People and/or patients *co-produce* their own health, being actively involved in their own treatment, which would require the transformation of professionals' expertise, and ultimately the nature of employed interventions [15].

This latter point can be illustrated by the management of intermittent claudication. Traditionally, this was a choice between surgery and angioplasty. Nowadays, walking exercises are the preferred approach, stimulating the production of collaterals resulting in symptom reversal [16]. Both, surgical interventions and simple walking exercises have one aspect in common—both achieve recovery. Whereas the former is "high-tech" and requires a highly trained surgeons, the latter is "low-tech" and merely requires commitment, as well as social network pressures, either positive or negative, to "*co-produce one's own recovery*".

Similarly, evidence is emerging that the treatment of non-insulin-dependent (type 2) diabetes by lifestyle modification can achieve full recovery in most patients [17]. Lastly, physiotherapy achieves low back pain resolution in most patients, and physiotherapists teaching patient-specific exercise programmes can prevent most recurrences [18].

Facilitating the conditions to heal, with or without full recovery, requires a professional support system. In addition to professional care, people help themselves and each other by learning to cope (*deal*) and recover (*heal*) or to adapt to disability (*deal*). Finding a balance between relative dependence and independence is an ongoing process; however, the skills to expose patients to the possibilities of healing and dealing remain underdeveloped. The latter begs for attention—especially given the unsustainability of most healthcare systems worldwide. When people can better rely on themselves and keep themselves more fit, they will consume less cure and care services.

## 4 The Health System Quartet

Given the relevance and urgency of heal and deal, it is now timely to explore and operationalise the relationships and interactions with the professional-led cure and care systems. The latter are well-described in the literature. In its simplest form, we conceptualise cure as professional-led causal interventions aiming at the full recovery from a problem, e.g. reducing and fixating a broken leg. The care system entails professional-led services aiming at the care for people recovering from curative interventions or for whom cure is no longer possible to overcome a problem, e.g. home nursing, running therapy or activities-of-daily-living support. On the other hand, prevention can entail professional-led interventions to remove or ease risk factors that have the potential to ultimately result in disease requiring cure and care system interventions.

Professional-led cure and care are developed on the basis of scientific methodologies and are continuously under development. Interventions are discovered by causal relationships and statistical significance. The direction of the action is causal (Fig. 3).

The person-led *heal* and *deal* systems are of a very different nature. In line with complexity science thinking, both can be considered as self-organising. The co-evolving processes within these systems can result in growth, development, learning, resilience and recovery. Desired outcomes are more difficult to achieve than those within the cure and care systems. Based on the principles of complex adaptive systems, heal and deal are *autonomous, sensitive to initial conditions* and *attractors*. A better understanding of the "dynamic causes" of heal and deal conditions is crucial to enable health professionals to steer patients towards their desired outcomes.

The delivery of relational services incorporating positive feedback will benefit the majority of patients by enabling them to act as co-producers of health. Here,

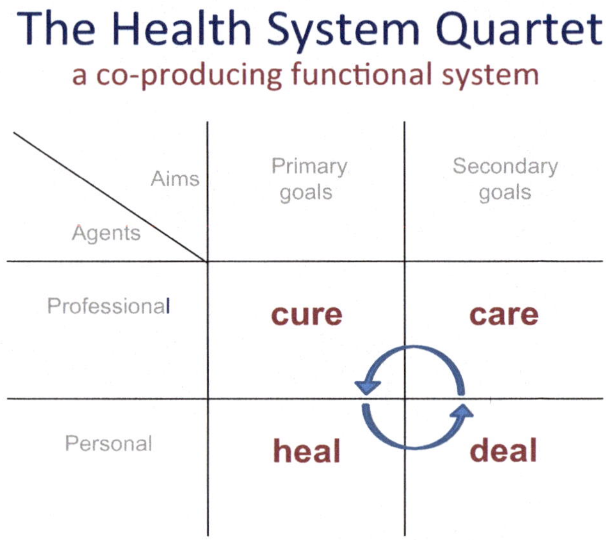


**Fig. 3** The health system quartet

healthcare providers and patients behave like adaptive agents, and the focus thus is on better understanding their interactions and their emergent potentials. Put differently, how can we—as health professionals—mobilise the huge potential of biological and mental properties inherent in every individual to enhance "their ability to adapt and to self-manage" [19]?

Both acute and time-limited conditions as well as chronic diseases can be studied within this model. More importantly, it provides the conceptual basis for shifting the focus to ***health*** rather than disease, as one key lever to more sustainable healthcare systems and healthier societies in general. Supportive professionals' coaching and enabling will help patients to better use their *heal* and *deal* abilities and to become healthier as well as easing current pressures on our healthcare systems.

Paying attention to the dynamics of healthcare delivery within the framework of the Health Quartet has society-wide implications—it will achieve better health and lower the burden of care on health professionals and it will make health systems more effective, more efficient and also more sustainable.

To illustrate this point, consider a person who had a car accident. The surgeon can *cure* the fractures and allow the patient to let his wounds heal. Rehabilitation services provide *care* during the recovery phase, but the patient has to *deal* with the ongoing consequences like the need to adapt to a stiff leg. The patient becomes independent again after dealing with his physical and mental shock—only then has he managed to *heal* as a person.

Until now, health professional intervention predominantly focuses on physical cure, care and recovery. Giving greater attention to the personal participation in care and developing greater coping capacities by dealing with the person's illness allows the emergence of true healing. Making this process explicit will allow the person to enhance his recovery.

## 5 Discussion

The ideas outlined in the Health Quartet will not be realised overnight. They will result from studying possibilities that appear achievable. This can be seen as "trend watching", i.e. placing a point at the horizon for orientation guiding the direction to search for solutions. The reality is that progress can only be made step by step. We regard as important those initiatives that focus on well-being, positive health and system approaches that promote personal health development. The focus on personal growth might show more success and sustainability for health than—still prevailing—approaches to behaviour change based on "do's and don'ts". Nevertheless, there always will be specific cases in which to demand a patient to change his/her attitudes and approach to his/her care.

The dynamic processes between behaviour, mind and biology are continually evolving, preferably in such a way that they are mutually reinforcing. Positive support by health professionals will enhance these dynamics in a positive way and reflects the human relational level for self-sustainability.

Adaptive and self-organising learning makes growth possible. The relationships in the figure show the evolving processes which—hopefully—will be recognised by practitioners and policy makers in due course as they are requirements for keeping the health system affordable. Only awareness strives for a fit. Think of a string quartet—the beauty emerges from co-adaptive self-organisation.

The output of professional interventions can lead to sustainable outcomes by positive co-operation between behaviour, biology and mind amongst co-producing people. This positive co-operation will become increasingly important to make health systems effective and sustainable. In the Netherlands, we see positive developments exemplified by "Buurtzorg", "Institute for Positive Health", "Immunowell" and the dynamic description of "Health as the ability to adapt and to self-manage". The co-adaptive self-organising synergy is promising better health and the sustainability of the health system.

In this paper, well-being and behaviour were the focus. As a next step, we want to include mental health, biological health and the environment in this framework. We believe that this will not only sustain personal health but also has the potential to substitute professional level care with personal level self-care and personal growth. This outcome can be expected when health professionals not only provide best possible curative interventions but simultaneously act as change agents to facilitate their patients to *heal*. As part of a system where self-confidence and competence can grow, substitution between professional and self-care may be expected.

## 6 Conclusions

The natural healing capacity and the ability of people to adapt and to self-manage should be given a much greater prominence in the healthcare system. The initiatives for this deserve systematic attention in research, policy and practice. Given that the functions *cure*, *care*, *heal* and *deal*, being partly independent, when acting together can provide added value (emergence) to patient care and health system organisation—the Health System Quartet offers a coherent framework for such an endeavour. In practice, a relative contribution of the four functions will must always be considered and need to be adjusted in the course of a treatment. The promise is that it will relieve the pressures on healthcare systems as people will better use their own abilities, arguably leading to less healthcare use, and thus contributing to the imperative of making our healthcare systems more person-centred, equitable and sustainable [20].

**Acknowledgements** The authors like to acknowledge the useful comments and edits of Joachim Sturmberg on earlier drafts of this chapter.

## The Transformative Aspects of This Study

The chapter proposes the juxtaposition of "heal and deal" next to the existing "cure and care" based focus of healthcare systems. In its simplicity, it unifies key dynamics within health policy for the future sustainability of health care: (1) the focus on prevention and health promotion, (2) more integrated and holistic approaches towards health and disease and (3) the empowerment of people and patients.

**Take Home Message**

- The healthcare system's ***Cure*** and ***Care*** focus can cooperate with people's agency to ***Deal*** with their biological and mental dynamics to ***Heal***.
- The interactions of Cure, Care, Deal and Heal are at the heart of the ***Health Systems Quartet***, a framework to form a simple basis for the complex transdisciplinary approaches to achieve "health".
- It opens a new perspective for sustainable health policy, health system organisation and health praxis.
- The intrinsic emerging powers of life and well-being have a huge potential to guide health system redesign.

## References


1. Rutter H, Savona N, Glonti K, Bibby J, Cummins S, Finegood DT, et al. The need for a complex systems model of evidence for public health. Lancet. 2017;390(10112):2602–4
2. Plsek PE, Greenhalgh T. The challenge of complexity in health care. Br Med J. 2001;323: 625–8
3. Ahn A, Tewari M, Poon C-S, Phillips R. The limits of reductionism in medicine: could systems biology offer an alternative? PLoS Medicine. 2006;3(6):e208. Available at: http://medicine.plosjournals.org/perlserv/?request=get-document&doi=10.1371%2Fjournal.pmed.0030208
4. Kurtz CF, Snowden DJ. The new dynamics of strategy: sense-making in a complex and complicated world. IBM Syst J. 2003;42(3):462–83
5. Friel S, Pescud M, Malbon E, Lee A, Carter R, Greenfield J, et al. Using systems science to understand the determinants of inequities in healthy eating. PLoS ONE. 2017;12(11):e0188872. Available at: https://doi.org/10.1371/journal.pone.0188872
6. Mitchell M. Complexity: a guided tour. Oxford: Oxford University Press; 2009
7. Sturmberg JP, Martin CM. Complexity in health: an introduction. In: Sturmberg JP, Martin CM, editors. Handbook of systems and complexity in health. New York: Springer; 2013. p. 1–17
8. Hammond RA. Complex systems modeling for obesity research. Prev Chronic Dis. 2009;6(3):A97
9. Seale P, Lazar MA. Brown fat in humans: turning up the heat on obesity. Diabetes. 2009;58(7):1482–4
10. Huber M. Towards a new, dynamic concept of health. Its operationalisation and use in public health and healthcare, and in evaluating health effects of food. Doctoral Thesis, Maastricht University. Enschede: Ipskamp Drukkers; 2014
11. Adelaide Recommendations on Healthy Public Policy. Second International Conference on Health Promotion, Adelaide, South Australia, 5–9 April 1988. http://www.who.int/healthpromotion/conferences/previous/adelaide/en/
12. Sturmberg JP. The personal nature of health. J Eval Clin Pract. 2009;15(4):766–9.
13. Sturmberg JP, Topolski S, Lewis S. Health: a systems- and complexity-based definition. In: Sturmberg JP, Martin CM, editors. Handbook of systems and complexity in health. New York: Springer; 2013. p. 251–3
14. Kamp Jan van der. Managing health promotion as an open process: holistic and ecological tools for managing and marketing of innovations. In: Evers A, Farrent W, Trojan A, editors. Healthy public policy at the local level. Colorado: Westview; 1990
15. Plochg T, Klazinga NS, Starfield B. Transforming medical professionalism to fit changing health needs. BMC Med. 2009;7:64. Available at: https://bmcmedicine.biomedcentral.com/articles/10.1186/1741-7015-7-64
16. Norgren L, Hiatt WR, Dormandy JA, Nehler MR, Harris KA; Fowkes FGon behalf of the TASC II Working Group. Inter-society consensus for the management of peripheral arterial disease (TASC II). J Vasc Surg. 2007;45(1 Suppl):S5–67
17. Battjes-Fries MCE, Patijn ON, Voshol PJ. Tweede tussenrapportage groepsprogramma Keer-Diabetes-Om. Louis Bolk Institute. December 2017 [In Dutch]
18. Foster NE, Anema JR, Cherkin D, Chou R, Cohen SP, Gross DP, et al.; Lancet Low Back Pain Series Working Group. Prevention and treatment of low back pain: evidence, challenges, and promising directions. Lancet 2018;391(10137):2368–83
19. Huber M, Knottnerus JA, Green L, Horst HVD, Jadad AR, Kromhout D, et al. How should we define health? Br Med J. 2011;343:d4163
20. Sturmberg JP. Health system redesign. How to make health care person-centered, equitable, and sustainable. Cham: Springer; 2017

# Humans and Big Data: New Hope? Harnessing the Power of Person-Centred Data Analytics

**Carmel Martin, Keith Stockman, and Joachim P. Sturmberg**

According to the Oxford English Dictionary the term 'Big Data' was first used in 1941 to describe what now is popularly been known as the information explosion [1]. And, there are high hopes that Big Data can improve what we do as exemplified by these two quotes:

> Hiding within those mounds of data is knowledge that could change the life of a patient, or change the world.—Atul Butte, Stanford School of Medicine

> The goal is to turn data into information, and information into insight.—Carly Fiorina, CEO

Big Data is a term used to encompass the expanding information systems including the 'internet of things' that are increasingly pervasive in society internationally. While many ideas are linked under this umbrella term, the major themes include the 'three V's'—*Volume* (vast amounts of data), *Variety* (significant heterogeneity in the type of data available in the set), and *Velocity* (speed at which a data scientist or user can access and analyse the data) [2]. Defined as such, health care has become one of the key emerging users of 'big data'.

Big Data can create both major opportunities and major challenges for health services. In order to make sense, data must be translated into information that informs the personal nature of health care, and the individual heterogeneity of

C. Martin (✉)
Department of Medicine, Nursing and Allied Health, Monash University, and Monash Health, Clayton, VIC, Australia

K. Stockman
Operations Research and Projects, General Medicine Program, Monash Health, Clayton, VIC, Australia
e-mail: Keith.Stockman@monashhealth.org

J. P. Sturmberg
School of Medicine and Public Health, University of Newcastle, Wamberal, NSW, Australia

International Society for Systems and Complexity Sciences for Health, Waitsfield, VT, USA



J. P. Sturmberg (ed.), *Embracing Complexity in Health*,
https://doi.org/10.1007/978-3-030-10940-0_8

illness dynamics and responsiveness to illness interventions [3]. Data science predominantly focuses on the metrification of human health and the biomedical or natural sciences, particularly in clinical cardiology and neuroscience with their disease-oriented goals [4]. Vast patient genomic data promise to deliver even greater personalised medicine. The 'internet of things' and the 'quantified self' together with health system data collections present a tsunami of data which provides major challenges for analysis and sense-making. The IT industry is pressured to deliver processing, networking and database infrastructures that are capable of handling the data volumes and variety of information fast enough for real-time decision-making.

While such Big Data might be manageable, is it useful or necessary? There is a tendency to associate Big Data with data mining techniques to encompass every possible facet of human existence to identify patterns. Researchers and scientists, however, still need to ask critical questions:

- What is the nature of human-centric care systems in the context of Big Data?
- How are data likely to reflect and influence individual personal health?
- What are the implications?

Many hold that Big Data in health care will create improved health outcomes and contain costs [5]. On the other hand, there has been much historical and contemporary concern about the utility of Big Data as stated by Tilly: "*the investigators tend to lose their wit, grace, and sense of proportion in the pursuit of statistical results, that none of the big questions has actually yielded to the bludgeoning of the big-data people*" [6]. Alternatively, there are concerns about privacy and how big data analytics might be used for profit, surveillance or other nefarious purposes. Increasingly, the public are raising concerns over privacy, confidentiality and control of shared personal data with the potential for 'intrusive inferences'. On the other hand, the IT industry and other organisations are acquiring 'big data' by stealth with little scrutiny for various purposes other than improving quality of life or health [7].

This chapter explores data analytics in human-centric health care and science in potentially preventable hospitalisations.

## 1 Modelling Health Journeys

This work is situated in the context of prevention of avoidable hospitalisation. Patients classified as 'avoidable hospitalisation cases' are on one hand a vulnerable cohort of poorly managed people, intractable chronic diseases such as heart failure and COPD and frailty, and on the other a problem for hospitals in terms of their inability to cope with their needs and cost inefficiency without making people worse [8]. The big question is how to provide *anticipatory care* that firstly *meets the needs of this cohort* and secondly applies *limited resources* in a more *cost-effective way*.

## 1.1 The Need for a Model

Frames are the mental structures that shape the way we see the world [9]. Theories, facts, data and models only have meaning in the context of their frame. Most data collected for the purpose of health care has some type of relationship to the real world and an implied anticipation of outcomes, so that there is an ability to update or refine care. Rosen calls this the modelling relationship. He identified anticipation as a fundamental characteristic of all living complex systems [4] and subsequently provided a relational model of living complex systems [5]. Anticipation is both a "*specification of what the system is like at any particular instant of time, with the associated concept of the instantaneous state of the system, and a specification of how the system changes state, as a function of present or past states and of the forces imposed on the system*" [10].

All systems have in their trajectories information about their future trajectories. However, the model representing the natural system constantly needs to adapt and refine the formal system. This concept underpins artificial intelligence and machine learning; however, it is most importantly the basis for human systems who are able to use constructivist and open learning rather than reductionist and rigid protocols.

## 1.2 Complex Adaptive System Dynamics and Health

Complex adaptive systems describe the interconnected and interdependent nature of phenomena. Complex adaptive systems exhibit many-to-many relationships that typically create feedback loops which define the dynamic behaviour of the system. Changes to the configuration and/or relationships within the system alter its behaviours and its observable characteristics (or outcomes) in predictable or almost unpredictable ways. Emergence is thus based on feed-forward and feed-backward dynamics.

Complex adaptive systems are layered with each layer describing the features of the system at a different scale and at a different level of detail. This has been described as every system (or system level) being part of a larger supra-system and itself being constituted by any number of smaller subsystems.

Ellis [11] stated: "*complexity* [in biological systems] *consists of modular hierarchical structures, leading to emergent levels of structure and function based on lower level network* [function]". Top-down influences provide contextual constraints on possible bottom-up functions. Biological systems behaviour is neither linear nor random.

Complex adaptive system dynamics result in unpredictable outcomes which form discernible patterns. Importantly though, one cannot deduce from the observed outcomes which system component or which interaction has caused this outcome, a point already emphasised in 1976 by Harvard epidemiologist Rothman [12] who termed it *sufficient causes*.

> A cause is an act or event or a state of nature which initiates or permits, alone or in conjunction with other causes, a sequence of event resulting in an effect. A cause which inevitably produces the effect is sufficient. The inevitability of disease after a sufficient cause calls for qualification: disease usually requires time to become manifest, .... Common usage makes no distinction between that constellation of phenomena which constitutes a sufficient cause and the components of the constellation which are likewise referred to as "causes". Another qualification for sufficient causes is restriction to the minimum number of required component causes; this implies that the lack of any component cause renders the remaining component causes insufficient.

Health is the outcome of complex adaptive processes across the scale from the micro-level of biology and physiology through to the macro-level of the physical and sociocultural environments. Health thus is a balanced experiential state—between the physical, emotional, social and cognitive (sense-making) domains [13, 14]. Perturbations in each of these domains can result in illness (or non-health) experiences, and adaptation to these disturbances restores the experience of health (Fig. 1).

In line with Ellis's logic, health and illness are '*caused*' by top-down political/socioeconomic contextual constraints that limit the bottom-up biological/physiological potential. At the functional level of the person, the '*causative pathways*' responsible for the health and illness experience as well as the development of overt diseases are principally regulated by the psycho-neuro-immunological pathways [15], and responsible as much for disease production as the person's illness behaviour [16]. Figure 1 schematically summarises how health results from the interplay between the perturbations resulting from our social situatedness with that of our biological and physiological blueprint.

## 2 The Human Dimension

Ian McWhinney's 1989 paper '*An Acquaintance with Particulars* ...' highlighted an important weakness of reductionist science—namely, that its efforts to produce abstractions strip away the all-important contextual dimensions. However, context matters greatly, especially in the domain of caring for people/patients. In his paper, McWhinney provides a different approach to understanding patients—as particulars [17]. As particulars they "*occup*[y] *a region of space,* [that] *persists through time, has boundaries and has an environment*" [18]. Besides, they have a history that persists and impacts on future behaviours [18]. Therefore, a better understanding of people and their health experiences requires an understanding of the complex adaptive nature of health, and the need to respond to each person's needs for care in an adaptive way [17].

McWhinney described five features that distinguish human from natural sciences all of which entail key characteristics that place medicine in the realm of complex adaptive system sciences (CAS), although he never explicitly used the term:

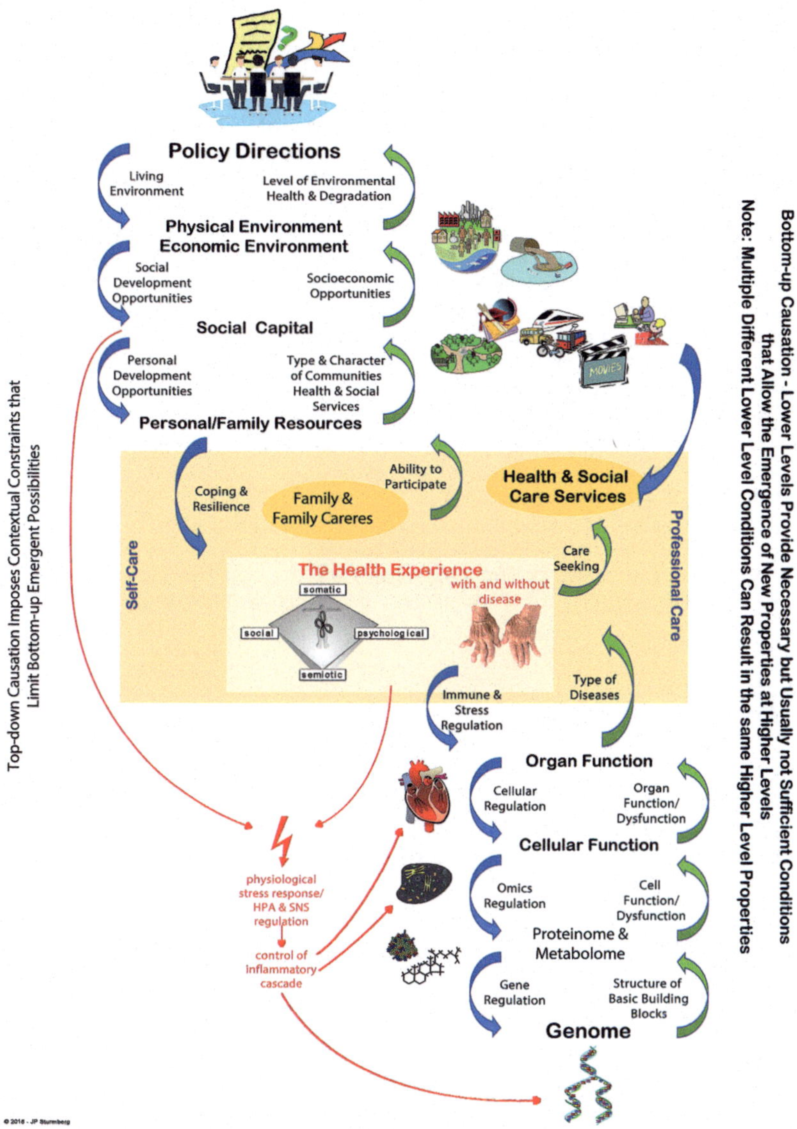


**Fig. 1** Health and illness are experienced within the constraints of one's social situatedness limiting one's biological and physiological potentials. A framework for multi-layered systems influencing human health from the genomic to the whole person to the care system nested in the socio-political-economic. Health ultimately results from the interplay between the perturbations resulting from one's social situatedness with that of one's biological and physiological blueprint. *Note* that the hierarchical nature of the system results in the higher levels constraining the emergent possibilities of the lower levels

1. Human science is about meaning—the meaning of events, experience, symbols, utterances, and behaviour. There is no objective test for meaning. The only way to establish what an experience means to a person is to enter into a dialogue with him or her, from which the meaning gradually emerges.
2. The scope for generalization in human science is limited. No human event ever recurs in exactly the same way. ... Complex natural systems are "particulars." To make general inferences from studies in these sciences we must have good descriptions of the contexts in which they were conducted.
3. In human science, causality is not linear and unidirectional. A complex, self-organizing system does not respond to change in a simple unidirectional manner. Reciprocal effects and feedback loops are circular, not linear processes. As Gregory Bateson observed, when causal systems become circular, any event in the circle may be both the effect of a previous event and the cause of a subsequent event anywhere in the circle. ... it does require a change from simplistic causal thinking to thinking about how change can be facilitated in complex systems.
4. ... prediction is not the prime objective in human science. ... The goal of human science is understanding. Human science helps us by deepening our understanding of the "particulars" we see every day in our practices.
5. Human science is interactive–person to person. Natural science relies on objective methods for validation. ... There is no ... test for the meaning of experience. This can be established only inter-subjectively, by a dialogue between people from which the meaning gradually emerges. Both participants may be changed by the dialogue: the investigator revising original interpretations, the subject gaining new insights.

## *2.1 Personal Dynamics*

Multiple dynamics of internal and external network interactions result in the emergent observable state of a person's health [13, 14]; however, despite the availability of Big Data we cannot fully predict what specific intervention will result in a change in health.

Essentially, healthcare professionals provide patterned responses to pattern-recognised conditions, i.e. as health professionals we are generally good in managing the uncertainties and unpredictability of *individual condition variability*, which is '*hidden*' in 'his personal Big Data set'. Critically, in an environment of great *interpersonal condition variability* evaluating healthcare achievements would require the measurement of changes in health at the subjective and objective levels.

The personal dynamics of one's state of health have been shown to be reliably measurable by the single-item measure of *self-rated health* [19], and self-rated health has emerged as a reliable predictor of one's future health service utilisation [20] and mortality [21].

# 3 Big Data Disturbing Human-Centric Health Care

Healthcare delivery is at a crossroad between its traditional—and widely accepted—approaches and the emerging drive to treat—and prevent—disease pushed by the precision medicine and pharmacogenomics movements, often underwritten by big business. Are these approaches compatible and in the best interest of people/patients? And if so, who will most likely benefit?

## *3.1 Competing Frameworks for Care*

New models of integrated *disease care* seek to enhance continuous, coordinated access to a comprehensive array of specialist care [22, 23], but have neglected to describe—and deliver—whole-person focused care [22]. In so doing, they are contributing to new problems like overwhelming treatment burden [24], over-diagnosis [25], and problematic polypharmacy [26] in ageing populations living with multimorbidity; as well as underdiagnosis and management of the growing phenomenon of symptoms without clear biomedical explanations [27].

In contrast, *person-centred care* is a model of health care that prioritises the goal of supporting '*a life for living*'. Recognising health as a necessary resource for daily living [28], the goal for health care is to enable—certainly not undermine—that outcome.

The rapid technological and computing advances enabled genome and gene-regulation research and has opened the promises to improve health care through precision medicine and pharmacogenomics:

> There is a lot of overlap between the terms "precision medicine" and "personalized medicine." According to the National Research Council, "personalized medicine" is an older term with a meaning similar to "precision medicine." However, there was concern that the word "personalized" could be misinterpreted to imply that treatments and preventions are being developed uniquely for each individual; in precision medicine, the focus is on identifying which approaches will be effective for which patients based on genetic, environmental and lifestyle factors. The Council therefore preferred the term "precision medicine" to "personalized medicine." However, some people still use the two terms interchangeably [29].
>
> Pharmacogenomics is a part of precision medicine. Pharmacogenomics is the study of how genes affect a person's response to particular drugs. This relatively new field combines pharmacology (the science of drugs) and genomics (the study of genes and their functions) to develop effective, safe medications and doses that are tailored to variations in a person's genes [30].

These competing frameworks raise important issues for the future of medical care.

# 4 Hype *and* Hope: Tensions and Contradictions in Real-World Clinical Practice. The Case of Preventable Hospitalisations

A real threat to the sustainability of western health systems is the burgeoning problem of avoidable hospitalisations, overdiagnosis, problematic polypharmacy and ineffective medical, surgical and allied health professional care. Equally threatening for the patient are increasing instances of underdiagnosis and missing opportunities for cure with aggressive treatments. These problems are rarely evident from routine collated hospital performance reports—in fact, they are lost in the inefficient and coarsely grained analytical approaches of routinely collected hospital and other clinical data sets. More sophisticated data collection and analytics are needed.

## *4.1 Measure (and Analyse) What Matters*

What really matters in health care is simply: **does the care we receive help us *experience healthy again* regardless of the nature of our diseases**. In that regard, as already alluded to, the metric of *self-rated health* has emerged as the most reliable measure of one's *whole state of health*.

Self-rated health perceptions are based on interoception—our sense of the internal state of our body—and helps us to make sense of our ever-changing personal health journey [19]. Self-rated health emerged as being a more sensitive measure than the objective findings of the presence or absence of diagnosable diseases or their level of control. Determining one's personal health state (and anticipated health) is a consciously reflective process and involves the processing of information about one's bodily state (based on diagnosis, functional status, level of personal control and prognosis) and one's personal interpretation of meaning [13, 14] and takes into account one's socio-cultural environment [19, 31].

In addition, self-rated health measures one's adaptive capacity associated with ageing and increasing morbidity [32, 33]. In particular, these adaptive changes show nonlinear relationship—older people with greater pre-existing multiple morbidities typically have a smaller drop in self-rated health compared to younger, healthier individuals, and diseases with a major impact on life like the diagnosis of a malignancy, paralysis or dementia have far greater impacts [34].

Loss of self-rated health is not alone caused by the mere presence of a condition (yes/no) but related to the condition severity and likely contextual factors such as other morbidities, frailty and family and social support [35–38].

In short, **self-rated health is a measure about what matters**, and should be in the forefront of studying the *efficacy and effectiveness* of healthcare delivery.

Self-rated health is a predictor of mortality, morbidity and is highly correlated with hospital admission [39]—it is "*a condensed summary of information about* [one's] *bodily condition that in one way or another* [is] *involved in* [the causal] *biological chains* [of decline]" [19]. Hence, the observation of a negative change in self-rated health can indicate the approach of a tipping point in health and the need for medical intervention.

### 4.2 *Case Study of Predicting Avoidable Hospitalisations: Improving Human-Centric Health Care by Harnessing the Power of Person-Centred Data Analytics*

Monash Health is the largest public hospital and community care system in Victoria servicing one of the lowest socioeconomic and ethnically diverse areas of Melbourne. Its 15,000 staff work at more than 40 sites, providing over 3 million occasions of service, admitting more than 238,000 hospital patients, and handling more than 206,000 emergency presentations. Over 3000 patients had 4+ admissions, and a proportion of the over 12,000 with 3+ admissions had at least one potentially avoidable admission per year [40].

The challenge for Monash Health remains how to best detect those patients at high risk of readmission or worsening health in a low-cost flexible manner. To that end Monash Health implemented the Patient Journey Record System (PaJR) methods, a tool that applies a complex adaptive person-centred approach to understand and manage potentially avoidable hospitalisations. Lay telecare guides regularly converse with "at risk" individuals to track their concerns and self-perceived health (for a detailed description of the PaJR model see [41]; Fig. 2 shows a schematic overview).

Three cases were randomly selected to illustrate human-centric health care augmented by the power of collecting, analysing and acting upon person-centred data. Table 1 summarises the study design which has been described previously in reference [42].

#### 4.2.1 Three Case Studies

Three cases—patient identifiers (PID) 20, 1024 and 1040—with more than 25 calls were randomly selected to demonstrate distinct patterns of health journeys 'hidden' in the person's health data time series. Understanding the dynamics of individual patterns may allow anticipation of the need for pre-emptive care interventions immediately or in the near future and achieve both, better personal health experiences and reduced avoidable hospital attendances. The MW team assess needs and provide some direct services but mainly provide brokerage across a broad spectrum of clinical, social, welfare, financial, legal and any other appropriate services.

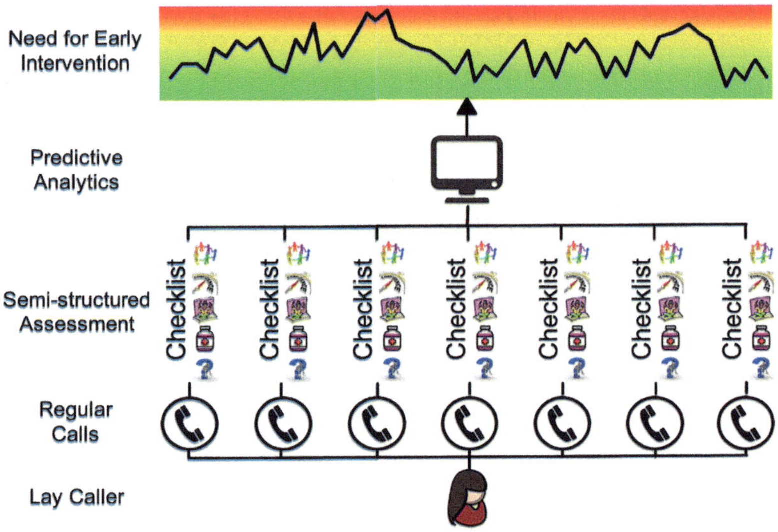


**Fig. 2** Schematic view of the PaJR model. A lay telecare guide calls a patient at regular intervals, using a semi-structured assessment guide to record data relating to self-rated health experience, medication, drug and alcohol use, available support and changes in health. Predictive analytics compute a score indicating the likely need for early intervention

- PID 20 is a 60-year-old male who had multiple brief admissions to hospital for gastroenterological conditions related to his previous alcohol and depressive history with concerns about his partner's health. He lives with his partner.
- PID 1024 is a 76-year-old male who did not have any admissions during the period of study. His main problems relate to his eyes, his arthritis, his tremor and lack of transport. His partner is overseas during the study period.
- PID 1040 is a 86-year-old female ex-smoker who has respiratory problems—chronic obstructive pulmonary disease and recurrent chest infections. She lives alone as a widow and her family lives nearby.

PID 20 had the worst average self-rated health, and more changes in his health care needs. PID 1024 had the most medication changes, while PID 1040 had the most change in social support arrangements. PID 1040 was away for a trip for 3 weeks and therefore had fewer calls.

Table 2 provides an overview of the main journey characteristics of the 3 cases over an approximately 6-month study period. '*Self-Rated Health*' (SRH—0 excellent, 1 very good, 2 good, 3 fair, 4 poor and 5 very poor); '*Health/Care Change*' (0 no, 1 yes); '*Medication/Drug/Alcohol Change*' (0 no, 1 yes) and '*Support Structure Change*' (0 no, 1 yes) were extracted from the dataset.

What is the meaning of these average values over time? Only health and health care change was similar across all the 3 cases which is not unexpected. This is confirmatory of the unstable nature of these selected health journeys.

**Table 1** The MonashWatch model

| Model elements | MonashWatch cohort |
|---|---|
| Case finding through 'Big Data' | Health links chronic care algorithm [43] identifies people at risk of 3+ potentially preventable hospitalisations using state-wide public hospital data |
| Setting | Monash Health Dandenong Hospital Catchment (low socioeconomic status urban) |
| Participants | 300 intervention; 195 control—systematically 3:1 allocation before recruitment |
| Time | 18 months (ongoing) |
| Phone calls | 12,000+ using the PaJR system |
| Age (median) | 65 years (31–91) |
| Gender | 55% female |
| | Baseline profiles are described previously and represent a group with frailty, poor physical health and fluctuating quality of life [41] |
| Lay care (telecare) guides | 3 full-time equivalents |
| Clinician coaches | 3 full-time clinicians—nursing, physiotherapy and occupational therapy |
| Service model | Integrated community sector—hospital outreach with guides and clinician coaches with general practitioner remaining as main medical provider with a back-up from hospital internal medicine/geriatrics and psychiatry |
| Process | In-time monitoring and brokerage of resources in a rapid and timely manner including clinical, drug and alcohol, community, volunteer and family resources |

To describe the patterns that generated these statistical summaries, we plotted the indices of '*SRH*', '*Health/Care Change*', '*Medication/Drug/Alcohol Change*' and '*Support Structure Change*' over time from monitoring information acquired via the PaJR programme.

**PID 20**

The trajectory of PID 20 demonstrates a change in SRH pattern around 10th of May 2017 with a shift to worse health experience associated with persistently high levels of healthcare changes (i.e. he repeatedly sought medical care services—GP, Emergency Department care and other medical care), high levels of alcohol and medication changes (repeated drinking bouts and then needing medication) and ongoing problems in the relationship with his wife due to persistent concerns about her illness (Fig. 3). His trajectory included >20 days in an acute admission in hospital with 9 episodes, the first being just before he entered the program (Table 3).

**Factors Triggering PID 20's Hospital Admission**

The factors that probably triggered admission were severe pain in a backdrop of good to fair self-rated health with pain being the most consistent reason for change in health and health status reported consistently before admissions. PID

**Table 2** Overview of the main journey characteristics of the 3 cases over an approximately 6-month study period

| Calls | Mean | Std. deviation | *P*-value differences |
|---|---|---|---|
| **PID 20** ($n = 71$ calls) | | | |
| SRH | 1.93 | 0.99 | *** |
| Health/care change | 0.746 | 0.438 | ** |
| Med/drug/alcohol change | 0.761 | 0.43 | * |
| Support structure change | 0.817 | 0.39 | |
| **PID 1024** ($n = 87$ calls) | | | |
| SRH | 2.816 | 0.518 | *** |
| Health/care change | 0.644 | 0.482 | ** |
| Med/drug/alcohol change | 0.874 | 0.334 | ** |
| Support structure change | 0.816 | 0.39 | |
| **PID 1040** ($n = 58$ calls) | | | |
| SRH | 2.948 | 0.804 | *** |
| Health/care change | 0.552 | 0.502 | ** |
| Med/drug/alcohol change | 0.621 | 0.489 | * |
| Support structure change | 0.983 | 0.131 | ** |

Average values of '*Self-Rated Health (SRH)*' (SRH—0 excellent, 1 very good, 2 good, 3 fair, 4 poor and 5 very poor); '*Health/care change*' (0 no, 1 yes); '*Medication/drug/alcohol change*' (0 no, 1 yes); '*Support structure change*' (0 no, 1 yes) in a case study of 3 patients—PID20, 1024 and 1040. ****p*-value > 0001; ***p*-value > 001; **p*-value > 0.05 using *t*-test for 2 samples repeated among samples (https://www.xlstat.com/en/solutions/premium)
ANOVA (analysis of variance) demonstrated statistical significant differences among the different parameters in each of these three journeys in the patterns of '*SRH*', '*Health/care change*', '*Medication/drug/alcohol change*' and '*Support structure change*'; and across all journeys for the domains '*SRH*', '*Medication/drug/alcohol change*' and '*Support structure change*' ($p$-value $< 0.005$). Only '*Health/care change*' was not statistically significantly different across all patients ($p > 0.5$) (http://www.openepi.com/Mean/t_testMean.htm)

20 had consistent changes in his medication/drug/alcohol use before admission (in this case, a relapse of alcohol misuse and changes in prescriptions to deal with his pain related to reflux oesophagitis and pancreatitis; and post-admission this fluctuated even more than before admission with reduced alcohol consumption). His social support structure (relationship with his wife and concerns about her illness) remained very changeable in the days before and after admissions.

**PID 1024**

The trajectory of PID 1024 demonstrates a change in his SRH pattern around 12th of October 2017 with a shift to worse health with persistently high levels of healthcare changes (repeatedly seeking medical care services—GP, Emergency and other medical care) and frequent changes of medications. While health/care change and medication/drug/alcohol change were at high levels (1024 was not an alcohol misuser), there was no time during this period that he had an admission. His daughter moving away around 22nd of February 2017 and reducing his support

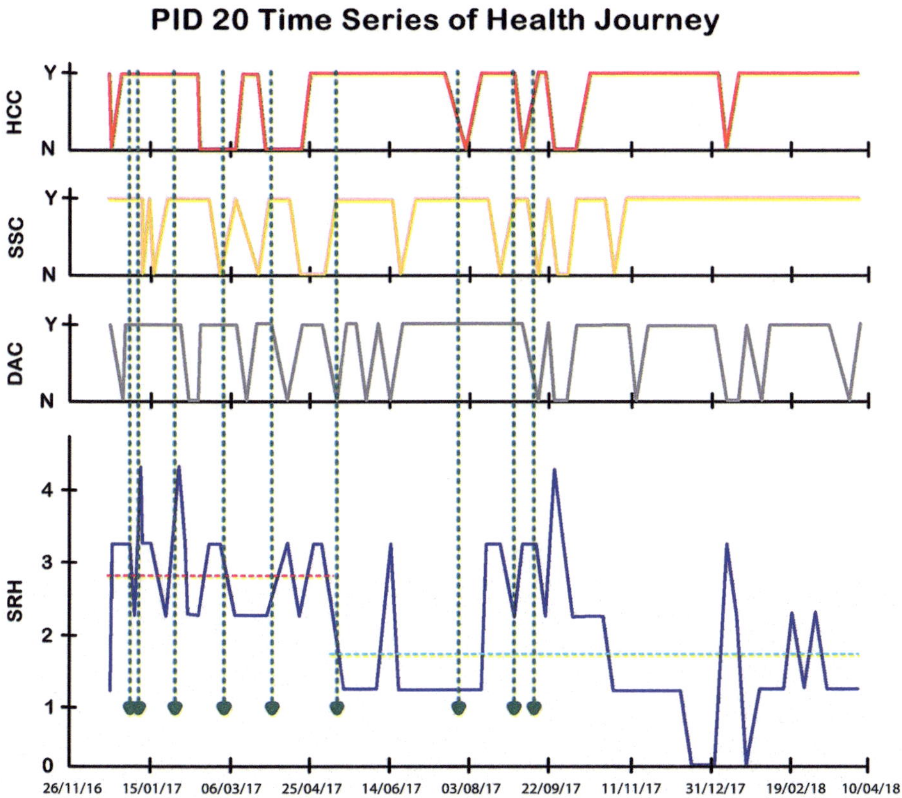


**Fig. 3** Health trajectory of PID 20. SRH Self-Rated Health (SRH—0 excellent, 1 very good, 2 good, 3 fair, 4 poor and 5 very poor); DAC Medication/Drug/Alcohol Change (0 no, 1 yes); SSC Support Structure Change (0 no, 1 yes); HCC Health/Care Change (0 no, 1 yes); arrows indicate hospitalisation

**Table 3** PID 20 profile of admissions and diagnostic related group (DRG)s

| Admission date | Discharge date | DRG description |
|---|---|---|
| 14/12/16 | 16/12/16 | Disorders of pancreas, except malignancy, major complexity |
| 17/12/16 | 20/12/16 | Disorders of the biliary tract, major complexity |
| 30/01/17 | 01/02/17 | Disorders of pancreas, except malignancy, minor complexity |
| 03/03/17 | 05/03/17 | Disorders of pancreas, except malignancy, minor complexity |
| 06/04/17 | 10/04/17 | Disorders of pancreas, except malignancy, major complexity |
| 06/05/17 | 08/05/17 | Disorders of pancreas, except malignancy, major complexity |
| 29/07/17 | 31/07/17 | Disorders of pancreas, except malignancy, minor complexity |
| 23/08/17 | 24/08/17 | Other digestive system disorders, minor complexity |
| 10/09/17 | 10/09/17 | Trauma to skin, subcutaneous tissue and breast, minor complexity |

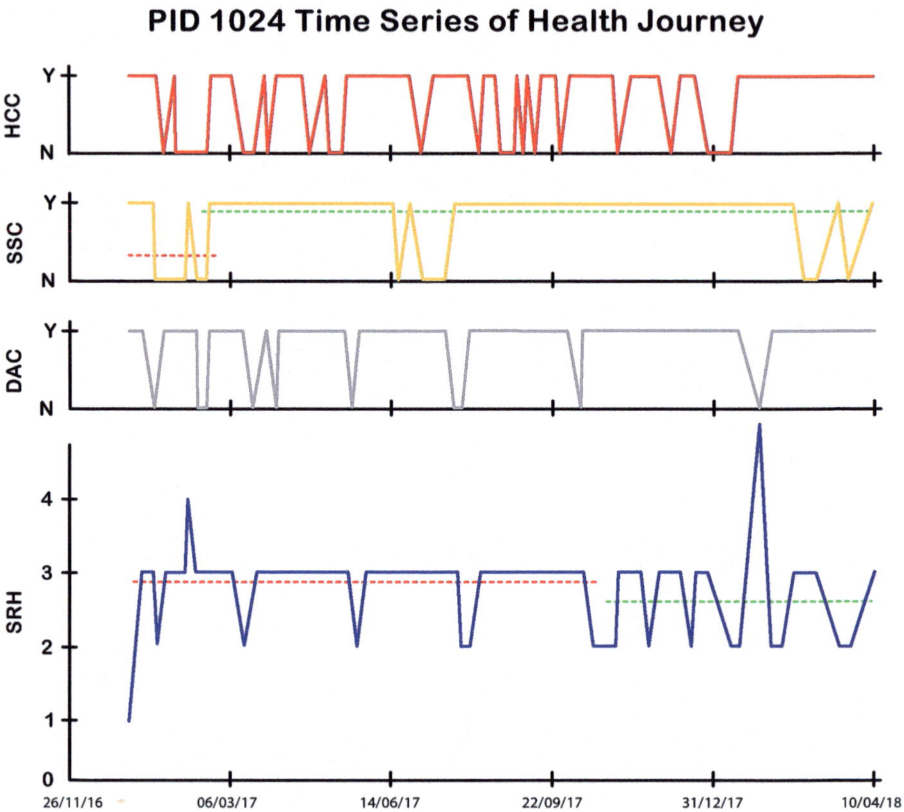


**Fig. 4** Health trajectory of PID 1024. SRH Self-Rated Health (SRH—0 excellent, 1 very good, 2 good, 3 fair, 4 poor and 5 very poor); DAC Medication/Drug/Alcohol Change (0 no, 1 yes); SSC Support Structure Change (0 no, 1 yes); HCC Health/Care Change (0 no, 1 yes)

another was associated with a general worsening of SRH but did not significantly affect his overall trajectory into an admission. PID 1024 did not have an admission during the period of observation (Fig. 4).

**PID 1040**

PID1040, generally, reported very good to good SRH with several dips to fair health related to her disease fluctuations. Her social support was very problematic except on one occasion. Her frequent changes in health and health care and medication (she only used prescription medication) indicate very unstable health and continual changes of medication. However, support structure change did significantly alter at one point in time when one of her children (daughter) came to stay with her from interstate to assist her in her worsening condition (Fig. 5). Her 3 admissions were for her COPD and were only for 1 day in duration (Table 4).

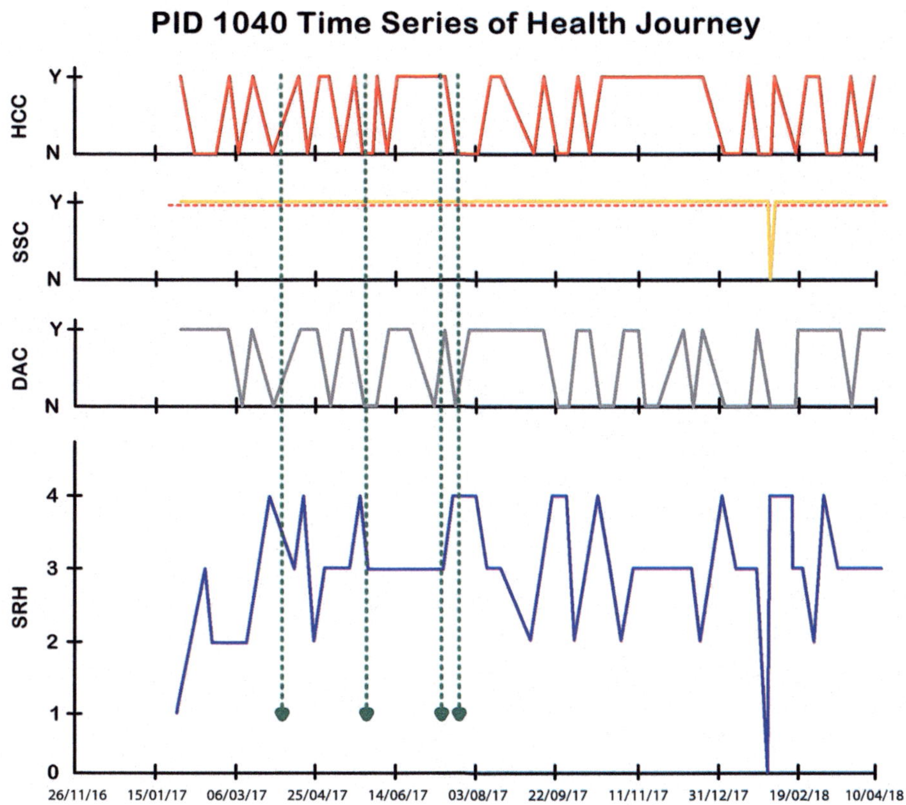


**Fig. 5** Health trajectory of PID 1040. SRH Self-Rated Health (SRH—0 excellent, 1 very good, 2 good, 3 fair, 4 poor and 5 very poor); DAC Medication/Drug/Alcohol Change (0 no, 1 yes); SSC Support Structure Change (0 no, 1 yes); HCC Health/Care Change (0 no, 1 yes); arrows indicate hospitalisation

**Table 4** PID 1040 profile of admissions and diagnostic related group (DRG)s

| Admission date | Discharge date | DRG description |
|---|---|---|
| 05/04/17 | 05/04/17 | Chronic obstructive airways disease, major complexity |
| 19/05/17 | 19/05/17 | Chronic obstructive airways disease, minor complexity |
| 22/07/17 | 26/07/17 | Other respiratory system disorders, minor complexity |
| 31/07/17 | 31/07/17 | Chronic obstructive airways disease, minor complexity |

# 5 Discussion

These three case studies demonstrate the variability in data of unstable individual health journeys. In none of the cases was it clear when and why an admission would be triggered.

Prediction would seem to be a very imprecise activity in a patient with nonlinear multiple unstable trajectories in different domains—'*SRH*', '*Health/Care Change*', '*Medication/Drug/Alcohol Change*' and '*Support Structure Change*'. Anticipatory care, i.e. care that recognises the nature of the living organism's journey moving forward, is a highly nuanced clinical activity [44]. These cases demonstrate that admissions occur in the context of fluctuating self-rated health triggered by apparent progressive disease processes, compounded by persistent health and care service changes and frequently exacerbated by lacking and/or discontinuous social support. Many admissions occur as a consequence of early life lifestyle choices—e.g. alcohol binges and smoking in PID 20 and smoking in PID 1040.

At a more systemic level, these dynamics are emergent from multiple interconnected nonlinear processes that are occurring and have occurred at different times as identified in Fig. 1—the framework of multi-layered systems influencing human health from the genomic to the whole person to the care system nested in the socio-political-economic environment. The concept of allostatic load—a gestalt of multiple stresses and adaptive and maladaptive responses—aims to quantify some of these processes and their effects, and requires further exploration in the context of our broader framework [45, 46].

## *5.1 How Data Can Depict an Individual's Personal Health Journey?*

### 5.1.1 Person-Centric Data

The three cases presented illustrate how the theoretical framework of health and illness care 'plays out' in real life. They highlight the phenomenon of unstable illness journeys and their effects on 'potentially preventable hospitalisations' which have been linked to increasing allostatic load arising from the dynamics within the patient's physical, treatment and social support domains [45]. These individual patterns emerge from the types of dynamics depicted in the multi-level framework in Fig. 1.

These cases also demonstrate that in each context, the circumstances surrounding each person's health and biopsychosocial situatedness are unique. The prevailing approach of exploring cohorts defined by a one-dimensional feature like 'avoidable hospitalisation' places significant limitations on a '*one size fits all*' predictive approach—each of these three individuals from the 'avoidable hospitalisation cohort' are likely to require different care and social support brokerage as well as tailored interventions to alter their journey and ultimately avert potentially avoidable hospitalisations.

Indeed, for those with the most unstable health journeys, it is difficult to see how monitoring any of the specific parameters—'*SRH*', '*Health/Care Change*'; '*Medication/Drug/Alcohol Change*' and '*Support Structure Change*'—on their own would be sufficient, even though they are based upon everyday reality. In longitudinal studies, SRH has been shown to reflect a sense of current and expected wellbeing with links to epigenetics, internal circulatory systems and total load of stress on an individual's *system as a whole* [18–20, 45, 47]. The levels of social structure and support are similarly linked to health outcomes (https://www.xlstat.com/en/solutions/premium).

What is more real and different from previous studies is the addition of the dynamics of '*Health/Care Change*', i.e. changes in perceived health and health service use and/or '*Medication/Drug/Alcohol Change*', i.e. substance ingestion whether it be prescribed, self-medicated, licit or illicit alcohol and drug use. In practical terms, as evidenced by the dynamics demonstrated in the cases studies, they are highly important in triggering or maintaining stability or instability.

Unravelling the demonstrated complex dynamics of highly variable and perhaps feed-forward and/or feed-backward loops in an individual trajectory, even by the PaJR close monitoring approach, is highly challenging. They did not allow highly precise predictions of deterioration to allow for quick fix linear interventions.

Do we need to measure everything at all times? Does big data provide more or better information for decision-making than judicious '*small data*' at the '*right level*' with '*human science*' that is interactive—person to person and experiential. To paraphrase Rosen: anticipation requires a 'simple' model of the future at any one time $t_1$ that can be acted on today in order to optimise one's current trajectory at a future time $t_2$ [9]. Anticipation is a process of living systems-not a mechanistic process [48], and the relationship between the real world and the model needs to be organic and dynamic [48][1].

### 5.1.2 Big Data

In contrast, MW participants were identified from a big data program with an entirely different model based on generic disease and service profiles in hospital administrative datasets.

Such big data analytics identified the HLCC cohort in real time and are a very important contribution [43] and with the predictive analytics that underpin the PaJR system should form an information system that enables human sensemaking [41]. Arguably, the collection of individual trajectories over time in different settings would itself become a form of big data.

[1]The closer the $t_1$ model is to actual reality (the modelling relationship), the more likely anticipatory actions are to be useful. Of course 'simple' models in dynamic systems are constantly being adjusted with feedback. For example, my body tells me 'I am thirsty' at $t_1$ so I drink water; however, I am thirsty because I need increased intravascular volume despite increasing dependent oedema which more oral fluids will not fix. Hence, I need to reframe my anticipatory model at $t_1$ else I will be worse off at $t_2$.

### 5.1.3 The Future

Multi-layered information systems need to be generated to capture the detail of each of the levels indicated in Fig. 1. Only then can the role of biomarkers in the very unstable phases of health journeys be fully explored. In the interim, biometrics may be useful in better managing the preceding phases of a health journey when they are still more amenable to genomic, proteonomic and anti-inflammatory interventions. These include greater understandings of how human biological systems and human sensemaking work together.

No doubt, big data analytics, artificial intelligence and deep learning will improve exponentially ensuring better predictive capacity. However, will our respect for the capacity of the '*human science*' of sensemaking and our human capacity to support, care and anticipate changes in wellness and illness be disregarded, blinded by our overwhelming fascination with any form of '*hype*'—here the technical buzz and brilliance of informatics.

## *5.2 What Are the Implications for Health Care and Health System Planning?*

A model is, in ideal terms, a *simplified external and explicit representation of our mental model* about the world, it is not the *real world* itself [49]. Data—'*big*' and/or '*human centric*'—are needed to provide the necessary input to validate a model and its dynamic behaviours observed in the real world. If the data do not validate the model, either the *mental model* is wrong, or we collected the *wrong data*. On the other hand, data driven models without theory, have problems of validity and coherence.

No one approach fits all clinical problems of concern. The PaJR model, while both model-based and data-driven, still requires '*human sensemaking*' input to help appropriate decision-making in the context of the *particulars* of each individual's health journey. In other words, in order to make sense data must be translated into information that apprises the personal nature of health care, and the individual heterogeneity of illness dynamics and responsiveness.

Hence, the best of all worlds would be an agile approach to modelling health journeys with the most appropriate '*big data*', '*small data*' and '*human sensemaking*' to answer the questions being posed. The question or problem to be solved should drive which data need to be collected rather than vice versa—the still dominant '*one size fits all*' approach to solving complex health care and health system problems will never fit all.

'*Big data*' brings information that generally speaking provides greater detail about an individual or cohort. A major critique of this data-based approach to strategy is that it is based on the underlying assumption that more data will provide the necessary information that ultimately will lead to greater success. Clearly, this assumption is embedded in the move to '*big data*'—it may provide the material to support, but not create, greater knowledge and wisdom for human action [50]. At this stage, it remains unclear if '*big data*' may create nothing more than an industry of data collection, with little real value to human health and clinical decision-making.

## 6 Conclusions

Using a complex adaptive systems framework builds on the works of intellectual leaders including McWhinney, Ellis and Rosen. *Anticipation* is a feature of living systems, while *prediction* is a feature of big data analytics. These approaches may be contradictory; however, the emergence of the sciences of *human sensemaking*, which encompasses human perceptions and experiences as central in data models, provides new hope to improve best possible individualised care.

Our case studies on data use in preventing avoidable hospitalisations in the MonashWatch program describe the potential of data in human sensemaking. Personal health monitoring was conducted in patients with unstable health journeys leading to repeated hospitalisation. For the MW care team, personal journey monitoring provided insights related to *when*, *how* and *why* deteriorations were likely to occur, allowing for anticipatory care based on patterns but not precise predictions. The implementation described in this chapter highlights the dynamics amongst the four different domains of '*Self-rated health*', '*Health/Care Change*', '*Medication/Drug/Alcohol Change*' and '*Support Structure Change*' that arguably have significant impact on patients' vulnerabilities and risk for hospitalisation. A first step to understanding the *specific systemic nature* behind the *particulars of an individual* can emerge from mapping various features of the person's presenting state.

'*Big data*' **and** '*human-centric data systems*' **and** '*human sensemaking*' are all equally needed to understand and manage unstable health journeys that otherwise may lead to potentially preventable hospital admissions. To that end, '*big data*' should be an adjunct and enabler, not the objective fact.

While hospital and public health systems can use '*big data*' analytics to identify cohorts at risk of avoidable hospitalisations. The analytics provide little information about *when*, *how* and *why* to intervene in the care of a *particular* patient. Ultimately, patients, their networks and their health professionals have to make everyday decisions about individualised care, and no information system can replace these human-to-human interactions, given that no data system can truly anticipate human behaviours.

**Acknowledgements** The collaboration in the development, trialling and evaluation of the PaJR project by our colleagues Narelle Hinkley and Donald Campbell at Monash University, Australia, Carl Vogel and Lucy Hederman at Trinity University, Dublin, Ireland and Kevin Smith and John-Paul Smith, University of Queensland is kindly acknowledged.

## The Transformative Aspects of This Study

The implementation of a data system that takes a human science perspective in the context of big data analytics is a step forward to an integrative approach to clinical information systems.

**Take Home Message**

- A model is ideally a *mental representation* of the *real world*, not the real world itself. If data do not validate a model, either the *mental model* is wrong or we collected the *wrong data*.
- Data systems that closely model the realities of everyday human systems are likely to be useful for clinical care. This approach is novel as much emphasis is placed on large-scale 'objective' data systems which can provide information but little insight into the dynamic realities that underpin an individual's health journey.
- While data can provide information, knowledge and wisdom arise from the human capacity of *sensemaking*.

## References

1. Oxford University P. Merriam-Webster Online Dictionary. The New Oxford dictionary of English; 1998.
2. Dimitrov DV. Medical internet of things and big data in healthcare. Healthc Inform Res. 2016;22(3):156–63.
3. Norbury A, Seymour B. Response heterogeneity: challenges for personalised medicine and big data approaches in psychiatry and chronic pain. F1000 Res. 2018;7:55.
4. Hollar D. Trajectory analysis in health care. New York: Springer; 2018.
5. Smith A. The big data revolution: from drug development to better health outcomes? Am J Manag Care. 2014;20(8 Spec No.):E4.
6. Tilly C. The old new social history and the new old social history. Ann Arbor: Center for Research on Social Organization. Harvard; 2007.
7. Kostkova P, Brewer H, de Lusignan S, Fottrell E, Goldacre B, Hart G, et al. Who owns the data? Open data for healthcare. Front Public Health. 2016;4:7.
8. Krumholz HM. Post-hospital syndrome—an acquired, transient condition of generalized risk. N Engl J Med. 2013;368(2):100–2.
9. Lakoff G, Johnson M. Metaphors we live by. Chicago: The University of Chicago Press; 1980.
10. Rosen R. Anticipatory systems: philosophical, mathematical, and methodological foundations. 1st ed. Oxford: Pergamon Press; 1985.
11. Ellis GFR. Top-down causation and emergence: some comments on mechanisms. Interface Focus. 2012;2(1):126–40.
12. Rothman KJ. Causes. Am J Epidemiol. 1976;104(6):587–92.
13. Sturmberg JP. The personal nature of health. J Eval Clin Pract. 2009;15(4):766–9.
14. Sturmberg JP. Health: a personal complex-adaptive state. In: Sturmberg JP, Martin CM, editors. Handbook of systems and complexity in health. New York: Springer; 2013. p. 231–42.

15. Sturmberg JP, Picard M, Aron DC, Bennett JM, Bircher J, deHaven MJ, et al. The emergence of health - how top-down environmental and social contexts constrain bottom-up biological potentials. A consensus framework. Front. Med. 2019;6:59. https://doi.org/10.3389/fmed.2019.00059.
16. Dantzer R. Cytokine-induced sickness behavior: where do we stand? Brain Behav Immun. 2001;15(1):7–24.
17. McWhinney IR. An acquaintance with particulars .... Fam Med. 1989;21(4):296–8.
18. Gorovitz S, MacIntyre A. Toward a theory of medical fallibility. J Med Philos. 1976;1(1):51–71.
19. Jylhä M. What is self-rated health and why does it predict mortality? Towards a unified conceptual model. Soc Sci Med. 2009;69(3):307–16.
20. DeSalvo KB, Jones TM, Peabody J, McDonald J, Fihn S, Fan V, et al. Health care expenditure prediction with a single item, self-rated health measure. Med Care. 2009;47(4):440–7.
21. Idler EL, Benyamini Y. Self-rated health and mortality: a review of twenty-seven community studies. J Health Soc Behav. 1997;38(1):21–37.
22. Lewis S. The two faces of generalism. J Health Serv Res Policy. 2014;19(1):1–2.
23. Reeve J, Byng R. Realising the full potential of primary care: uniting the 'two faces' of generalism. Br J Gen Pract. 2017;67(660):292–3.
24. May C, Montori VM, Mair FS. We need minimally disruptive medicine. BMJ. 2009;339:b2803.
25. Too much medicine. https://www.bmj.com/too-much-medicine.
26. Duerden M, Avery T, Payne R. Polypharmacy and medicines optimisation. Making it safe and sound. London: The King's Fund; 2013.
27. Burton C. Can we explain medically unexplained symptoms? Fam Pract. 2014;31(6):623–4.
28. WHO. Ottawa charter for health promotion. First International Conference on Health Promotion. Ottawa, 21 November 1986. 1986: WHO/HPR/HEP/95.1. Available from, http://www.who.int/hpr/NPH/docs/ottawa_charter_hp.pdf.
29. A Primer on Precision Medicine: US National Library of Medicine; 2018. Available from, https://ghr.nlm.nih.gov/primer/precisionmedicine/precisionvspersonalized.
30. What is pharmacogenomics? US National Library of Medicine. 2018. Available from, https://ghr.nlm.nih.gov/primer/genomicresearch/pharmacogenomics.
31. Benyamini Y. Why does self-rated health predict mortality? An update on current knowledge and a research agenda for psychologists. Psychol Health. 2011;26(11):1407–13.
32. Ferrucci L, Giallauria F, Schlessinger D. Mapping the road to resilience: novel math for the study of frailty. Mech Ageing Dev. 2008;129(11):677–9.
33. Gijzel SMW, van de Leemput IA, Scheffer M, Roppolo M, Olde Rikkert MGM, Melis RJF. Dynamical resilience indicators in time series of self-rated health correspond to frailty levels in older adults. J Gerontol Ser A. 2017;72(7):991–6.
34. Heller DA, Ahern FM, Pringle KE, Brown TV. Among older adults, the responsiveness of self-rated health to changes in Charlson comorbidity was moderated by age and baseline comorbidity. J Clin Epidemiol. 2009;62(2):177–87.
35. Oosterveld SM, Kessels RP, Hamel R, Ramakers IH, Aalten P, Verhey FR, et al. The influence of co-morbidity and frailty on the clinical manifestation of patients with Alzheimer's disease. J Alzheimers Dis. 2014;42(2):501–9.
36. Lutomski JE, Baars MAE, Boter H, Buurman BM, den Elzen WPJ, Jansen APD, et al. [Frailty, disability and multi-morbidity: the relationship with quality of life and healthcare costs in elderly people]. Ned. Tijdschr. Geneeskd. 2014;158:A7297.
37. Geessink N, Schoon Y, van Goor H, Olde Rikkert M, Melis R. Frailty and quality of life among older people with and without a cancer diagnosis: findings from TOPICS-MDS. PLoS One. 2017;12(12):e0189648.

38. Haaksma ML, Vilela LR, Marengoni A, Calderon-Larranaga A, Leoutsakos JS, Olde Rikkert MGM, et al. Comorbidity and progression of late onset Alzheimer's disease: a systematic review. Plos One. 2017;12(5):e0177044.
39. Martin CM. Self-rated health: patterns in the journeys of patients with multi-morbidity and frailty. J Eval Clin Pract. 2014;20(6):1010–6.
40. MonashWatch: Keeping people healthy at home: Monash Health; 2016. Available from, http://monashhealth.org/page/monashwatch.
41. Martin CM, Vogel C, Grady D, Zarabzadeh A, Hederman L, Kellett J, et al. Implementation of complex adaptive chronic care: the Patient Journey Record system (PaJR). J Eval Clin Pract. 2012;18(6):1226–34.
42. Martin C, Sturmberg JP, Stockman K, Campbell D, Hederman L, Vogel C, et al. Supporting complex dynamic health journeys using conversation to avert hospital readmissions from the community: an ecological perspective incorporating interoception. In: Sturmberg J, editor. Putting systems and complexity science into practice. Cham: Springer; 2018.
43. Ferrier D, Diver F, Corin S, McNair P, Cheng C. HealthLinks: incentivising better value chronic care in Victoria. Int J Integr Care. 2017;17(3):A129. Available from, https://www.ijic.org/articles/abstract/10.5334/ijic.3241/.
44. Staiger TO, Kritek PA, Blakeney EL, Zierler BK, O'Brien K, Ehrmantraut R. A conceptual framework for applying the anticipatory theory of complex systems to improve safety and quality in healthcare. In: Nadin M, editor. Anticipation and medicine. Cham: Springer; 2016. p. 31–40.
45. Goldwater D, Dharmarajan K, McEwen BS, Krumholz HM. Is posthospital syndrome a result of hospitalization-induced allostatic overload? J Hosp Med. 2018;13(5). https://doi.org/10.12788/jhm.2986.
46. Martin C, Hinckley N, Stockman K, Campbell D. Post-hospital syndrome (PHS) and potentially preventable hospitalizations (PPH) in adults. MonashWatch adult cohort patient telehealth journeys. JMIR Preprints 2018. Available from, http://preprints.jmir.org/preprint/11952.
47. Martin CM, Stockman K, Campbell D. Resilience, health perceptions, stressors and hospital admissions - observations from the real world of clinical care of unstable health journeys in Monash Watch (MW), Victoria, Australia. J Eval Clin Pract. 2018;24(6):1310–18.
48. Rosen R. An interview with Robert Rosen. In: Rosen J, editor. (This is a corrected version [July 14, 2000], thanks to the help of Esther Wieringa). Available from, http://www.people.vcu.edu/~mikuleck/rsntpe.html1997.
49. Mikulecky DC. The emergence of complexity: science coming of age or science growing old? Comput Chem. 2001;25(4):341–8.
50. Sturmberg JP. Knowledge translation in healthcare - towards understanding its true complexities; comment on "using complexity and network concepts to inform healthcare knowledge translation". Int J Health Policy Manag. 2018;7(5):455–8. Available from, http://ijhpm.com/article_3415.html.

# Is Decision-Making of Women Concerning Their Violent Relationships Truly Nonlinear . . . and Why Is That?

**David Katerndahl, Sandra Burge, Robert Ferrer, Johanna Becho, Robert Wood, and Maria Del Pilar Montanez Villacampa**

## 1 Introduction

Intimate partner violence (IPV) is a blight upon human civilization. Globally, 30% of women report having ever experienced IPV [1]. Over 35% of American women experience IPV or stalking, with 15–42% sustaining injuries and 8–12% requiring medical care [2]. The impact of assault is long term and not limited to injury. Battered women are 2–7 times more likely to suffer somatization, anxiety, depression, and phobias compared to women who report no abuse [3, 4]. Victims of violence also report poorer physical and mental health overall [2]. Victims' health costs are higher with more frequent hospitalizations and more visits to emergency departments, outpatient clinics, and mental health services [4]. Yet, our understanding of women's decision-making about IPV is still rudimentary.

## 2 Nonlinearity of Partner Violence

Dynamics of day-to-day violence can be characterized in two ways: (1) the degree of nonlinearity (nonlinear phenomena are characterized by irregular trajectories, dynamic and variable relationships, and a disproportional response to interventions,

D. Katerndahl (✉) · S. Burge · R. Ferrer · R. Wood · M. D. P. Montanez Villacampa
Department of Family and Community Medicine, University of Texas Health Science Center San Antonio, San Antonio, TX, USA
e-mail: katerndahl@uthscsa.edu; burge@uthscsa.edu; ferrerr@uthscsa.edu; wood@uthscsa.edu; MontanezVill@uthscsa.edu

J. Becho
Department of Psychiatry, University of Texas Health Science Center San Antonio, San Antonio, TX, USA
e-mail: becho@uthscsa.edu

 
J. P. Sturmberg (ed.), *Embracing Complexity in Health*,
https://doi.org/10.1007/978-3-030-10940-0_9

leading to unexpected events and changing patterns), or (2) dynamical pattern (categorical description of periodic, chaotic, random dynamics).

When system dynamics are "nonlinear," they are unpredictable. Three types of nonlinearity measurements are available [5] (see Table 1 for details). In addition to sensitivity to initial conditions (speed with which two adjacent points diverge over time) as measured by the largest Lyapunov's exponent [6], nonlinearity can

**Table 1** Types and sources of nonlinearity

| Types of nonlinearity | Sources of nonlinearity |
|---|---|
| **Chaos-based**<br>*Lyapunov's exponent*—indicates the rate at which information about the initial conditions is lost<br>*Interpretation*<br>positive: system is chaotic and unstable<br>negative: system attracts to a fixed point<br>0: system is in a steady-state mode | **Nonlinearity of underlying predictor(s)**<br>*Measure of predictor nonlinearity*—irregular trajectories, dynamic and variable relationships, and a disproportional response to interventions lead to unexpected events and changing patterns (e.g., nonlinearity of his violence reflects the nonlinearity of her feelings of emotional distance from him) |
| **Algorithmic complexity**<br>*LZ complexity*—indicates the repetitiveness of a particular characteristic (e.g., alcohol consumption) over a time period<br>*Interpretation*<br>0: fixed point<br>low positive periodic<br>increasing positive: increasingly random | **Interdependence among predictors/ circular causality**<br>*Vector autoregression*—uses multiple concurrent predictors' time series to develop models explaining each other's variable time series (e.g., his violence is predicted by prior-day levels of her feelings and hassles, of distance, her degree of upset, but distance, upset, and hassles predict each other/distance predicts his violence but his violence predicts her distance) |
| **Degree of irregularity**<br>*Approximate entropy*—indicates the amount of regularity and the unpredictability of fluctuations in time-series data (e.g., prior day alcohol consumption and occurrence of violence escalation)<br>*Interpretation*<br>0: fixed point<br>low positive periodic<br>increasing positive: increasingly random | **Catastrophic phenomenon**<br>*Cusp catastrophe modeling—applies* catastrophe theory to model the discontinuous relationship between predisposing factors and outcomes due to variables that distort the relationship (e.g., relationship between violence burden and behaviors her use of negative coping distorted by her use of violence |

Measures of nonlinearity fall into one of three types, each having several ways of measurement. In addition, nonlinearity in general can develop from a variety of sources, each having unique ways of assessment be measured as algorithmic complexity or irregularity. Algorithmic complexity is a measure of the amount of information needed to describe the data and can be measured by statistics such as Lempel-Ziv (LZ) complexity [7]. Degree of irregularity of time series can be measured by statistics such as approximate entropy (ApEn) [8]. Previous work on IPV found that most couples' violence is nonlinear and that violence nonlinearity is a significant predictor of women's negative coping strategies, positive violence appraisals, as well as hope and social support, and it can be a stronger predictor of outcomes than either violence frequency or severity. In addition, there is a curvilinear relationship between violence nonlinearity and symptoms, function, and readiness-for-change [9]. Prior research has found that violence in these relationships generally follows nonlinear trajectories [9].

Dynamics can also be classified into three dynamical patterns.

- *Periodic dynamics*, in which the system cycles its behavior, results when actions and outcomes are tightly coupled, and when current behavior is dependent on previous behavior. Periodic systems have strong attractors (repeating patterns of phenomena) influencing possible behaviors and are stable and insensitive to small changes in their state. Periodic systems are predictable and respond predictably to interventions.
- In *chaotic dynamics*, the overall pattern of behavior recurs but the specific path is unpredictable; this results when actions and outcomes are separated in time, and when feedback within the system varies in strength and direction. Chaotic systems also have attractors influencing their behavior but they are sensitive to small changes in terms of the specific path they follow. Chaotic systems are unpredictable, long-term, and do not respond predictably to interventions.
- A type of *random dynamics* (pink noise or criticality) is common in complex systems. Criticality results from constant stress on a system composed of interdependent components with varying predilections to respond, yielding a random pattern of responses of varying intensity. Systems characterized by criticality have no attractors influencing their behavior, and may or may not be sensitive to initial conditions. Random systems are unpredictable and do not respond predictably to interventions [10].

Hence, dynamical patterns can range from linear and predictable (*periodic*) to mid-level nonlinear (*chaotic*) to extremely nonlinear and unpredictable (*random*). Prior work on IPV found that, while 12% of couples exhibit periodic dynamics, 30% show chaotic dynamics and 58% demonstrate random dynamics [11]. Nonlinearity itself suggests either chaotic or random dynamics.

Prior research on the dynamics of violent relationships suggests that such relationships may have both predictable and unpredictable components (see Table 2):

- predictable in their lack of emotional reaction to relationship dynamics and stress [12],
- but unpredictable in the shifting power dynamics within the relationship [13].

The prevalence of nonlinear chaotic and random violence within couples creates a challenge as we attempt to understand and intervene in these relationships.

**Table 2** Types and sources of nonlinearity

| Variables | Key findings from previous studies |
|---|---|
| **Background (B)** | |
| Demographics<br>Relationship and violence history<br>Childhood abuse<br>Relationship history and function<br>Depression<br>Social network<br>Prior experience with actions | • Social networks of women in violent relationships are smaller, less interconnected and less support received than given<br>• 70% of women in violent relationships taken prior action, with both positive and negative results; few women have gone to shelters |
| **Factors affecting progress through stages (B, E)** | |
| Violence appraisal<br>Hope<br>Support/stress<br>Coping strategies<br>Awareness | • Just participating in the study resulted in better sense of control of the violence, less use of denial to cope and more readiness to leave the relationship, but no change in awareness |
| **Daily violence and environment (D)** | |
| Level of husband/wife violence<br>Husband's stalking<br>Violence escalation<br>Perceived violence control<br>Husband's/wife's alcohol intake<br>Level of stress<br>Level of marital harmony<br>Forgiveness sought/given<br>Concern: children, safety, finances<br>Desire: move on, keep family together<br>Need: leave, coping, legal | • Daily levels of violence and perceived needs-for-action depend on a variety of prior-day predictors<br>• Although association between his violence and alcohol use is consistent, the nature of its relationship remains unclear<br>• Although forgiveness by her is publicly condemned, it is associated with less marital distance, alcohol use by her, stress, argument frequency on the following day, but NO effect on her decision-making |
| **Readiness-for-action (B, E)** | |
| Help counseling<br>Legal assistance<br>Leaving | • Taking action depends upon a combination of prior experience with taking action, readiness-to-act and immediate perceived need-to-act, varying depending upon the specific action |
| **Action taken (W)** | |
| Counseling<br>Legal action<br>Leaving | • Action can happen without immediate sense-of-need |

Frequency of measurement: **B** baseline; **D** daily; **E** end-of-study; **W** weekly
As a complex system, to understand the violence of women's decision-making process requires in-depth assessment of background, context, and events measured at different frequencies. This table presents the wealth of variables assessed during this study

## 3 A Focus on Decision-Making in Partner Violence

"Decision-making" is the process of making a choice between a number of options and committing to a future course of action. Hence, it is a process over time that may involve a series of steps, beginning with a perceived need to make a change. For a decision to be made, more than one option must be available and choice is based upon inputs, values, and constraints. Finally, the decision-making process involves action, even if that action is to delay the change [14].

### *3.1 Decision-Making of Women in Violence Relationships*

In addition to seeking informal support, formal actions among women in violent relationships can be grouped into three categories: (1) leaving the household, (2) seeking help or counseling, or (3) taking legal action, with leaving the relationship being the most studied. Studies on action-taking among women in violent relationships have generally used quantitative methods to document events (i.e., leaving) with cross-sectional correlates of those events or qualitative methods to study factors women consider important in those decisions. Qualitatively, the process of taking action for these women is described as a nonlinear, fluctuating process [15], reflecting a sequential process of "two steps forward and one step back" [16]. Leaving an abusive partner may be considered the initial step in recovery [17], and the beginning of a gradual but difficult process [18]. However, leaving may not represent the only path to recovery. Bell et al. [19] found that, among 206 women seeking general help for IPV, over the course of a 1-year period, 57% women left the relationship soon after seeking help and never returned, while an additional 15% left within 9 months of help-seeking. The remaining women either remained in the relationship (15%) or spent time in and out of the relationship (13%). Cattaneo et al. [20] found that victims of IPV commonly seek both legal and non-legal help repeatedly over the course of a year. Those who leave soon after seeking help reported the highest quality-of-life and lowest frequencies of physical or psychological abuse or stalking 1 year later [19]. The complexity of this decision-making trajectory suggests the presence of a variety of factors in tension.

In general, decision-making processes include social, cognitive, and cultural factors as well as perceptions, interpretation, judgment, motivation, and post-action reflection [21]. A woman's decision to separate from her violent partner or seek help from the health care or legal systems is related to a number of internal and external factors, such as the level of violence and alcohol consumption of both partners in the relationship [22, 23], the man's stalking behavior [24], pragmatic factors such as financial independence [25], partner infidelity [26], relationship quality and safety [26–29], perceived barriers and support [27, 30], and her prior experience with taking action [31]. Personal attitudes concerning the violence may also play a role [32], and perceived or real external family pressures, relationship investment, and alternatives are important [33]. The presence of children can be critical to the woman's decision to take action, creating conflict between concern for the child's well-being [26, 27] and desire to keep the family together [34]. These stressors and risks may represent important factors in building the perception of need-for-action (and eventually taking action) in the abused woman, contributing to its nonlinearity.

## 3.2 Studying Decision-Making in Partner Violence

To date, the framework mostly used to study action-taking among abused women is the Transtheoretical Model [15] because the stages of moving from no perceived need-for-action to taking action correspond to the five stages in the model [35]. The Transtheoretical Model of Change [36] states that behavior change moves through five stages: precontemplation, contemplation, preparation, action, and maintenance. Those in the "precontemplation" stage are characterized by disinterest in change, perceiving that there is no need for change; those in "contemplation" are considering a change, and ambivalent about the "pros" and "cons." In "preparation," abused women are convinced that change is necessary and are actively preparing to make a change (they are ready for change), taking small steps in that direction. In the "action" stage, they make key changes and wrestle to maintain them, dependent upon many forces that push toward and pull away from the change. "Maintenance" differs from "action" in that the change has been maintained for at least 6 months. Those in action and maintenance are at risk for returning to the abusive relationship, especially under stress [15].

Several contextual factors appear important in fostering the perceived need-for-action that moves women through these stages, including awareness of the violence and the reality of their situation [26]. Awareness is the primary factor in moving women from precontemplation to contemplation [35]. Two factors that encourage action-taking among abused women are insight into the violence [22], and a sense of empowerment to act [27]. While consciousness-raising is important at all stages of the process, self-evaluation is particularly relevant during the contemplation–preparation–action stages [37]. Social support also correlates with seeking legal assistance [38] and leaving the relationship [31, 39]. Hence, while awareness and appraisal may be important in promoting perceived need-for-action, coping style and support may be critical in spurring her into action once a decision is made. Action-taking is dependent on problem recognition and support factors [40] along with the recognition of important individual, interpersonal, and sociocultural influences. But decision-making, in general, and specifically for IPV is qualitatively nonlinear. Is it quantitatively nonlinear as well? If so, it has important implications for healthcare providers encouraging women in abusive relationships to take action.

### 3.3 *Potential Sources of Nonlinearity*

Measuring nonlinearity quantitatively in IPV is challenging. This requires complete time series data of sufficient length to result in stable measures, difficult to achieve from women scrutinized by a controlling, abusive partner. If present, nonlinearity could have a variety of sources. Nonlinearity in taking action could be due to nonlinearity of perceived need-for-action, which may in turn be due to (1) the nonlinearity of underlying partner-perpetrated violence as observed in prior studies [9], or (2) the presence of multiple, interdependent predictors or (3) circularly-causal predictors [41]. Or nonlinearity in taking action could be present if readiness-for-change is (4) a catastrophic phenomenon ("Catastrophe theory" seeks to explain sudden, large changes in behavior based upon small, continuous changes in one or more control variables; cusp catastrophe theory is one of the simpler catastrophic models of change). Determining the source of the nonlinearity in decision-making could suggest action-specific interventions to promote action-taking among women.

## 4 Research Approach

To determine the degree of nonlinearity involved in women's decision-making and its source(s), we used methods similar to those of a prior study [42], enrolling women from primary care clinics who had a recent history of IPV. At baseline, all 143 women completed measures designed to assess background characteristics as well as factors which may affect the decision-making process. Prior work found that religious variables [43], awareness [35], depression and hope, childhood abuse, coping and violence appraisal, and partner's controlling behaviors contribute to violence dynamics and outcomes, including healthcare utilization [44]. To provide contextual information concerning subjects' support, we asked subjects to describe their social networks (immediate social contacts), using a social network analysis matrix. The effect of social support on women's actions is complex. While victims of IPV are more likely to seek legal assistance when they receive adequate social support [38], they are more likely to leave the relationship if support is inadequate [39], especially if support is sought but not received [31]. Finally, women completed measures of decision-making and behavioral change at baseline and end-of-study. The Transtheoretical Model of Change is appropriate for describing the decision-making process of leaving an abusive partner [37]. "Readiness-for-change" includes "readiness-to-leave," "readiness-for-help-coping," and "readiness-for-legal-assistance." While "readiness-for-leaving" included leaving relationship, entering a women's shelter, or moving in with a friend or family member, "readiness-for-help" included seeking counseling or seeking help through the Family Justice Center. "Readiness-for-legal-action" involved getting a lawyer, filing a police report, applying for a protective order, filing for child custody, or filing for divorce. In addition, women were asked to complete a daily assessment using Interactive Voice Response (IVR) via telephone for 8 weeks, describing the previous day's experience. In addition to reporting on violence severity and alcohol use by both partners, women assessed violence escalation and stalking behavior. Women also assessed daily potential predictors of abuse, including arguments, stress, marital distance, and forgiveness sought and given. In addition, the woman's perceived need-for-action (seeking help, taking legal action, leaving) was assessed as well as factors that could potentially affect this need, such as perceived control of the violence, concerns for children's safety, the effect of violence on the children and/or about money, and desires to move on and/or keep the family together.

## 5 Analysis

To compute nonlinearity measures, complete time series data is needed. While study completers reported an average of 75% of days, missing data was imputed, using an approach shown to least distort nonlinear characteristics of time series when compared to traditional methods [45]. Using these complete time series, we calculated nonlinearity scores with higher scores indicating a greater degree of nonlinearity, using two measures of nonlinearity: LZ complexity and approximate entropy. These were applied to each subject's time series for partner-perpetrated violence, and each assessment of perceived need-for-action.

To predict severity of violent events and environmental variables, vector autoregression (VAR) was applied to the IVR time series. Vector autoregression seeks predictors of each dependent variable (i.e., need-for-help) from prior (lagged) measures of itself and other independent time series variables (i.e., his violence, her alcohol use, stress). In the example above, variables A, B, and C are predicted by the two prior A scores as well as the two prior levels of B and C. Because predictors of need-for-action were analyzed individually for participants, to combine results across participants, we applied methods traditionally reserved for meta-analyses. Individual study statistics were combined across studies to estimate overall statistics; thus, statistics were combined rather than the raw data, using weighted coefficients (weighted by SE) [46].

Finally, readiness-for-action was modeled using cusp catastrophe modeling (CCM). In CCM analysis, the impact of the asymmetry (variables expected to linearly predict the outcome) and bifurcation (variables that could distort the asymmetry–outcome relationship) variables on the outcome is modeled using regression analysis, comparing the CCM against linear models to determine which model accounts for the most variance in the outcome. Based on theory, asymmetry variables focused on violence burden including husband-perpetrated violence frequency and mean episode severity, partner's controlling behaviors, and mean daily level of need specific to the action being modeled (i.e., leaving). To reduce the number of asymmetry variables used in the analysis, a principal component analysis with varimax rotation was performed using these variables. One asymmetry factor ("violence burden") was extracted for each readiness-to-take-action outcome, accounting for 38–40% of the variance. Bifurcation variables were chosen based upon their potential to yield both positive and negative reactions; these included social support (betweenness, indegree), hope and positive coping (hope, active coping, reinterpretation coping), forgiveness (frequency of his asking forgiveness, frequency of her forgiving), and number of children at home. To reduce the number of bifurcation variables, a principal component analysis with varimax rotation was performed using these eight potential bifurcation variables. Four factors were extracted, accounting for 75% of the variance, corresponding to "hope and cope," "support," "forgiveness," and "number of children." Outcome variables included the three readiness-for-action variables from the baseline and end-of-study surveys.

To determine whether CCM explained more outcome variance than linear methods, CCM was compared against two linear models. For each dependent variable three models were compared, using the asymmetry factor and the four bifurcation factors. To establish that CCM explained an outcome, the CCM had to be statistically significant, and both the $Y_1^3$ term and at least one bifurcation term had to be significant [47]. To conclude that CCM was at least as good as linear modeling in explaining an outcome, the CCM had to account for at least as much of the variance as both linear models.

## 6 Results

Of the 143 women enrolled, 105 completed the end-of-study interview and 93 provided enough daily reports to be included in nonlinearity analysis. Those who completed were very similar demographically to those who enrolled. Overall, the sample was predominantly low income and Hispanic. The mean duration of the relationship was $14.8 \pm 12.2$ (SD) years with the mean duration of abuse being $10.6 \pm 11.2$ (SD) years.

Women provided 4696 daily reports which included 1005 (21%) reports of partner-perpetrated abuse and 622 (13%) reports of wife-perpetrated abuse. Table 3 compares nonlinearity measures across perceived needs. Both the mean level of perceived need-for-legal-action and its nonlinearity were less than those for either need-for-help or leaving. Using datasets of known dynamics as benchmarks, most approximate entropies were more nonlinear than known chaotic time series while most of the LZ complexities were in the ranges seen in random dynamics. To assist in identifying the source of nonlinearity of needs, regression analyses were performed to predict measures of nonlinearity for all three perceived needs. The nonlinearity of violence only predicted nonlinearity of need-to-leave.

VAR is useful in addressing questions of causality. In complex systems, causality may be difficult to determine due to issues of (1) circular causality and (2) the presence of multiple, interconnected predictors [41]. First, nonlinearity of need could be a product of circular causality in which predictors of need are themselves predicted by the need. Need-for-help and for-legal-action (see Figs. 1 and 2) predict the perception that violence is increasing which, in turn, predicts both needs. In

**Table 3** Types and sources of nonlinearity

| Nonlinearity | Partner's violence | Need-for- Help | Legal action | Leaving |
|---|---|---|---|---|
| Mean level of need[a] | – | 2.66 | 2.05 | 2.75 |
| Nonlinearity of violence | | | | |
| LZ complexity[b] | 0.861 | 0.853 | 0.693 | 0.885 |
| Approximate entropy[b] | 0.450 | 0.453 | 0.362 | 0.480 |

Differences in level and nonlinearity of needs-for-help, legal action and leaving among women in violent relationships showing that both the level of need-for-legal-action and its degree of nonlinearity are less than those of the other needs.
[a]Legal Action < Help/Leaving
[b]Legal Action < Others

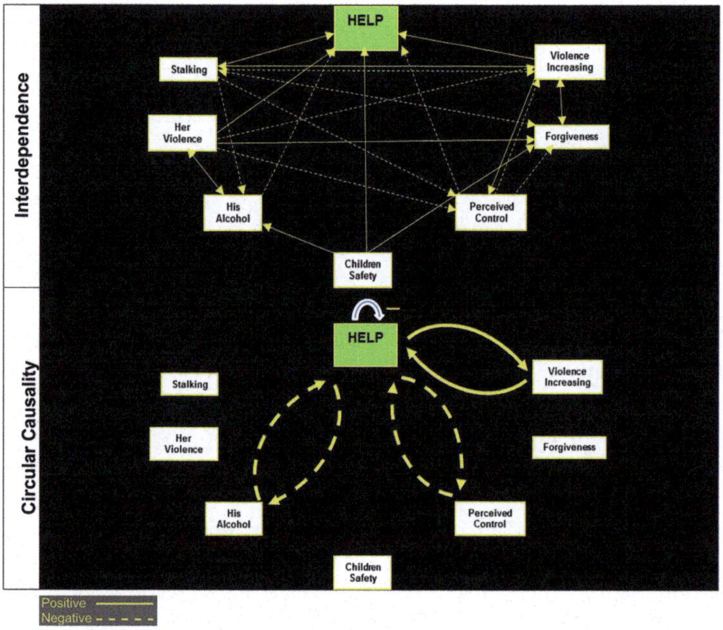


**Fig. 1** Significant relationship between prior-day predictors and the need-for-help. Interrelationships among prior-day predictors of need-for-help (Adapted from Katerndahl et al. [48])

addition, lower perceived control and husband's lower alcohol intake predict lower next-day need-for-help which, in turn, predicts lower next-day perceived control and his alcohol intake. Lower perceived control is also circularly-causal with need-for-legal-action, but no such circular causality exists for need-to-leave. In addition, four predictors (his violence, her readiness to move on, her forgiveness, and her concern about the effects of violence on children) have a negative feedback relationship with need-to-leave (see Fig. 3). Second, all three perceived needs have interdependent prior-day predictors. Of the seven predictors of need-for-help, 20 (48%) of the

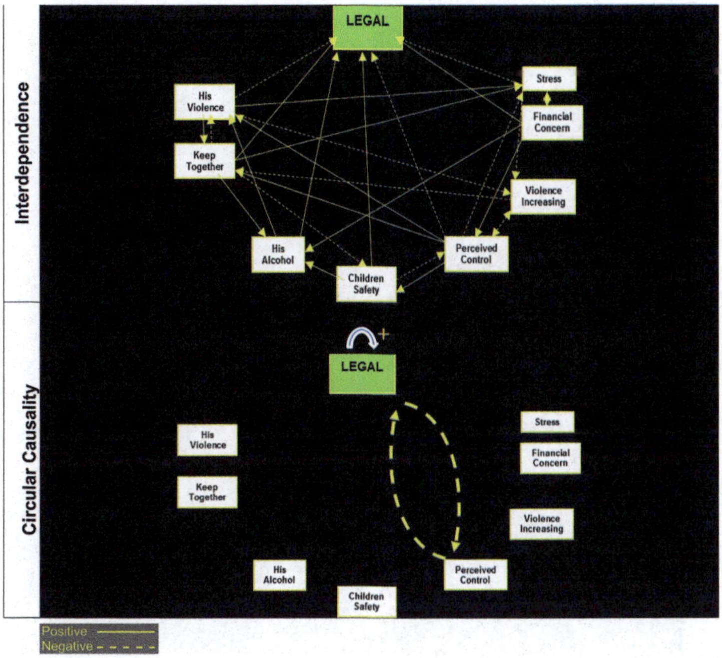


**Fig. 2** Significant relationship between prior-day predictors and the need-for-legal action. Interrelationships among prior-day predictors of need-for-legal action (Adapted from Katerndahl et al. [48])

42 possible links among them are actually observed. In need-for-legal-action, 21 (38%) of the 56 possible links among its eight predictors are statistically significant. Finally, for the six prior-day predictors of need-to-leave, 12 (40%) of the 30 possible links are observed.

Table 4 presents the results of the CCM analyses along with their linear model comparisons; in all three actions, CCM accounted for more variance than the linear comparisons. Violence burden was not significant in CCMs of readiness-for-legal-action and readiness-to-leave, suggesting that the CCMs were not complete and other asymmetry factors may be important. The CCM for readiness-for-help did find that violence burden contributed to the variance, and forgiveness was an important bifurcation factor. Number of children served as the bifurcation factor for readiness-for-legal-action. Readiness-to-leave was more complex; both number of children and hope-and-cope were bifurcation factors in this analysis.

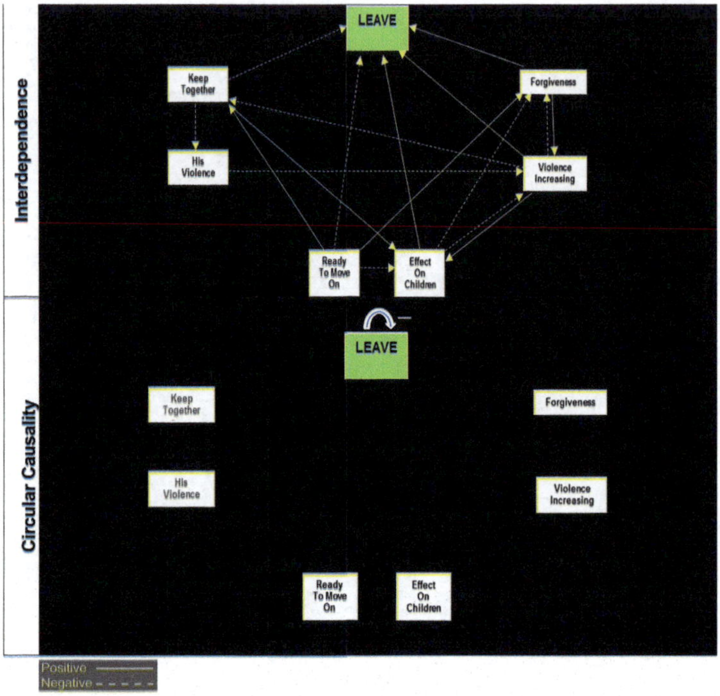


**Fig. 3** Significant relationship between prior-day predictors and the need-to-leave. Interrelationships among prior-day predictors of need-to-leave (Adapted from Katerndahl et al. [48])

## 7 Interpretation

Quantitative assessments of nonlinearity using daily IVR reports of needs-for-action show wide variation in their day-to-day nonlinearity measures, but generally indicate that the patterns are nonlinear. The mean level of perceived need-for-legal-action was less than that for either need-for-help or need-for-leaving, and its nonlinearity measures were also lower. Yet, needs-for-help and leaving exhibited negative feedback from day-to-day [48], which should minimize nonlinearity [41]. For example, if need-to-leave increases 1 day, the tendency is for it to decrease the next day, preventing rapid, progressive increases in perceived need. In contrast, nonlinearity of need-for-legal-action was lower (more predictable), but displayed feedforward dynamics which should promote greater nonlinearity [41]. Such positive and negative feedback would serve to keep nonlinearity for all three needs at a midrange. In general, while linear periodic dynamics implies predictable response to intervention, it also suggests limited options. Extreme nonlinear (random) dynamics implies many possible states but unpredictable response to intervention. Hence, midrange nonlinearity may be optimal in terms of combining adaptability with enough variability to permit adaptation [49]. In fact, previous work with women in

**Table 4** Cusp catastrophe modeling of readiness-for-action compared with linear modeling

| Model | Help | | | Legal action | | | Leaving | | |
|---|---|---|---|---|---|---|---|---|---|
| | $\mathbf{R^2}$ | Coefficient | F | $\mathbf{R^2}$ | Coefficient | F | $\mathbf{R^2}$ | Coefficient | F |
| Cusp catastrophe | **0.321** | | **4.94**$^{****}$ | **0.460** | | **8.11**$^{****}$ | **0.480** | | **8.69**$^{****}$ |
| $Y_1^3$ | | −0.527$^{****}$ | | | −0.687$^{****}$ | | | −0.751$^{****}$ | |
| Asymmetry | | | | | | | | | |
| Violence burden | | 0.245$^{*}$ | | | 0.188 | | | 0.145 | |
| Bifurcations@ | | | | | | | | | |
| Hope and cope | | 0.030 | | | 0.165 | | | 0.276$^{*}$ | |
| Support | | 0.183 | | | 0.215 | | | 0.173 | |
| Forgiveness | | −0.256$^{*}$ | | | 0.100 | | | −0.045 | |
| Number of children | | −0.035 | | | −0.367$^{***}$ | | | −0.269$^{*}$ | |
| Linear models | | | | | | | | | |
| PrePost | 0.231 | | 3.50$^{***}$ | 0.035 | | 1.30 | 0.378 | | 6.06$^{****}$ |
| Linear change | 0.000 | | 0.92 | 000 | | 0.88 | 0.000 | | 1.63 |

Adapted from Katerndahl et al. [51]
Comparisons of fit modeling readiness-for-help, legal action, and leaving using CCM versus two linear models
BOLD values indicates the best fitting model
@ = Bifurcation interaction term
$^{*}p \leq 0.05$; $^{**}p \leq 0.01$; $^{***}p \leq 0.005$; $^{****}p \leq 0.001$
Predictor Factors:

- Violence burden (frequency of husband's violence, severity of husband's violence episodes, mean need-for-action, total ABI score)
- Hope and cope (Hope, active coping, reinterpretation coping)
- Support (Betweenness centrality, indegree)
- Forgiveness (Frequency of husband requesting forgiveness, frequency of wife forgiving)
- Number of children

violent relationships found that, when violence nonlinearity was indeed midrange, those women reported fewer psychiatric symptoms and better emotional functioning while recognizing that the violence was not her fault [11, 44].

Using regression analysis of baseline characteristics, the degree of nonlinearity, or (unpredictability), of need-for-action generally depended upon a few factors. The unpredictability of all three needs was greater when partners attempted to isolate the women. Yet, social network variables particularly predicted nonlinearity especially for needs-for-help and legal action, suggesting that the interplay between his attempts to isolate her and her interactions with her social network were important to the nonlinearity, or unpredictability, of her need to take action. Lack of awareness was important to the unpredictability of needs-for-help and leaving. Only nonlinearity of need-to-leave was predicted by the nonlinearity of the underlying violence [50].

## *7.1 Explaining Nonlinearity of Action in IPV*

The nonlinearity of action may be related to nonlinearity of perceived need-for-action due to (1) the nonlinearity of the underlying partner-perpetrated violence, (2) the presence of multiple, interdependent predictors, and/or (3) circularly-causal predictors; or it could be due to (4) an underlying cusp catastrophic phenomenon in which the relationship between violence burden and readiness-for-action is distorted by factors affecting the violence–readiness relationship. By combining analyses [48, 50, 51], we can determine which of these explanations best explains the nonlinearity of action.

### 7.1.1 Nonlinearity Due to Nonlinear Nature of Underlying Violence

If perceived need is linked to his violence, then same-day and prior-day violence should correlate with perceived need, and the level of nonlinearity (unpredictability) should be similar for both violence and need. In this scenario, perceived need would be nonlinear because his violence is nonlinear. Prior analysis found that, although same-day violence is associated with all three perceived needs, prior-day violence is not [48]. This study found that the degrees of nonlinearity of violence and need-for-help are similar, but regression analysis found that violence nonlinearity was not predictive of nonlinearity of need-for-help. The level of nonlinearity of need-for-legal-action is significantly lower than (more predictable than) that of the violence. And prior-day violence is inversely-related to need-for-legal-action [48]. The nonlinearity of need-to-leave may well be due to the nonlinearity of his violence for the following reasons. Both same-day and prior-day violence are associated with need-to-leave [48], and the degree of nonlinearity is similar to that of violence. Furthermore, the nonlinearity of violence predicts the nonlinearity of need-to-leave.

Hence, only for need-to-leave can we make a strong case for its nonlinearity being due to the nonlinearity of the underlying violence.

### 7.1.2 Nonlinearity Due to Dependence upon Multiple, Interdependent Predictors

Based on prior analysis [48], all three perceived needs have interdependent prior-day predictors. Of the seven predictors of need-for-help, 48% of the possible associations among predictors are actually significant predictors. In need-for-legal-action, 38% of the links among its eight predictors are statistically significant. Finally, for the six prior-day predictors of need-to-leave, 40% of the possible links were significant [48]. Hence, the case for nonlinearity of need being due to the interdependence of its predictors is strongest for need-for-help, but could be made for all three needs.

### 7.1.3 Nonlinearity Due to Dependence upon Circularly-Causal Predictors

Nonlinearity of need could also be a product of circular causality in which predictors of need are themselves predicted by the need. Based on prior analysis [48], a strong case for this explanation can be made for need-for-help in which three predictors (perceived control, his alcohol use, increasing violence) are circularly-causal relationships with the need itself. Needs-for-legal-action and leaving predict each other. Although need-for-legal-action has two other circularly-causal predictors (perceived control, increasing violence), it also has two predictors (stress, his alcohol use) with negative feedback relationships with need-for-legal-action. Such relationships would be expected to dampen nonlinearity. In the case of need-to-leave, there is little evidence that circular causality is responsible for its nonlinearity; other than the circularly-causal relationship with need-for-legal-action, none of its other predictors have such a relationship. In addition, four predictors (his alcohol use, desire to move on, concern for effect of violence on children, forgiveness) have a negative feedback relationship with need-to-leave [48]. Hence, only for need-for-help can a strong argument be made that circular causality may explain its nonlinearity.

### 7.1.4 Nonlinearity Due to Catastrophic Nature of Decision-Making

Finally, the existence of sudden, reversible changes in readiness-for-change suggests that action-taking may be best modeled as a catastrophic phenomenon using cusp catastrophe modeling. Indeed, based on prior analysis of readiness-for-action [50], such catastrophic models accounted for more variance in readiness-for-action than either of the two linear models. For readiness-for-help, forgiveness (a key prior-day predictor) was the significant bifurcation variable, distorting the linear relationship between violence burden and readiness-for-help. However, the presence of children

**Table 5** Support for potential causes of nonlinearity of perceived need-for-action

| | | Action | | |
|---|---|---|---|---|
| Potential cause | Measure | Help | Legal action | Leaving |
| Nonlinearity of violence | Need-for-action | + | 0 | +++ |
| Interdependent predictors | Need-for-action | +++ | ++ | ++ |
| Circular causality | Need-for-action | +++ | + | 0 |
| Cusp catastrophe | Readiness-for-action | + | +++ | ++ |

Levels of evidence supporting the potential sources of nonlinearity for need-for-help, legal action, and leaving
0 no evidence, + minimal evidence, ++ moderate evidence, +++ strong evidence

at home was important for readiness-for-legal-action and leaving (with wanting to keep the family together and concern for child safety important prior-day predictors), while hope and positive coping were also important as bifurcation variables for readiness-to-leave [51]. Hence, the nonlinearity of all three actions could be due to an underlying catastrophic relationship.

Overall, the cause of nonlinearity of help-seeking can be made for all explanations except the first one (due to a relationship with nonlinear violence), but interdependent predictors and circular causality are the most strongly supported. While the nonlinearity of need-for-legal-action is lowest of the three, it is still nonlinear. Yet, the best explanation for nonlinearity of seeking legal action is that it is a catastrophic phenomenon. This may explain the suddenness of legal action without same-day correlates [48]. Finally, for the nonlinearity of leaving, nonlinearity of need-to-leave is best linked to the nonlinearity of the underlying violence (see Table 5).

## 8 Discussions

Prior studies suggest that women want nonjudgmental, nondirective, individualized intervention from providers [52]. If we want women in violent relationships to make quality decisions, such decision-making should involve clarifying values, identifying alternatives, obtaining necessary information, combining them to balance heart-and-head factors to make a sound decision, and then committing to act [53]. This framework is compatible with the IPV-specific approaches of Liang et al. [40].

Can we intervene to assist these women with their decision-making? Three factors that appear to be important in spurring abused women into action are insight into the violence and their own decision-making [22, 26], and a sense of empowerment to act [27]. Empowerment programs for victims of IPV promote awareness of violence patterns, engagement in developing safety strategies, and practice of behaviors designed to reduce violence [54], and social support correlates with both seeking legal assistance [38] and leaving the relationship [31, 39].

However, this study found that need-for-action among women in violent relationship was nonlinear and unpredictable, making optimal decision-making (and efforts to encourage it) difficult. We should expect that women's actions will seem sudden and unexpected, and that our interventions will produce unpredictable results. If we choose to intervene in such nonlinear phenomena, then the nature of the intervention should match the potential source(s) of the nonlinearity.

Women in violent relationships tend to cope through minimizing the abuse, increasing defenses, or relinquishing parts of themselves [18]; in the face of increasing or severe violence, these strategies do not work and need-for-action builds. Her choice of which particular action to consider may be a sequential narrowing process. Most women (72%) experiencing IPV report prior having taken action in the past, most commonly seeking counseling (54%), leaving the relationship (41%), moving in with others (32%), or filing police reports (33%); with the exception of police contact, these actions were generally rated by women as positive [55]. Once, she has narrowed her choice, then specific factors seem to reinforce particular needs. Thus, to assist a woman in promoting her need-for-help through counseling, discussing those factors that predict need-for-help (i.e., increasing violence, her violence, his stalking, forgiveness and child safety) may help, while to promote her need-to-leave, discussing level of violence, increasing violence, forgiveness, and effects of violence on children might promote leaving. But establishing need is only the first step (and not that helpful if she is considering legal action). Once she perceives a need-for-action, the next step is to prepare her for action by focusing her on those prior-day factors that were significant (control for help-seeking, stalking and concern for child safety for legal action, his alcohol use, and increasing violence for leaving).

The recognition that readiness-for-legal-action was best modeled as a catastrophic phenomenon with number of children as its bifurcation variable means that we should expect sudden extreme changes rather than progressive linear changes in readiness-for-action in response to progressive changes in violence burden. Second, current decision-making theory supports such modeling because several characteristics important in the decision-making process involve factors that could result in sudden reversals. For example, decision quality depends upon sound reasoning based upon the weighing of information, values, and alternatives. Thus, the process represents a balancing of "head and heart," susceptible to the distorting effects of unstable interpretation, due to fluctuating rationalization, wishful thinking, egocentric effects, and mental illness [53]. Based upon these findings, if we try to intervene with these women, not only should we expect sudden changes in readiness, but our efforts to facilitate decision-making should focus on addressing those factors that may distort her interpretation of reality (her children).

Finally, the nonlinearity of need-to-leave depends upon the nonlinearity of the violence itself. If we could lessen such nonlinearity, it may create an opportunity for predictable intervention. Constraints can reduce a system's nonlinearity; such constraint in a relationship could take the form of minimizing couple interaction or introducing a factor known to limit the perpetrator's behavior (i.e., a parent). An alternate method of reducing the nonlinearity of violence could be to use interventions under the woman's control (i.e., limiting her behaviors known to trigger his violence). Hence, she may minimize arguments, her alcohol intake, or her violent responses.

## 9 Conclusions

While all three needs-for-action were nonlinear, the level of women's perceived need-for-legal-action and its degree of nonlinearity were lowest compared with needs-for-help and leaving. Positive feedback of need-for-legal-action coupled with negative feedback for both need-for-help and need-to-leave serve to maintain the nonlinearity of all three needs. Of the four possible explanations for nonlinearity of need-for-action, need-for-help is best explained by its multiple, interdependent predictors and circular causality, while need-for-legal-assistance is best understood via cusp catastrophe modeling; nonlinearity of need-to-leave is best explained by its dependence upon the underlying nonlinear violence itself. Tailoring provider intervention to the source of action-specific nonlinearity may maximize predictability of response and promote women's action-taking for IPV.

**Acknowledgements** This project was funded by a grant from the National Science Foundation (#1260210).

## The Transformative Aspects of This Study

This work can transform how we study violence and care for its victims. This project has demonstrated that it is indeed possible to quantitatively determine the degree of nonlinearity of a *variable* whether it is the level of violence or perceived need for action. And, once identified, it is possible to assess the source(s) of that nonlinearity using quantitative approaches. These realizations can enable investigators to pursue studies they deemed impossible before, leading to new (and transformative) knowledge.

In addition, the observation that needs-for-help and leaving (both very nonlinear) display negative feedback upon themselves while need-for-legal-action (less nonlinear) shows feedforward dynamics suggests that all three needs are inherently kept at midrange levels on nonlinearity. Such optimal variability has often been seen in complex systems and suggests that it provides enough predictable linearity as a foundation to build upon while providing enough flexible nonlinearity to adapt; rigid periodicity minimizes options and ephemeral randomness lacks the consistency needed as a base for the development.

Finally, this study has transformative practice implications. First, it explains the frustration many clinicians experience when dealing with women in violent relationships and why simple interventions rarely work in these situations. Second, as mentioned above, interventions that target the source of nonlinearity may foster more predictable responses to intervention. Third, the study suggests that tailoring intervention to the dynamic pattern the woman displays (if it can be determined) may yield the best results. While women whose perceived need varies cyclically may respond to simple interventions, those exhibiting random fluctuations in need will not. Random dynamics may only respond to constraints designed to reduce nonlinearity (i.e., limited options) or mindfulness activities (i.e., journaling) to improve self-awareness of her situation and future. When perceived need variability is neither cyclic nor random, the woman may respond to timed interventions which foster epiphany moments or interventions targeting attractors that discourage action.

**Take Home Message**

- Decision-making of women in violent relationships is qualitatively and quantitatively nonlinear.
- Nonlinearity of need-for-help is primarily due to its numerous, interdependent, and circularly-causal predictors.
- Nonlinearity of readiness-for-legal-action is a catastrophic phenomenon, distorted by the number of children at home.
- Nonlinearity of need-to-leave is largely due to the nonlinearity of the underlying violence.
- Intervening with women to encourage action needs to focus on the source of the action-specific nonlinearity.

## References

1. Devries KM, Mak JYT, Garcia-Moreno C, Petzold M, Child JC, Falder G, Lim S, Bacchus LJ, Engell RE, Rosenfeld L, Pallitto C, Vos T, Abrahams N, Watts CH. Global prevalence of intimate partner violence against women. Science. 2013;340:1527–8.
2. Black MC, Basile KC, Breiding MJ, Smith SG, Walters ML, Merrick MT, Chen J, Stevens MR. The national intimate partner and sexual violence survey (NISVS): 2010 summary report. Atlanta: National Center for Injury Prevention and Control, Centers for Disease Control and Prevention; 2011.
3. Coker AL, Smith PH, Bethea L, King MR, McKeown RE. Physical health consequences of physical and psychological intimate partner violence. Arch Fam Med. 2000;9:451–7.
4. Roberts AL, Gillman SE, Breslau J, Breslau N, Koenen KC. Race/ethnic differences in exposure to traumatic events, development of posttraumatic stress disorder, and treatment-seeking for posttraumatic stress disorder in the United States. Psychol Med. 2011;41:71–83.
5. Land B, Elias D. Measuring the "complexity" of a time series. 2005. Retrieved from http://www.nbb.cornell.edu/neurobio/land/PROJECTS/Complexity/index.html.

6. Wolf A, Swift JB, Swinney HL, Vastano JA. Determining Lyapunov exponents from a time series. Physica. 1985;16D:285–317.
7. Ziv J, Lempel A. Compression of individual sequences via variable-rate coding. IEEE Trans Inform Theory. 1978;IT-24:75.
8. Pincus SM. Approximate entropy as a measure of irregularity for psychiatric serial metrics. Bipolar Disord. 2006;8:430–40.
9. Katerndahl DA, Burge SK, Ferrer RL, Becho J, Wood R. Dynamics of violence. J Eval Clin Pract. 2014;20:695–702.
10. Morrison F. Art of modeling dynamic systems. New York: Wiley; 1991.
11. Burge SK, Katerndahl DA, Wood RC, Becho J, Ferrer RL, Talamantes M. Using complexity science to examine three dynamic patterns of intimate partner violence. Fam Syst Health. 2016;34(1):4–14.
12. Umberson D, Anderson KL, Williams K, Chen MD. Relationship dynamics, emotion state, and domestic violence. J Marriage Fam. 2003;65:233–47.
13. Ristock JL. Exploring dynamics of abusive lesbian relationships. Am J Commun Psychol. 2003;31:329–41.
14. Higson P, Sturgess A. Uncommon leadership. New York: Kogan Page; 2014.
15. Anderson C. Evolving out of violence. Res Theory Nurs Pract. 2003;17:225–40.
16. Stork E. Understanding high-stakes decision making. J Fem Fam Ther. 2008;20:299–327.
17. Landenburger KM. Dynamics of leaving and recovering from an abusive relationship. J Obstet Gynecol Neonatal Nurs. 1998;27:700–6.
18. Merritt-Gray M, Wuest J. Counteracting abuse and breaking free. Health Care Women Int. 1995;16:399–412.
19. Bell ME, Goodman LA, Dutton MA. Dynamics of staying and leaving. J Fam Violence. 2007;22:413–28.
20. Cattaneo LB, Stuewig J, Goodman LA, Kaltman S, Dutton MA. Longitudinal helpseeking patterns among victims of intimate partner violence. Am J Orthopsychiatr. 2007;77:467–77.
21. Pijanowski JC. The role of learning theory in building effective college ethics curricula. J Coll Character. 2009;10(3):1–13.
22. McDonough TA. Policy capturing investigation of battered women's decisions to stay in violent relationships. Violence Vict. 2010;25:165–84.
23. Chabot HF, Tracy TL, Manning CA, Poisson CA. Sex, attribution, and severity influence intervention decisions of informal helpers in domestic violence. J Interpers Violence. 2009;24:1696–713.
24. Logan TK, Walker R, Shannon L, Cole J. Factors associated with separation and ongoing violence among women with civil protective orders. J Fam Violence. 2008;23:377–85.
25. Kim J, Gray KA. Leave or stay? J Interpers Violence. 2008;23:1465–82.
26. Chang JC, Dado D, Hawker L, Cluss PA, Buranosky R, Slagel L, McNeil M, Scholle SH. Understanding turning points in intimate partner violence. J Women Health. 2010;19:251–9.
27. Ballantine MW. Decision-making processes of abused women. Diss Abstr Int A Humanit Soc Sci. 2005;65(11-A):4346.
28. Duterte EE, Bonomi AE, Kernic MA, Schiff MA, Thompson RS, Rivara FP. Correlates of medical and legal help seeking among women reporting intimate partner violence. J Women Health. 2008;17:85–95.
29. Barrett BJ, St. Pierre M. Variations in help seeking in response to intimate partner violence. Violence Against Women. 2011;17:47–70.
30. Burton SJ. To go or not to go. Diss Abstr Int B Sci Eng. 2004;64(9-B):4605.
31. Koepsell JK, Kernic MA, Holt VL. Factors that influence battered women to leave their abusive relationships. Violence Vict. 2006;21:131–47.
32. Gordon KC, Burton S, Porter L. Predicting the intentions of women in domestic violence shelters to return to partners. J Fam Psychol. 2004;18:331–8.
33. Stork EP. Analyzing decision making. Diss Abstr Int A Humanit Soc Sci. 2005;65(10-A):3994.
34. Rhodes KV, Cerulli C, Dichter ME, Kothari CL, Barg FK. I didn't want to put them through that. J Fam Violence. 2010;25:485–93.

35. Burke JG, Gielen AC, McDonnell KA, O'Campo P, Maman S. Process of ending abuse in intimate relationships. Violence Against Women. 2001;7:1144–63.
36. Prochaska JO, DiClemente CC. Toward a comprehensive model of change. In: Miller WR, Heather N, editors. Treating addictive behaviors. New York: Plenum Press; 1986.
37. Burke JG, Denison JA, Gielen AC, McDonnell KA, O'Campo P. Ending intimate partner violence. Am J Health Behav. 2004;28:122–33.
38. Wright CV, Johnson DM. Correlates for legal help-seeking. Violence Vict. 2009;24:771–85.
39. Wilcox P. Me mother's bank and me nanan's, you know, support! Women's Stud Int Forum. 2000;23:35–47.
40. Liang B, Goodman L, Tummala-Narra P, Weintraub S. Theoretical framework for understanding help-seeking processes among survivors of intimate partner violence. Am J Community Psychol. 2005;36:71–83.
41. Erdi P. Complexity explained. Berlin: Springer; 2008.
42. Burge SK, Becho J, Ferrer RL, Wood RC, Talamantes M, Katerndahl DA. Safely examining complex dynamics of intimate partner violence. Fam Syst Health. 2014;32:259–70.
43. Katerndahl DA, Burge SK, Ferrer RL, Becho J, Wood R. Effects of religious and spiritual variables on outcomes in violent relationships. Int J Psychiatr Med. 2015;49:249–63.
44. Katerndahl DA, Burge SK, Ferrer RL, Becho J, Wood R. Do violence dynamics matter? J Eval Clin Pract. 2014;20:719–27.
45. Kreindler DM, Lumsden CJ. Effects of the irregular sample and missing data in time series analysis. NDPLS. 2006;10:187–214.
46. Greenland S. Quantitative methods in the review of epidemiologic literature. Epidemiol Rev. 1987;9:1–30.
47. Clair S. Cusp catastrophe model for adolescent alcohol use. NDPLS. 1998;2:217–41.
48. Katerndahl DA, Burge SK, Ferrer RL, Becho J, Wood R. Predictors of perceived need for and actual action taking among women in violent relationships. J Interpers Violence. 2016;September issue:1–28. Retrieved from https://doi.org/10.1177/0886260516669543.
49. Guastello SJ. Self-complexity and the interpretation of entropy and information statistics. Soc Chaos Theory Psychol Life Sci Newsl. 2012;19(2):5–10.
50. Katerndahl DA, Burge SK, Ferrer RL, Becho J, Wood R. Is perceived need for action among women in violent relationships nonlinear and, if so, why? J Interpers Violence. 2017;August issue. https://doi.org/10.1177/0886260517727495.
51. Katerndahl DA, Burge SK, Ferrer RL, Becho J, Wood R. Is readiness to take action among women in violent relationships a catastrophic phenomenon? J Interpers Violence. 2017;March issue:1–25. Retrieved from https://doi.org/10.1177/0886260517698280.
52. Feder GS, Hutson M, Ramsay J, Taket AR. Women exposed to intimate partner violence. Arch Intern Med. 2006;166:22–37.
53. Kedin T, Shoemaker P, Spetzler C. Decision quality. Palo Alto: Decision Education Foundation; 2009.
54. Islam N. Exploring the development of psychological empowerment among survivors of intimate partner violence. Diss Abstr Int A Humanit Soc Sci. 2010;70(8-A):3190.
55. Katerndahl DA, Burge SK, Ferrer RL, Wood R, Becho J. Decision dynamics among victims of violence (Final Report). Washington, D.C.: National Science Foundation; 2016.

# Co-producing Healthcare Interventions: Transforming Transdisciplinary Research to Develop Healthcare Services to Meet the Needs of Patients with Complex Problems

**Susanne Reventlow, Alexandra B. R. Jønsson, Marlene C. R. Møller, Annette Sofie Davidsen, and Line Olsen**

## 1 Introduction

Patient-centred health care must take a starting point in people's experiences of health [1–3], and involvement of patients in co-production of healthcare service has gained increased focus during the last decades [4]. Co-producing healthcare interventions at various stages of the process have been shown to improve the quality and feasibility of interventions [5]. Particularly concerning the complex care for people with multiple chronic diseases, so-called multimorbidity, co-production holds the potential for comprehensive responsiveness to the needs of both patients and health care providers [6]. This chapter deals with the experiences from an on-going study, The Phy-Psy Trial (PPT), co-producing a healthcare intervention for patients with severe mental illness (SMI) and concurrent physical diseases. This group of patients has particularly complex health problems, requiring collaboration between primary health care, municipal social psychiatry, and hospital-based psychiatry. In the longer term, we anticipate that an intervention developed to help this group of patients with SMI will also prove useful for other patients with somatic multimorbidity.

Using the PPT as a case, we aim to describe and discuss the co-producing processes in developing an intervention for patients with complex health problems. The intention of the PPT is to lower the mortality and increase the quality of life for people with SMI by using a co-produced, coordinated care plan as well as including

S. Reventlow (✉) · A. B. R. Jønsson · A. S. Davidsen · L. Olsen
Section of General Practice and Research Unit for General Practice, Department of Public Health, University of Copenhagen, Denmark
e-mail: susrew@sund.ku.dk; a.joensson@sund.ku.dk; adavid@sund.ku.dk; liol@sund.ku.dk

M. C. R. Møller
Research Unit for General Practice, Department of Public Health, Aarhus University, Denmark
e-mail: mcr.moller@ph.au.dk



J. P. Sturmberg (ed.), *Embracing Complexity in Health*,
https://doi.org/10.1007/978-3-030-10940-0_10

information and communication technology (ICT) to support collaboration across sector borders. The development of the intervention uses a co-production approach building on the perspectives and experiences of all actors involved, including patients, healthcare professionals, and policy makers. In this chapter, we address possibilities and complexities that may occur when planning or taking part in the co-production of interventions for patients with SMI, including a discussion on the challenges associated with practising co-production.

In the PPT, co-production takes place on two levels: firstly, in the interdisciplinary research group; secondly, in the encounter with and collaboration between the involved actors from the care settings, the patients and their networks, and the researchers. Inspired by Frodeman's [7] distinction between inter- and transdisciplinarity, we use the term 'transdisciplinary' for the research practices that we have started to develop through creative co-production between clinical, social, technology sciences and the humanities, an approach that extends beyond academia. In the PPT, co-production denotes the involvement of patients, their network, the health professionals working in the healthcare services, and policy makers. The project is currently at its second year out of a 9-year period. The first 2 years are devoted to the development of the intervention; afterwards, the intervention will be run in a randomized controlled trial followed by a process- and effect evaluation.

## 2 Complex Health Problems: Patients with Severe Mental Illness and Physical Co-morbidity, and the Care They Need

Multimorbidity is most often defined as the co-occurrence of two or more chronic conditions in a person [8, 9]. Among patients with multimorbidity, patients with SMI have the greatest burden of illness [10, 11], and their excess mortality is mainly due to physical diseases [12], which are under-diagnosed and under-treated in this group of patients [13]. Because of these particularly complex health problems, patients with SMI and physical co-morbidities are used as a critical case of multimorbidity. Studies reveal the complexity in living with mental and physical multimorbidity [14]. The diversity of the comorbid diseases, the limited personal resources, and the severe social challenges of these patients increase the complexity of their life situation [15] and their care [16]. One of the major reasons for this rests with the structure of the highly specialized healthcare system focusing on distinct diseases rather than intricate and complex combinations of diseases. Consequently, patients with several diseases are treated with a separate focus on each disease, leaving them with the feeling that they are not being treated as whole persons [17]. Furthermore, the independent treatments of the single diseases are only partly coordinated—if coordinated at all. Therefore, the various treatments and the lack of overview place a heavy burden on the individual, and the lack of coordination and cooperation across sector borders makes it difficult for the individual to navigate the system [18–20]. This is especially challenging for patients with SMI, because they often need additional support from municipal social psychiatry to adhere to their treatments. Different initiatives using integrated care models—developed with or without the partial involvement of patients and healthcare providers—have been tested, but with disappointing results due to difficulties in engaging both patients and general practices [21]. These experiences show that there is a need for critical examination of clinical practices, and a need to develop new care plans based on the principle of participatory research and action learning [22]. For patients with SMI and other complex health problems, there is an additional need to develop new care approaches that can secure collaboration across sectors involving the locally governed services.

## 3 Co-producing Healthcare Interventions: Theoretical Perspectives

According to Batalden et al., a doctor cannot per se make another person healthy. Health outcomes (good and bad) are co-produced as a consequence of the dispositions, capacities, and behaviours of both doctor and patient [4]. This makes the patient-centred approach essential. Co-production is therefore relevant both for the individual consultation and for the development of the healthcare services in order to ensure meaningful, sustainable, and health optimizing interventions.

Our work with co-production is inspired by Batalden et al.'s concept of co-production as a new way of relating to the healthcare service depending on both the individual and the healthcare professional. Earlier models of chronic care stress the importance of collaborative management of chronic diseases and personalized care planning, supported by responsive policy and governance. The organizational processes and workflows and the capacities, dispositions, and behaviours of individual healthcare professionals and patients are also significant [23]. Sturmberg and colleagues stress people-centredness as the driver of a complex-adaptive health system and the importance of taking a bottom-up approach [1, 24]. Batalden et al. propose a model for co-producing healthcare services in which patients and professionals interact as participants within a local healthcare system in their community. According to this model, co-production is the interdependent work of all users—patients, relatives, and professionals—to design, create, develop, deliver, assess, and improve the relationships and actions that contribute to the health of individuals and populations [4].

From a *post hoc* analysis of the randomized trial Diabetes Care in General Practice (DCGP), we have evidence that supports the value of co-production between patient and general practitioner. DCGP showed that an intervention structured around individualized personal care greatly reduced the mortality of patients with diabetes and SMI [25]. In the DCGP intervention model, the GP and the patient worked together to identify the patient's major health problems and goals and determine which treatment and care plan the patient had the capacity to follow

[26]. This co-production approach of structured, individualized, goal-oriented care in general practice has served as an inspiration for the PPT, pointing to the need of personalized care planning in which patients, health professionals, and social workers from the municipality engage as co-productive partners. The results from the above-mentioned study highlight that finding a balance between the patient's 'capacity' (i.e. time, resources, and health literacy) and the 'workload' associated with care is essential [27] and may be strengthened by a patient-centred approach that enhances patient involvement.

Hence, healthcare services should provide a framework for the patient and health care professionals to co-produce in the individual consultation. However, in the PPT, we want to develop an intervention model that can embrace and support co-production both in the individual consultation and in the coordinated care across sector boundaries to optimize the overall outcome of care.

We use the term co-production to designate the inclusion of all aspects and perspectives of all the different actors involved in the development of the intervention. We regard patients, healthcare professionals, social workers, and researchers as equal contributors to the intervention. On-going dialogue between the actors is employed as a systematic tool in the process of developing the intervention. The dialogue is stimulated by input from the literature, observations, interviews, and register studies, which intend to substantiate the evidence base for the intervention. Interactive methods such as cross-sectorial and cross-disciplinary focus groups and workshops are applied to stimulate reflection on the different elements of the intervention, e.g. care plan, communication, collaboration, and ICT. These methods, combined with repeated pilot testing of intervention elements, will enable us to address potential unintended consequences during the design phase. The results will drive the development of the final intervention model, including the supporting ICT care platform.

## 4 Co-producing the Phy-Psy Trial: The Interdisciplinary Research Level

The PPT is a broad, interdisciplinary collaboration coordinated by the Section of General Practice, University of Copenhagen, and involving research groups from three Danish universities, representing different perspectives and competences within medicine, science, humanities, social sciences, economy, and design and IT engineering. This complex healthcare intervention, which is the goal of the research collaboration, is developed during these first 2 years of the project and will combine medical, social, technology sciences, and clinical practices (Fig. 1). Both qualitative and quantitative research methods are used in the co-production process. Researchers from different backgrounds work together within and across different work packages, focusing on areas supporting the development of the final intervention, e.g. user needs, technology solutions, preparation of the clinical trial,

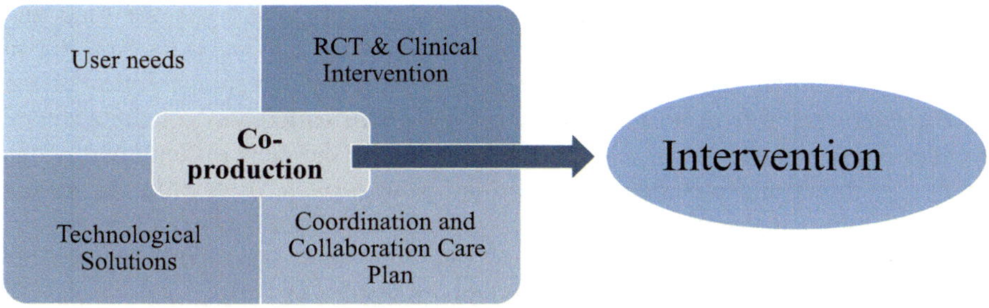


**Fig. 1** The Phy-Psy Trial working groups

care planning, coordination, and support. The research team meetings have been tape recorded, and notes have been taken to document the interdisciplinary work of the co-production processes.

The User Needs group is responsible for exploring the experiences, needs, preferences, and values of all users. This is done by ethnographic methods, taking into account both situational and cultural contexts. The researchers in this group are anthropologists, sociologists, and medical doctors from general practice. In the co-production research meetings, this group keeps a particular focus on participatory design and the development of outcomes that are relevant for and requested by both patients and health professionals. During the early interdisciplinary research meetings, it became clear that the gathered knowledge about user needs was required immediately for the other working groups to initiate their work, and that data, experiences, and produced knowledge had to be shared early in the process of analysing and contemplating. This inopportune timeline has turned out to be one of the most frequent challenges of the scientific PPT co-production work, which has to focus both on the exchange of knowledge for the intervention development to progress and on the production of the scientific knowledge base for the work.

The group responsible for the RCT and the clinical intervention involves researchers with medical backgrounds, bio-statisticians, and medical pharmacologists. They employ epidemiological methods to develop the knowledge base for the RCT, describe the profile of the intervention target group and the recruitment procedures as well as making suggestions for the clinical content of the intervention based on previous research. Their work also involves defining measurable outcomes. At the research meetings, the group exchanges plans, needs, and results with the other groups. For example, the other working groups help define the specific patient group for the intervention and offer their suggestions to the clinical content of the intervention. This work is challenged by the needs of the epidemiological research discipline for providing a study design which enables a scientific evaluation of the impact of the intervention, while at the same time ensuring a framework that complies with national laws, ethics, and the interest of the multiple stakeholders creating and receiving the intervention.

The group responsible for the development of care plans has the time and resource demanding challenge of finding and meeting professionals working in different contextual settings. Their focus is on roles and responsibilities of the different actors as well as on communication and coordination between these actors. Previous studies have shown that this could in fact be the most difficult part of the study—to gather and include all the relevant professionals from different sectors in responsible collaboration [28]. At research meetings, discussions addressed the aspiration level of a coordinated care plan involving actors across different sectors and its implementation in the forthcoming randomized trial.

The ICT group consists of engineers and software developers, among others. This group aims at developing tools to support the intervention. This could be a platform engaging both the care team and the patients in monitoring and treating the diseases or a tool to help support cooperation and communication. Their work depends both on knowledge of healthcare system procedures and current technologies, and on results from the User Needs group—the ICT group must identify and solve these challenges prior to the start of the PPT. At research meetings, the members of the ICT group have repeatedly brought up the difficulties they were experiencing, arguing that their work depends on the delivery of inputs from the other research groups.

## *4.1 The Challenges of Research Collaboration*

The activities of the different working groups run in parallel. Hence, while the co-production of the intervention elements is initiated and begins to evolve, other PPT researchers prepare a catalogue of potential clinical intervention elements to be included in the co-production process. One challenge is that such parallel courses are not well suited for projects where the deliverables from group are required for the other groups to get started. Another challenge is the inherent tension in the interdisciplinary research group and in the work with the production of knowledge supporting the intervention. Different perspectives are put into play in this large jigsaw puzzle, covering epidemiology and the design of the RCT, the measurability of outcomes, and the goals of the co-production process, which is to include the patients' and the professionals' perspectives based on knowledge produced by more action-based research methods. Co-producing at the research level can at times be a chaotic, time consuming, and opaque process. Still, the process of co-production aims to find meaningful elements across disciplines and research groups and to integrate these fields of knowledge in the co-production process with all users.

While initiating the work of developing an intervention model, the project group has faced the challenges of forming and consolidating the team. From the beginning of the project, it has been the intention that the project team members should be able to work openly and across working groups. However, since the different groups of researchers are employed at different institutions and have specific competences and responsibilities, their interactions with other groups mainly take place at research meetings, seminars, and workshops. This challenges the need for a close collaboration and the feeling of 'being part of a group'. Hence, it is hard to facilitate the usual social forming processes of a project group and its group dynamics (i.e. project groups are physically co-located and constantly informally interacting).

Indeed, the need for momentum in the research working groups as well as the shifting needs for deliverables and exchange of knowledge across the working groups are challenged in the existing structure. The core element of learning from the first year of the PPT is that the research groups have to interact much more than anticipated to understand and learn from each other's pre-understandings and perspectives; that there must be clear and well-articulated shared purposes and values, sufficient available resources, and well-defined processes and workflows. Hence, a restructuring of meeting frequency with more face-to-face interaction between the groups and team members from the different groups is in progress. Furthermore, the structure of the research processes, partly defined by the initially developed protocols, may include the possibility to be re-organized.

## 5 Co-producing Healthcare Service Involving Both Health Professionals and Patients: The Practice Level

In order to be implemented in real life, a cross-sectorial care model must make sense for the involved patients, their networks, and the professionals involved in their care. This level concerns the co-production of the intervention with all the actors that are and will be involved in the practical work with the care model.

In the project, the co-production of the intervention involves patients and their networks along with actors from the different care services—covering general practice, hospital psychiatric services, and locally governed health authorities in social psychiatric services in the municipality (Fig. 2). The starting point is the investigation of the mechanism and practices that enable the improvement of care and patient health from the perspectives of all actors.

Coulter and Collins describe patient expertise as knowledge on how disease and treatment affect the patient's everyday life, attitude towards risk, and values and preferences [29]. It has been argued that living with mental disease provides a certain kind of experience-based expertise [30]. According to Jønsson and colleagues, patient knowledge contains both particular knowledge used to cope with the disease and knowledge and experiences in general that have a great influence on everyday health management—all aspects have to be considered [31]. Hence, understanding how people experience the complexities of mental and physical multimorbidity may be crucial when designing and delivering interventions to support successful self-management [14].

In interviews with patients, conducted as part of the PPT, patients with SMI often recount that health professionals fail to listen to their stories about physical symptoms, resulting in the patients not feeling heard and taken seriously. They feel

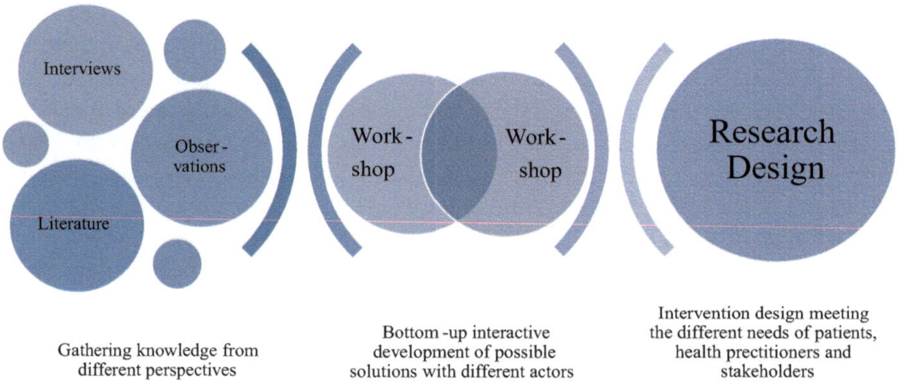


**Fig. 2** Overview of the potential healthcare providers that can be involved in the care of patients with psychiatric and somatic illnesses. The patient is placed at the centre of this model

that their mental disease overshadows the physical symptoms, and they tell stories of overlooked physical illness. Many of them say that they usually wait until there are visible signs of a disease before seeing a doctor, because otherwise they are afraid that they will not be believed. They also express that they have practical difficulties making an appointment. If, for example, they have to wait days or weeks for an appointment, they are uncertain if they will be able to show up. Some feel uncomfortable in the waiting room with other patients. In addition, they have problems with medications, for example, concerning whom to talk to about the side effects, how to administer them, and how to be able to pay for them. The informants' experiences that the different professionals do not share their information result in their belief that they have to manage the coordination of their treatments themselves. It is difficult for them to navigate the system without sufficient support.

Professionals from the municipalities have been interviewed and observed during their daily work routines at different places of residence for people with severe mental illness. They find that many different professionals are involved in the care and treatment of the patients, and that the lack of shared knowledge and coordination of care makes it difficult for both professionals and patients to know who is doing what—and when. They often experience errors and loss of information at the time of service sector transitions. They see a need for improving the levels of shared knowledge, so that all the professionals dealing with the patients should have the same knowledge base to act upon.

The professionals from the municipality support the experiences of patients about difficulties with fitting into the consultation system in general practice, e.g. with getting an appointment, showing up at a definite time, and waiting in the waiting room. In addition, the patients' problems are often too complex to be addressed in a normal 10-min consultation. Due to legal issues, there is no sharing of information between general practice and social psychiatry. Therefore, the social workers have no information about physical diseases and treatments. Moreover, the social workers recount that patients with low self-esteem, withdrawal, and cognitive impairments need support to make an appointment with the health care system and to overcome the transport difficulties, including costs. However, in some municipalities the approaches to physical recovery at times counteract the social workers' support. Regarding who should have the coordinating role in an integrated care plan, community-based professionals expressed doubt as to whether general practitioners would commit themselves to more intensive cooperation and a change in accessibility for these patients.

General practitioners participating in focus groups expressed that the most pressing challenge is to get an overview of their patients' suffering of SMI. Some expressed that the consultations with patients with SMI are often difficult and demanding. The patients frequently fail to turn up, are late, or have a different agenda when they show up. Furthermore, none of them have very good cooperation with the staff at municipal psychiatric facilities. Most of the GPs expressed frustration that there was no health-trained staff at these facilities, a fact that made the clinical observations and communication about physical symptoms and diseases more difficult.

In a focus group with staff from general practices, insecurities were expressed about how to deal with noisy and at times aggressive patients with SMI. The staff from general practices expressed frustration that even though a lot of the responsibility for coordination is on their shoulders, procedures on what to do and whom to contact in social psychiatry or psychiatric facilities are inconsistent and difficult.

These statements illustrate some of the differences—and parallels—in how professionals experience the challenges of working with patients with SMI and physical co-morbidity, how they view the cooperation across sectors from their position, but also what their attitudes are towards other professionals, pointing to the importance of defining and delineating roles and responsibility. The statements also emphasize the fact that the different professional groups do not know enough about each other's working conditions, and they all work with the patient from their specific theoretical standpoint and the goal defined by this. For example, as in regards to the concept of recovery, the difference between aiming at clinical or social recovery became clear. In order to be able to develop a cross-sectorial care model, one must understand and take a starting point in the diverse experiences and attitudes of the different actors involved [32, 33]. Furthermore, to develop patient-centred care, the needs of patients and their networks must come to the forefront when formulating shared intervention goals and the impact on the organizational level.

To include the views of the isolated clusters of actors in care management, we bring the disparate actors together in focus groups and workshops to address and connect their views, experiences, and perceptions, but most importantly to focus on possible solutions which can be developed in collaboration. Representatives for patients and their networks are equally represented at separate workshops focusing particularly on the patients' experiences. A specific challenge here is that patients themselves have difficulties attending such workshops. The most vulnerable

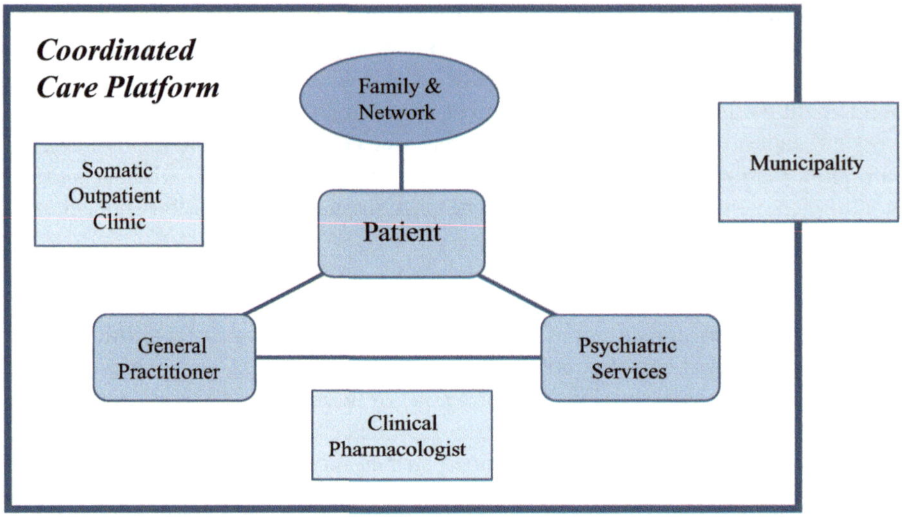


**Fig. 3** This figure illustrates how the co-production will be conducted through iteration of explorative studies followed by joint workshops involving all actors

patients' views are instead collected through ethnographic studies and individual interviews. Lastly, to make sure that the results from the workshops are feasible and supported at a policy level, we will invite strategically selected leaders in different managerial positions to participate in framing the ideas for the future care of patients with multimorbidity and SMI (Fig. 3).

## 6 Discussion

The experience of many healthcare reforms shows that it is often difficult and resource intensive to bring healthcare practices into line with externally formulated policies, recommendations, and standards [34, 35]. It is thus a major work to implement and anchor new knowledge and technology in a heterogeneous healthcare system. This is especially true when it comes to so-called complex interventions involving more active components, multiple types of actors, and relatively high demands on behaviour and competencies among actors performing and/or receiving intervention [36]. Recent health service research increasingly recognizes the complexity associated with developing, implementing, and evaluating new quality initiatives, and underlines the importance of exploring the processes and work needed to make these initiatives an integral part of practice in healthcare organizations [37].

The preliminary data from the PPT show that the complexity of both the internal research lines and the actual development of the intervention with many different actors and perspectives require continuous work and reflection on one's own practice and the development of knowledge, and on the definite work with the content of the intervention and its implementation. One challenge lies within the potentially conflicting goal of developing an intervention, which meets the needs of both the patients and the professionals across different sectors, while at the same time being suitable for an RCT, meaning that it has to meet the standards of medical knowledge generation and scientific research.

The PPT deals with patients with serious mental illnesses, requiring collaboration across both health care and social sectors. This calls for an extended co-production process to develop the collaboration between the parties, and for an agreement on roles, relationships, and purposes of actions as a prerequisite for a new way of delivering care that meets the needs of both patients and professionals, and which can be implemented in real life. Therefore, the question is if it is possible to integrate the perspectives of all actors in the emerging intervention, or—if not—which aspects to prioritize according to existing resources. Regarding the PPT, diversities between structures in the municipalities may require many resources to support the work with the implementation of an intervention.

Previous studies of the development of complex interventions have shown the importance of using a co-production process [10, 24, 38]. In a study of a primary care-based complex intervention for patients with multimorbidity living in deprived areas, Mercer and colleagues showed how the co-production process led to a system change involving longer consultations with relational continuity, change of patient–practitioner interaction, training and support for staff to deliver the intervention, and support for patient self-management [10]. The development of this intervention involved patients, patient representatives, and primary care providers working in areas of very high deprivation. However, many interventions have primarily focused on parts of the healthcare service, e.g. general practice, single hospital departments or sectors in the municipality, and have not involved patients.

According to Batalden, good service co-production requires civil discourse with respectful interaction and effective communication. Shared planning results in a deeper understanding of one another's expertise and values. Shared execution demands deeper trust, cultivation of shared goals, and mutual responsibility and accountability for performance [4]. The work with the development of the intervention in this study has shown the need for interactive work between the researchers to gain understanding of one another's view of problems, competences, and theoretical and methodological approaches as a starting point for the production of a knowledge base for a complex intervention. Furthermore, exploring experiences of involved actors and user needs have shown how they understood the problems from their perspectives and have exposed the need for interaction between actors and researchers to find solutions which can be part of the approaching implementation of the intervention.

The fact that co-producing is a new way of developing interventions means that there is still a lack of knowledge on how best to coordinate the work of the research groups that are at the same time working together and separately, and the co-production processes across sectorial boundaries, involving both patients, their relatives, and professionals on equal terms.

Patient involvement in health research is based on the rationale that patients and relatives are affected by implementation of research knowledge in health care and therefore have the right to influence; and their experiences and insights complement those of the researchers, contributing to more relevant research [39]. Patients' and relatives' involvement in research and in the development of the healthcare service has gained ground [29, 40] and is also asked for in research funding. However, in this project some of the patients are in a vulnerable position and do not have the capacity to participate in workshops or group meetings. We have tried to manage this by interviewing patients and involving them in alternative ways. Malterud and Elbakken suggest, from a systematic review of outcomes and experiences, that patient involvement does not necessarily lead to more advanced knowledge. Their analysis indicates that involving patients or relatives as co-researchers and peers with academic researchers will not guarantee the assumed deliverables [41]. Therefore, there is a need in co-production in health care to continuously reflect on the question who should be involved, why, when, and how. Furthermore, there is a need of more research in the area of co-production.

In our research group, we work towards the development of new knowledge in an interdisciplinary forum that integrates different facets of knowledge and thus ensures the emergence of new innovative ideas and opportunities. The research group aims specifically to enhance the interdisciplinarity among the researchers in order to ensure that instead of merely being juxtaposed, the different bodies of knowledge are synthesized [7, p. 35], whereby they help produce more sustainable knowledge. Frodeman uses the concept of transdisciplinary knowledge as knowledge that is developed partly across research disciplines, but which, in addition, involves experiences and knowledge from society. The process in our project is partly a co-production process in the interdisciplinary research team and the co-production of the intervention in various interactive processes with the involved parties, and therefore a case example of a process of transdisciplinary knowledge production.

## The Transformative Aspects of This Study

This study contributes to the development of methods and strategies for tackling complex health issues, both with regard to meeting the needs of individual patient through the development of coordination in across the healthcare system, with care coordination eventually being a dimension in patient-centred care. The present chapter emphasizes the different levels of co-producing and the issue of transdisciplinarity as being necessary to fully enabling the co-production of healthcare services for patients with complex health problems. At the same time, it stresses the importance of documenting the long term effects of an intervention on health and quality of life for patients, and more broadly, society. The case of the Phy-Psy Trial raises several reflections concerning methodology and how to involve different areas of knowledge, patients, their networks, and their caregivers in the development of new care models.

What is new in this study is the range of co-design, not only focusing on patients or healthcare providers, but also taking all other actors into account. Furthermore, this work implements transdisciplinarity—it takes the social science emphasis on co-design and involvement and brings it into the traditionally medical sphere of RCTs without compromising either. It is our belief that the PPT will benefit the treatment of multimorbid patients with concurrent mental illnesses—as well as patients on the whole—on more than one level.

**Take Home Message**

- For patients with severe mental illness and other complex health problems, there is a need to develop new care approaches involving patients, their networks, and professionals across health and social care sectors.
- Co-producing new interventions in healthcare service means to involve all aspects and perspectives of all parties involved, which, on the other hand, requires continuous reflection on one's own research practices.
- In the co-production process questions including who should be involved, why, when, and how must be repeatedly answered.
- Working transdisciplinarily in research is an inspiring learning process, it takes time and face-to-face interactions, and contributes to the development of new innovative ideas and opportunities.

## References

1. Sturmberg JP, O'Halloran DM, Martin CM. People at the centre of complex adaptive health systems reform. Med J Aust. 2010;193(8):474–8.
2. Searl M, Borgi L, Chemali Z. It is time to talk about people: a human-centered healthcare system. Health Res Policy Syst. 2010;8:35.
3. Plochg T, Klazinga NS, Starfield B. Transforming medical professionalism to fit changing health needs. BMC Med. 2009;7:64.
4. Batalden M, Batalden P, Margolis P, Seid M, Armstrong G, Opipari-Arrigan L, Hartung H. Coproduction of healthcare service. BMJ Qual Saf. 2015;25(7):509–17.
5. Mercer SW, O'Brien R, Fitzpatrick B, Higgins M, Guthrie B, Watt G, Wyke S. The development and optimisation of a primary care-based whole system complex intervention (CARE Plus) for patients with multimorbidity living in areas of high socioeconomic deprivation. Chronic Illn. 2016;12(3):165–81.
6. Sturmberg JP, O'Halloran DM, Martin CM. Understanding health system reform - a complex adaptive systems perspective. J Eval Clin Pract. 2012;18(1):202–8.
7. Frodeman R. Sustainable knowledge. A theory of interdisciplinarity. London: Palgrave Macmillan; 2014.
8. Barnett K, Mercer SW, Norbury M, Watt G, Wyke S, Guthrie B. Epidemiology of multimorbidity and implications for health care, research, and medical education: a cross-sectional study. Lancet 2012;380(9836):37–43.

9. Willadsen TG, Bebe A, Koster-Rasmussen R, Jarbol DE, Guassora AD, Waldorff FB, Reventlow S, Olivarius Nde F. The role of diseases, risk factors and symptoms in the definition of multimorbidity - a systematic review. Scand J Prim Health Care 2016;34(2):112–21.
10. Mercer SW, Gunn J, Bower P, Wyke S, Guthrie B. Managing patients with mental and physical multimorbidity. BMJ 2012;345:e5559.
11. Laursen TM, Nordentoft M, Mortensen PB. Excess early mortality in schizophrenia. Annu Rev Clin Psychol. 2014;10:425–48.
12. Lawrence D, Hancock KJ, Kisely S. The gap in life expectancy from preventable physical illness in psychiatric patients in Western Australia: retrospective analysis of population based registers. BMJ 2013;346:f2539.
13. De Hert M, Cohen D, Bobes J, Cetkovich-Bakmas M, Leucht S, Ndetei DM, Newcomer JW, Uwakwe R, Asai I, Möller HJ, Gautam S, Detraux J, Correll CU. Physical illness in patients with severe mental disorders. II. Barriers to care, monitoring and treatment guidelines, plus recommendations at the system and individual level. World Psychiatry 2011;10(2):138–51.
14. Coventry PA, Small N, Panagioti M, Adeyemi I, Bee P. Living with complexity; marshaling resources: a systematic review and qualitative meta-synthesis of lived experience of mental and physical multimorbidity. BMC Fam Pract. 2015;16:171.
15. Smith SM, Bayliss EA, Mercer SW, Gunn J, Vestergaard M, Wyke S, Salisbury C, Fortin M. How to design and evaluate interventions to improve outcomes for patients with multimorbidity. J Comorb. 2013;3(1):8.
16. Wallace E, Salisbury C, Guthrie B, Lewis C, Fahey T, Smith SM. Managing patients with multimorbidity in primary care. BMJ 2015;350:h176.
17. Sturmberg JP, Martin C, Katerndahl DA. Systems and complexity thinking in the general practice literature: an integrative, historical narrative review. Ann Fam Med. 2014;12(1):66–74.
18. Rosbach M, Andersen JA. Patient-experienced burden of treatment in patients with multimorbidity - a systematic review of qualitative data. PLoS One. 2017;12(6):e0179916.
19. Demain S, Gonçalves A-C, Areia C, Oliveira R, Marcos AJ, Marques A, Parmar R, Hunt K. Living with, managing and minimising treatment burden in long term conditions: a systematic review of qualitative research. PLoS One. 2015;10(5):e0125457.
20. May CR, Eton DT, Boehmer K, Gallacher K, Hunt K, MacDonald S, Mair FS, May CM, Montori VM, Richardson A, Rogers AE, Shippee N. Rethinking the patient: using Burden of Treatment Theory to understand the changing dynamics of illness. BMC Health Serv Res. 2014;14:281.
21. Speyer H, Christian Brix Nørgaard H, Birk M, Karlsen M, Storch Jakobsen A, Pedersen K, Hjorthøj C, Pisinger C, Gluud C, Mors O, Krogh J, Nordentoft M. The CHANGE trial: no superiority of lifestyle coaching plus care coordination plus treatment as usual compared to treatment as usual alone in reducing risk of cardiovascular disease in adults with schizophrenia spectrum disorders and abdominal obesity. World Psychiatry 2016;15(2):155–65.
22. Reeve J, Blakeman T, Freeman GK, Green LA, James PA, Lucassen P, Martin CM, Sturmberg JP, Weel C van. Generalist solutions to complex problems: generating practice-based evidence - the example of managing multi-morbidity. BMC Fam Pract. 2013;14:112.
23. Coulter A. Patient engagement–what works? J Ambul Care Manage. 2012;35(2):80–9.
24. Sturmberg JP, Njoroge A. People-centred health systems, a bottom-up approach: where theory meets empery. Journal Eval Clin Pract. 2017;23(2):467–73.
25. Larsen JR, Siersma VD, Davidsen AS, Waldorff FB, Reventlow S, de Fine Olivarius N. The excess mortality of patients with diabetes and concurrent psychiatric illness is markedly reduced by structured personal diabetes care: a 19-year follow up of the randomized controlled study Diabetes Care in General Practice (DCGP). Gen Hosp Psychiatry 2016;38:42–52.
26. de Fine Olivarius N, Beck-Nielsen H, Andreasen AH, Hørder M, Pedersen PA. Randomised controlled trial of structured personal care of type 2 diabetes mellitus. BMJ 2001;323:970–5.
27. Shippee ND, Shah ND, May CR, Mair FS, Montori VM. Cumulative complexity: a functional, patient-centered model of patient complexity can improve research and practice. J Clin Epidemiol. 2012;65(10):1041–51.

28. Rodgers M. Dalton J, Harden M, Street A, Parker G, Eastwood A. Integrated care to address the physical health needs of people with severe mental illness: a mapping review of the recent evidence on barriers, facilitators and evaluations. Int J Integrated Care 2018;18(1):9.
29. Coulter A, Collins A. Making shared decision-making a reality. No decision about me, without me. London: Kings Fund; 2011.
30. Gillard S, Simons L, Turner K, Lucock M, Edwards C. Patient and public involvement in the coproduction of knowledge reflection on the analysis of qualitative data in a mental health study. Qual Health Res. 2012;22(8):1126–37.
31. Jønsson ABR, Guassora AD, Freil M, Reventlow S. Patient knowledge. What the doctor doesn't know: discarded patient knowledge of older adults with multimorbidity. Chronic Illn. 2018; [E-pub ahead of print] https://doi.org/10.1177/1742395318796173.
32. Long JC, Cunningham FC, Braithwaite J. Bridges, brokers and boundary spanners in collaborative networks: a systematic review. BMC Health Serv Res. 2013;13:158.
33. Hunt CM, Spence M, McBride A. The role of boundary spanners in delivering collaborative care: a process evaluation. BMC Fam Pract. 2016;17:96–105.
34. Grimshaw JM, Shirran L, Thomas R, Mowatt G, Fraser C, Bero L, Grilli R, Harvey E, Oxman A, O'Brien MA. Changing provider behavior: an overview of systematic reviews of interventions. Med Care 2001;39(8 Suppl 2):II2–45.
35. Timmermans S, Berg M. The practice of medical technology. Sociol Health Illn. 2003; 25(3):97–114.
36. Craig P, Dieppe P, Macintyre S, Michie S, Nazareth I, Petticrew M. Developing and evaluating complex interventions: the new Medical Research Council guidance. BMJ 2008;337:a1655.
37. May C. A rational model for assessing and evaluating complex interventions in health care. BMC Health Serv Res. 2006;7(6):86.
38. Roberts G, Cornwell J, Locock L, Purushotham A, Sturmey G, Gager M. Patients and staff as codesigners of healthcare services. BMJ 2015;350:g7714.
39. Domecq JP, Prutsky G, Elraiyah T, Wang Z, Nabhan M, Shippee N, Brito JP, Boehmer K, Hasan R, Firwana B, Erwin P, Eton D, Sloan J, Montori V, Asi N, Dabrh AM, Murad MH. Patient engagement in research: a systematic review. BMC Health Serv Res. 2014;14:89.
40. Rowe J. Great expectations: a systematic review of the literature on the role of family carers in severe mental illness, and their relationships and engagement with professionals. J Psychiatr Ment Health Nurs. 2012;19(1):70–82.
41. Malterud K, Elbakken KT. Patients participating as co-researchers in health research: a systematic review of outcomes and experiences. 2019:(Forthcoming)

# Part IV
# Education and Leadership

The final part of this book describes a novel approach to sharing the experience of complexity—through art.

Why art? Art provides a means of expressing thoughts, feelings, and responses that may otherwise be difficult to communicate.

As Shelley Esaak[1] emphasised that a piece of art tells a story in context, here the shared understanding of the nature of systems and complexity sciences in health care.

The final art installation—co-produced through intermittent conversations between the artists and the scientists/health professionals/health system managers—reflected the three key functions of art:

- the physical artefact,
- the reflection of a collective understanding, and
- the stimulation of personal reflection.

[1]https://www.thoughtco.com/what-are-the-functions-of-art-182414.

# Coordinated Tension: The "Secret Sauce" to Enable Decision-Making in a Global Health Complex Adaptive System

**Robert C. Hausmann, Ferdinando Regalia, Emma Iriarte, and Jennifer Nelson**

## 1 Introduction

The theory and practice of complexity science has helped to create a new understanding of an organization as a complex adaptive system. Complex adaptive systems, a subset of non-linear system dynamics, are systems that have (1) many interacting heterogeneous people who (2) self-organize to (3) coordinate actions that lead to innovative solutions [1–4].

Global health innovations can be best described as a complex adaptive system [5], and health care was recently described as the most complex system, and that no other industry has the range or breadth due to numerous stakeholders, intricate funding models, options for treatment, and complicated client needs [6].

A global health system has many ***interactions*** among patients, families, clinicians, hospital staff, nurses, community health workers, program managers, development banks, donors, and many other partners who interact with the goal to reach mutual objectives such as high-quality effective care for at-risk populations. This objective has not yet been achieved through incentive systems that only focus on measurement and key performance indicators [6]. Instead, a system could be designed with learning as an explicit goal that enables clinicians, operators, and administrators to experiment with creative ***self-organization*** to achieve a collective agenda. In turn, this system could create feedback loops to try to build momentum

R. C. Hausmann (✉)
College of Education, The University of Houston, Houston, TX, USA
e-mail: rchausmann@uh.edu

F. Regalia · E. Iriarte · J. Nelson
Social Protection and Health, The Inter-American Development Bank, Washington, DC, USA
e-mail: ferdinandor@iadb.org; Emmai@iadb.org; jennifern@iadb.org



J. P. Sturmberg (ed.), *Embracing Complexity in Health*,
https://doi.org/10.1007/978-3-030-10940-0_11

for change [6]. With shared goals and learning established as a priority, ***coordinated tension*** is needed to enable others in the system to scale-up what has been learned. The coordination mechanisms of a complex adaptive system are the focus of this chapter and how we intend to get at what Hazy (2018 3rd International Conference for Systems and Complexity Sciences for Health, Auburn, VA) described as "simplicity on the other side of complexity."

## *1.1 Tension: The Go Behind the System*

Tension is seen as an inherent and essential feature of complex adaptive systems; it provides "*the go of the system, the force behind the elaboration and maintenance of structure*" [7, p. 99]. As organizations become more complex, "*adaptive tensions give rise to emergent self-organization*" [8, p. 343]. Hausmann [9] agrues, "*as adaptive tensions create a far-from-equilibrium state, the emergence of social innovations is more possible*" (p. 11). This definition of tension is compatible with theories of structuration [10–12] where actors in organizations reacting to the tension associated with the action (exploration) and institutional (exploitation) system stretch and break social structures. In a complex adaptive system, the agents' actions lead them to change, adapt, co-evolve, and transform their structures and practices in order to ensure their survival [13].

Tension is an important construct to complex adaptive systems and has been described as "adaptive tension" [14] or "opportunity tension" [15]. Tensions such as "stability-flexibility, commitment-change, and established routines-novel approaches have competing demands and pose challenges that require new practices that seek creative solutions that can enable fast-paced, adaptable decision making" [16, p. 58]. Hazy [17] suggests, "*the tension between the forces of exploitation and those of exploration is a constant of experience in life*" (p. 182). Hazy goes on to argue "*new possibilities emerge from exploration, and these demand resources. Thus, they conflict with established capabilities that may be losing their luster*" [17, p. 182].

We have found that a complex adaptive system requires coordination of ideas, resources, time, and people so that they can be recombined in such a way that new value is created for others in the system. Coordinated tension is created through a continuous cycle of pushing and pulling between exploiting what we believe we know and exploring what is possible which inherently involves learning. We came to understand that coordinating tension was the critical factor to enable innovation in a complex adaptive system. We share the practices that enable leaders to effectively coordinate tension in the following pages.

### 1.2 Coordinating the Tensions Between Exploration and Exploitation Systems

Coordinated tension mediates the interaction between exploration and exploitation. We call it coordinated tension because it focuses on the interaction between the exploitation system of rules and the exploration system of actors. The mechanism in the center coordinates how people will interact in order to create value together.

This coordination mechanism is like Hazy's [17] explanation of unified leadership in that it "*manages membership and boundaries internal and external to the system. It defines and maintains unity within the system* [18] *in the face of tension between convergent and generative activities within the system, and it makes sense of these tensions for the organization's members* [19] *to find meaning*." Furthermore, "*it creates and dissolves boundaries, determines the boundary's permeability to information* [20] *and establishes and enforces the rights and responsibilities of system membership*." (p. 175)

Coordinated tension is similar in that it creates and reinforces boundaries through which actors in the system will interact. However, it extends this in that it necessitates a requirement for learning among the actors. This learning component is what holds the system together so that members can make sense and negotiate a set of shared goals and measurements that define how they will reach their desired collective impact. In this case, the impact is to improve health outcomes for women and children. Using coordination tension as our framework, we describe the methods, tools, and approaches of the coordination unit of the Salud Mesoamerican Initiative.

## 2 Salud Mesoamerican Initiative as a Coordinated Learning System

In 2010, the Inter-American Development Bank, the Bill and Melinda Gates Foundation, the Carlos Slim Foundation, and the Government of Spain created a global partnership to improve the health of the poor in Mesoamerica, while testing out an innovative results-based financing (RBF) model, placing incentives at the national level, to generate evidence about RBF to increase aid effectiveness and reduce maternal and child health inequalities. This partnership resulted in the Salud Mesoamerica Initiative (SMI).

The SMI rules of the game include:

- Countries must work within the poorest 20% of their populations, selected based on poverty incidence data;
- SMI funds can only finance evidence-based, cost-effective interventions for maternal and child health;

- All projects are co-financed by SMI and countries (50% average cost-sharing); and
- All results are externally verified by an independent third party through both household and health facility surveys.

If countries meet 80% of their goals, they receive 50% of their original investment to use freely within the health sector.

In the region, SMI interventions are directly benefiting 1.8 million women of reproductive age and children less than 5 years of age. Indirectly 4.5 million people living in the poorest areas are also benefiting from these interventions. Through its RBF *plus* model, SMI has achieved results through a combination of national level incentives at the population outcome level, external verification, and technical assistance. Detail program description can be found in Eichler et al. [21] and baseline survey results and methodology can be found in Mokdad et al. [22]. A process evaluation conducted by El Bcheraoui et al. [23] found that regional competition, sense of a true partnership, technical assistance, and an experienced-based learning environment were drivers of success of the partnership.

The partnership has demonstrated impressive results. After 5 years of implementation, changes in coverage and quality of care were externally verified by the Institute of Health Metrics and Evaluation. The use of family planning methods went from 53% to 75%, which represents an increase of 22% points in 5 years in El Salvador. The typical acceleration rate in this indicator is less than 1% points every year [22]. Care for mothers and babies also improved: Early prenatal care increased by 31% in Nicaragua, institutional birth increased by 23% in Honduras, and early postpartum care increased in Belize by 81%. In Honduras, Nicaragua, and Belize, the quality of care during obstetric complications according to international standards improved between 17% and 61% and quality prenatal care in El Salvador improved by 24%. Children under 5 also benefited, coverage of measles, mumps, and rubella vaccination improved in El Salvador by 39%, and 95% of children with diarrhea were treated with both oral rehydration salts and zinc in Honduras and Belize, an innovation introduced to health systems by SMI. All four countries met 80% of their targets, resulting in $3.7 million in incentives for the Ministries of Health. Results from the remaining four countries will be available by January 2019.

In the SMI context, the main challenge proposed is not what to implement; cost-effective, evidence-based intervention packages exist in maternal and child health. Rather, the challenge is how to accelerate scale-up of implementation of these packages with quality in the hardest to reach areas of the region.

We believe this context qualifies SMI as a complex adaptive system. In complex systems, learning is imperative to creating and testing the innovations necessary to improve health outcomes. The complexity stemmed from the need to coordinate a collective agenda that included actors from a mult-lateral bank, two private sector foundations, one public agency, and multiple sovereign governments in order to have an effect on the poorest communities in the country. In complex development contexts, cause and effect do not exist in any meaningful way—and where such dynamic change exists, uncertainty, vague inter-relations, and problematic feedback loops also pose problems.

## 2.1 SMI's Coordinated Tension Model

SMI's coordination model has three elements:

- The exploitation system of rules;
- The exploration system of actors; and
- The coordination system of learning.

The exploitation system refers to the specific SMI rules of engagement and the boundaries put in place by the institutions involved, including incentives and control through policies and protocols. The exploration system of actors refers to all the many individual actions, perceptions, and experiences happening at various levels of the system, which create many weak signals throughout the system. The coordination system of learning refers to the system designed by SMI to manage the tension between exploitation and exploration. The system required a robust learning-performance feedback loop that coordinated specific data, the right actors and spaces for reflection within the programs infrastructure, resources, and incentives mechanism. This required enabling factors such as influential partners, timing of the Millennium Development Goals, and regional competition. Key adaptive coordination abilities were required including: creating a learning environment, experimentation, translation, and brokering.

The conceptual framework (presented in Fig. 1) provides a way of thinking about how the new value was created through the coordination mechanisms in a complex adaptive system.

Learning and performance functions are not done in isolation from other work: they support wider efforts to make progress. This means it is not possible to fully evaluate their success without assessing how successfully the learning was used. It also means that it is impossible to separate "pure" learning functions from the other project or program activities, especially due to the intrinsic nature of SMI in which learning is embedded in many processes triggered by the Initiative's components.

Learning was embedded in the everyday coordination practices of SMI operators, a process that was non-sequential, something other than an orderly march from intervention to success and results from many micro-interactions among participants over time. It included activities of both exploration and exploitation and needed to be systemically monitored before taking action.

## 2.2 Making Sense of Data in Coordination System

The ability to collect useful data, to achieve a thorough understanding of the problem, and to provide proper analysis is crucial to recommending effective interventions and programs. Operational leaders in global health settings have an array of approaches in which to make sense of the data that is coming their way about the efficacy of the efforts. The art is to know when to use which approach to make sense for the challenge.

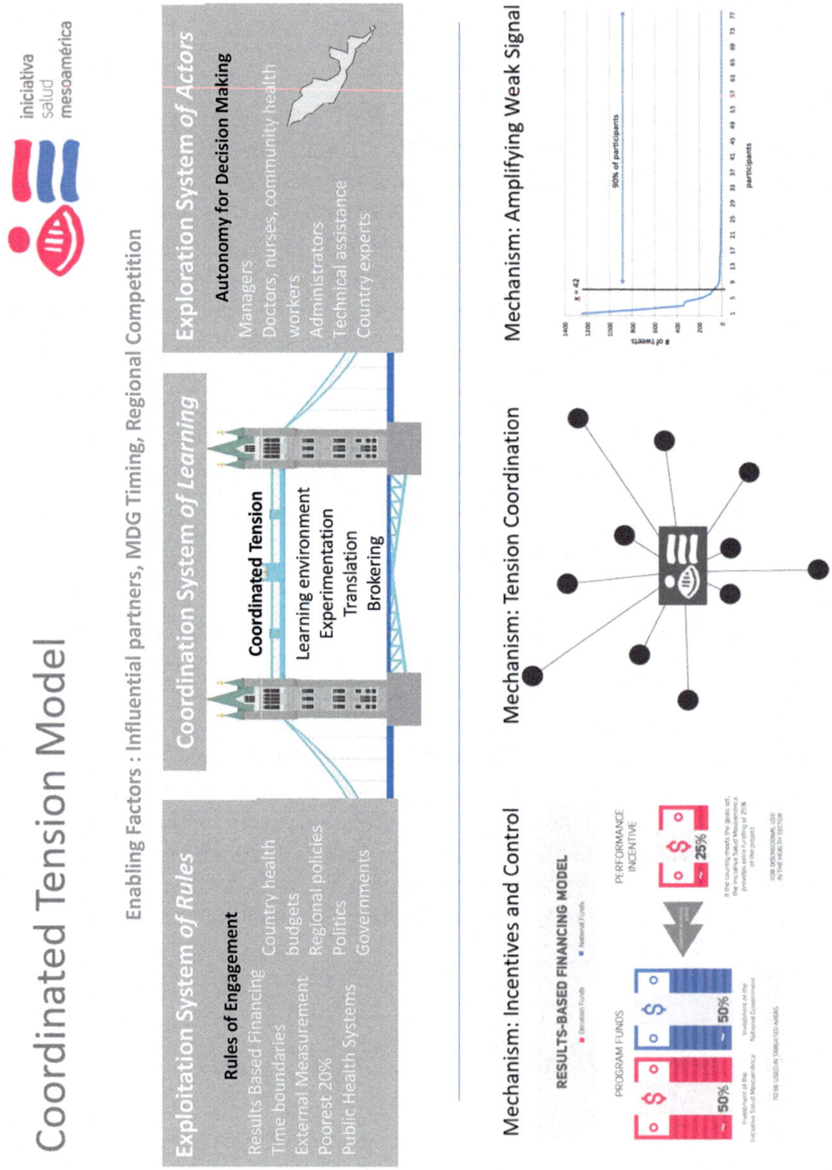


**Fig. 1** Coordination mechanisms in a complex adaptive system

SMI intentionally mixed quantitative and qualitative data in order *to understand the way in which people make decisions, and the context in which those decisions are made*. These two together support decision-making in a coordination system. This formed a rich dataset that permitted a combined qualitative–quantitative assessment for generating deep insights. Taken together, quantitative data (surveys, routine health information systems) and qualitative data (observations, stories and their meanings, discussions with experts) provided a perspective with both depth and breadth: broad enough to inform the regional program strategic thinking about the next years of operations, yet deep and real enough to provoke specific and immediate follow-up actions by the countries in planning their next year of operations. Each data source has a specific use case, audience and frequency, and was designed in an aligned and complementary fashion.

### 2.2.1 Quantitative Data Sources

SMI used three main sources of quantitative data: external household and health facility surveys; rapid household and health facility audits, and dashboards powered by routine health information systems. Some data sources, such as external household and facility data, were a program requirement. This data generated high-quality data from an externally credible source that was used for both policy dialogue and program design, in addition to determining if countries received the performance incentive. Some countries also used rapid household and health facility audits to measure progress prior to the external survey and to adjust their courses of action, in addition to providing sub-national performance incentives to primary healthcare teams. Lastly, countries used their routine health information systems to monitor progress towards their targets at local and aggregated levels using proxy indicators for external survey indicators. The frequency, quality, and use varied by source as outlined in Table 1; however, all indicators were related and aligned.

These data sources mainly answered complicated questions, for example, did countries meet targets or key milestones? Is implementation going as planned? What health facilities are the top/lowest performers? What household characteristics are associated with care seeking behaviors? This data helped to provide critical data about the program's theory of change of specific interventions. For example, surveys revealed if interventions were associated with behavior changes; households that were using micronutrient powders for point-of-use fortification of food to reduce anemia had also received counseling and had correct knowledge of their use, or if women who lived far from a health facility and opted for institutional birth were provided transportation vouchers.

### 2.2.2 Qualitative Data Sources

SMI also used three main qualitative data sources: observational data, expert opinion, and narrative data. Every 3 months, IDB/SMI staff and MOH personnel

**Table 1** Making sense of data from multiple sources in a global health initiative and intentionally creating spaces for reflective learning environment

| Data sources | | | | |
|---|---|---|---|---|
| Type of data | Data source | Description and use case | Audience | Frequency |
| Quantitative data | External household and health facility surveys | • Household and health facility data collected by external evaluator (Institute of Health Metrics and Evaluation)<br>• Generates high-quality data for policy dialogue, program design, and course correction<br>• Used to determine if countries receive the performance incentive as part of the program | Donors, IDB, countries, public | 18–24 months |
| | Rapid household and health facility audits | • Household and health facility surveys collected by external consultants within countries (BE, ES, HO, NI)<br>• Used to determine if local providers receive the performance incentive (BE, ES)<br>• Used by teams to course-correct during program implementation prior to external survey | IDB, national and local level implementers | Quarterly (BE) 6 months (ES) 1 time (NI, HO) |
| | Dashboards: routine information systems and program implementation data | • Dashboards were created to harness routine information systems. Proxies related to performance indicators were selected. Key implementation milestones related to implementation were also selected.<br>• Monthly targets were set and monitored by national level teams through supervision missions and local teams through their quality improvement process. | IDB, national and local level implementers | Monthly |

(continued)

**Table 1** (continued)

| Data sources | | | | |
|---|---|---|---|---|
| Type of data | Data source | Description and use case | Audience | Frequency |
| Qualitative data | Observational data | • Field visits are held every 3 months with IDB and national authorities to identify bottlenecks and propose solutions. | IDB, national and local level implementers | Quarterly |
| | Expert opinion | • SMI consulted with regional and local experts to gain insight on challenges and potential solutions | IDB, national and local level implementers | Ongoing |
| | Narrative data | • SMI ran an experiment to collect micronarratives about program successes and failures with local and national level program implementers (300 per country)<br>• Workshops were designed to analyze these micronarratives as part of the design of the second phase of the program. | Donors, IDB, countries, public | One time per country |
| Intentionally created spaces for reflective learning environment | | | | |
| Space | | Description | Actors | Frequency |
| SMI regional meetings | | • Meetings hosted by SMI to disseminate results from external surveys | Donors, IDB, countries, public | 3 years |
| (COMISCA) Meetings | | • SMI was invited to participate in COMISCA meetings every semester to share program progress with ministers of health and partners | IDB, COMISCA, regional partners | 6 months |
| Cross-country exchanges | | • SMI hosted cross-country exchanges between countries facing similar implementation challenges or policy dialogue decisions | IDB, countries | 4 in total |

(continued)

**Table 1** (continued)

| Intentionally created spaces for reflective learning environment | | | |
|---|---|---|---|
| Space | Description | Actors | Frequency |
| IDB supervision missions | • Every quarter, IDB and MOH authorities meet to review program progress, conduct field visits, identify bottlenecks, and make decisions | IDB, countries | Quarterly |
| Quality improvement meetings and collaboratives | • SMI provided technical assistance to countries to design or improve continuous quality improvement strategies.<br>• Quality improvement teams in health centers and hospitals collected and reviewed data as part of the PDSA cycle<br>• Collaboratives were hosted within countries to allow quality improvement teams to share data, best practices and challenges | Subnational and local country implementers | Monthly/ quarterly |

from the national level conducted field visits to program implementation areas to collect feedback by discussing issues with frontline providers and local managers and through direct observation. After-action reviews were held following field visits to discuss findings and next steps. SMI also called experts in the field to gather feedback on findings or implementation questions. Teams also held focus group discussions with beneficiaries to gather feedback regarding intervention processes, messaging, barriers, and perceptions as part of intervention design and implementation. SMI also piloted a micronarrative data collection trial using Sensemaker® to collect and analyze over 2000 micronarratives. These data sources were mainly used to answer complex questions, for example: How was an intervention implemented? Why did it work or fail? What were the challenges? What are recommendations for going forward? What was the context?

## 2.3 *Reflecting on Findings with the Right Actors*

The various stakeholders involved in the initiative already had several opportunities for interactions during the activities that are necessary to execute, monitor, supervise, evaluate, and share for implementing health and nutrition intervention at scale. SMI created and took advantage of existing spaces to intentionally use the data generated as part of the program for course correction summarized in Table 1. At the regional level, SMI hosted regional meetings to disseminate results of the external surveys at the end of each phase of the program. These meetings provided donors, IDB, and country implementers the opportunity to discuss both successes and failures and provide feedback to the RBF model. Countries also learned from each other's experiences, shared best practices and challenges. International partners also participated in these meetings. SMI also hosted cross-country learning visits between countries facing similar implementation challenges or policy dialogue decisions. For example, Panama visited Nicaragua to learn about the maternal waiting home and transportation voucher strategy. SMI also participated in existing spaces, including the Council of Ministers of Health from Central America and Dominican Republic (COMISCA) meetings every 6 months.

Every quarter as part of the SMI Supervision and Monitoring strategy, IDB/SMI conducted a supervision mission with the country to review financial and technical progress within the program. Both high level authorities and subnational and local implementers were invited to attend the meetings. The SMI rules of engagement put the focus on small voices in the proverbial "long-tail of innovation" by creating an intentional feedback loop between operators closest to the action and policy makers who control resources. By systemically probing for many small observations, or stories, from the local level, SMI was able to detect, make sense of, and amplify voices across the program.

Tools such as a dashboard and project execution plan were reviewed. Field visits were also conducted to collect insights from local program implementers. The SMI coordination unit assisted missions in all countries and provided program staff with a space to share lessons learned and demonstrate successful intervention strategies. This provided fertile ground for iterative design and cross-fertilization. For example, the *hoja filtro para mujeres en edad reproductiva* or *screening form for women of reproductive age* was first created by a local team in El Salvador and shared during a supervision mission with IDB and national levels. Given the team's success with the tool in increasing early prenatal care and family planning use, it was decided that it would be scaled-up to other primary healthcare teams in the SMI area. Within 1 week, the tool went through six iterations and was finalized for printing and training. SMI shared the tool with four other countries, who also thought the tool was promising and adapted and implemented it locally (Fig. 2).

Lastly, SMI supported countries in the design and implementation of continuous quality improvement strategies. SMI's QI approach has been a blend of total quality management and continuous quality improvement and seeks to create both system wide and sustainable change. SMI has approached this challenge at the national level by providing direct technical assistance to countries to create quality improvement strategies and standards. At points of service (in outpatient clinics, maternal clinics, and hospitals) SMI has provided technical assistance to identify, map, and optimize critical processes related to SMI targets; develop and measure standards; prioritize areas for improvement; and develop improvement plans. SMI has developed tools to facilitate data collection and analysis to support the creation of a reflective

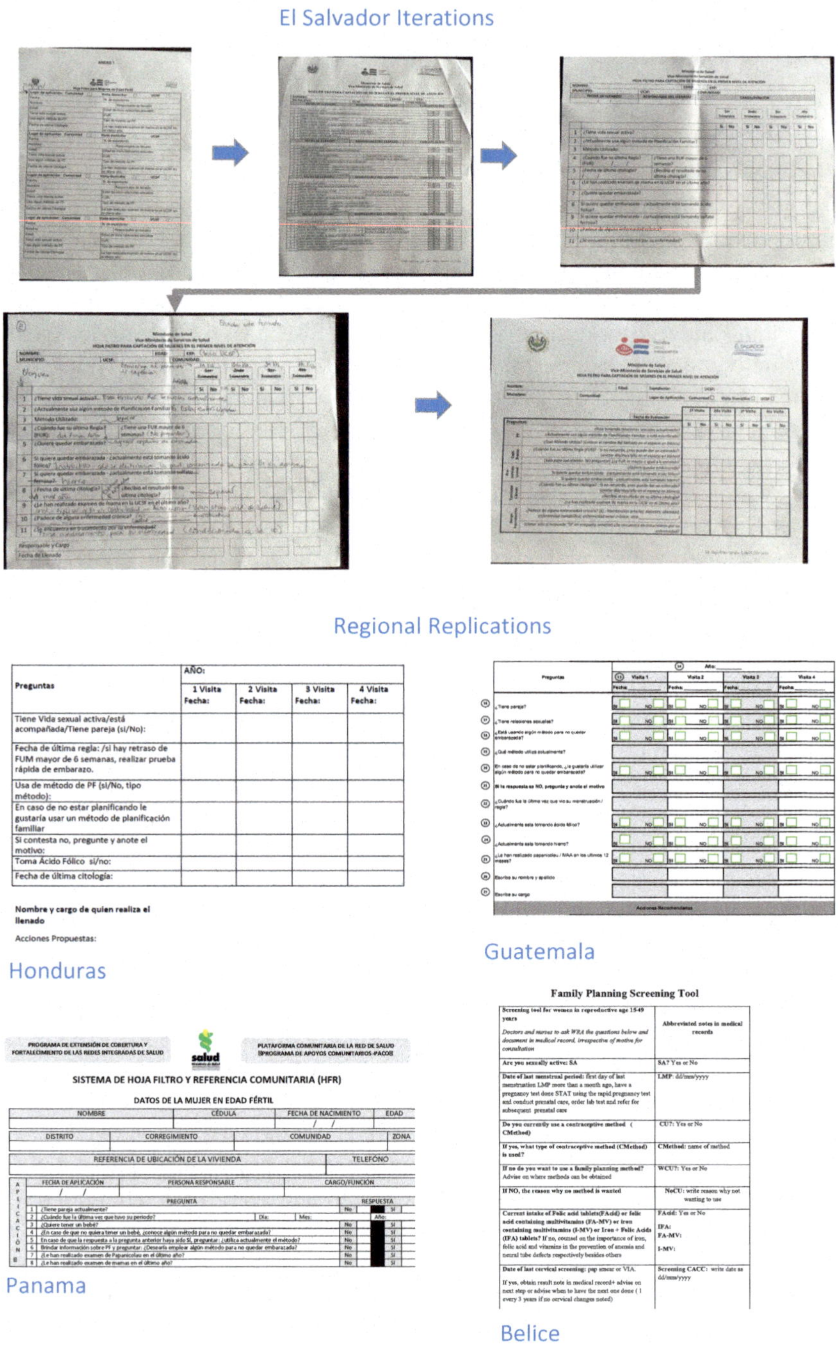


**Fig. 2** Rapid iteration and replication tool

environment. SMI has also facilitated collaboratives between health centers and hospitals to share learnings. This alone was a great challenge, and many teams for the first time are now running plan-do-study-act (PDSA) cycles and sharing successes. Table 1 describes the coordination mechanisms for reflective learning that were intentionally created.

SMI was able to make sure that the right people were in the room. For example, Minister of Health and Finance, the Director of Primary Health Care Services, the Director of Hospital Networks, or the Director of the Technology Department attended these meetings to review latest available data and to make strategic and operational decisions. IDB team leaders, fiduciary experts, technical experts, subnational managers and providers also participated to provide "***a holistic view***" of the system. In this process, SMI ensured that key decision makers and implementers could jointly discuss issues.

### 2.4 SMI Practices to Effectively Coordinate Tension

The SMI coordination unit embodied key practices to effectively coordinate tension. As mentioned, the team intentionally created learning environments for stakeholder interaction. The team also actively practiced experimentation and agile management within regional and country level strategies; many operational interventions, such as the *hoja filtro*, were emergent. Given their coordination role, vertical and horizontal translation between various levels of the systems was critical. For example, SMI assisted teams in translating findings from data from the Institute of Health Metrics and Evaluation (IHME) surveys or routine health information systems into action. The coordination unit also asked as a broker to detect local innovations and share them with actors from other countries facing similar challenges for adaptation.

In the case of SMI, this was achieved by creating a small, dedicated team with clear individual and collective roles for coordination and learning. All members had a commitment to a clear set of results and principals. The team operated with intentionality to solve problems; they applied their data and deep knowledge of local systems using a systems approach to intervention design and implementation.

## 3 What Did We Learn About the Mechanisms of Coordination in a Complex Adaptive System?

Our approach to coordinated tension focuses on resilience which allows a degree of failure and emphasizes learning as a priority. The system shifted from a tool for planning to a system that was open to emergent outcomes and creating the right environment where these outcomes could be capitalized on. This required designing a coordinated learning system that fits the context.

### 3.1 Coordinating the Long-Tail of Innovation

As discussed, coordination is needed to amplify and exploit the tensions that will create the energy to change the system in some way. As Boisot and Mckelvey [24] stated: "*Many events connected under tension … are often distributed according to a power law* (p. 416)". A power law suggests that in nature small events happen quite often, but large events are very rare.

The "long-tail" representation of data indicates that data are most likely distributed according to a power-law—our findings suggest that coordinating the action of the global health professionals across countries in the Mesoamerica Region was about amplifying the voices of the actors in the long tail (e.g., community health workers, doctors, nurses, local managers, country actors, etc.). These are the actors found in the exploration system of our model. In fact, the actors in the long-tail are often the ones that are breaking institutional norms often required to enact sustainable change. The mechanism of coordination is important in understanding the potential for scaling innovation by awaking the resources in the long-tail.

In SMI, we found local actors had the critical knowledge and resources to help solve problems and provided ideas and stories from the long tail (exploration system). The coordination unit saw patterns in those stories and experiences and saw that they were often disconnected from policy makers or program manager perceptions. The stories in the long tail sound like "this matters to me" or this "matters to us." This was in stark contrast to "They need this" that came from the 10% of people in the exploitation system creating rules and policies. SMI helped to translate these experiences to those making decisions.

For example, one story we labeled "The lawnmower." In the story, the community health worker talks about using the resources to "buy a lawnmower" to improve the look of the public health facility. As the facility improved, it attracted more women because it appeared to be a more beautiful place to convene and access care. That created an environment where they wanted to be and thus deliver their babies and come for pre- and post-natal care.

So, why would one give up 10% of the output value, especially if novel system change came from the other 90% of participants? If your system is designed where one must give up the value of the long-tail of innovation, the system should be re-engineered [25]. That is the value of "tension coordination." The coordination and scalable response does not ask "how do we manage these people," but "what is their contribution and how do we coordinate their action." Therefore, the point of the lawnmower story is not for the MOH to buy lawnmowers for every health facility. Instead, create a process for local teams to make changes to facilities or processes based on their local expertise and insights, which in Belize and El Salvador, was achieved by providing teams with additional resources for these types of efforts.

## 3.2 SMI's Lessons Learned Implementing a Coordination System of Learning

We find that SMI created a learning system within the global health complex adaptive system to achieve results which relied on three main elements: (1) System of rules (exploitation); (2) System of actors and variation (exploration); and (3) Coordinated system of learning. To manage the tension between exploitation and exploration systems, the learning system intentionally created a feedback mechanism that required specific data, the right actors, enabling factors, and adaptive coordination abilities. Based on this experience, we find that to manage complex adaptive systems and balance the tension between exploitation and exploration, it is necessary to create coordinated learning system with four critical objectives: creating a learning environment, experimentation, translation, and brokering. SMI is not the only system that has found these elements to be important; looking at achievements in healthcare delivery across 60 low, middle, and high income countries, other research has found four factors:

- Begin with small scale initiatives and build up (experimentation),
- Convert data and information into intelligence and give this openly to the appropriate decision makers (translation and learning environment),
- Remember the lone hero model does not work and that collaboration underpins all productive change (brokering), and
- Always start with the patient at the center of any reform measure [6].

However, SMI had three key learnings from implementation: (1) Trade-offs exist between data sources; (2) Context and culture must be taken into consideration; and (3) Learning must be planned and intentional.

### 3.2.1 Trade-offs Between Data Sources

Data is a very powerful tool to influence strategy, design, and implementation when used effectively. However, each of the data sources used by SMI had trade-offs related to quality, frequency, cost to collect, and effort to use. Table 2 summarizes the trade-offs observed and resulting decisions. These issues are important to consider when designing and selecting data for feedback in the coordination system.

### 3.2.2 Context and Culture

Elements of the SMI program play a key role in generating an incentive for data use. Time-bound targets, performance incentive, and regional reputation were found to create a sense of urgency to use data to track progress. Technical assistance provided by the IDB/SMI and data collection experts allowed for meaningful technical dialogue. Data was transformed into visualizations that made it more

**Table 2** SMI Data source trade-offs

| Data source | Quality | Frequency | Cost to collect | Effort to use | Insights generated | Decision |
|---|---|---|---|---|---|---|
| External HH and HF surveys | Extremely high | 6 months to collect; 6 months to process | High | Medium | Extremely high: course correction and policy change | N/A program requirement |
| Rapid HH and HF surveys | High | 3 months to collect; 1–2 months to process | Medium | Medium | High: course correction | Continue use |
| Dashboards | Medium-low depending on source and country | Monthly | Low | Medium | Medium: able to review local performance; improved data flow to local implementers, but quality sometimes an issue | Varies by country. In countries with higher quality routine data, use has been continued |
| Observational data | High, but limited in scope | Quarterly | Medium | Low | High: insight from local implementers critical to design and improve interventions. Additionally, provided insight to national level decision makers regarding local realities | Continue use |
| Micronarrative data | Medium | One time | High | High | High: shared both successes and failures. Helped teams to identify new interventions | Cost to collect, process, and use was very high. Use was discontinued, although valuable insights were generated |

useful for decision-making. SMI's regional nature played a role in allowing for cross-fertilization of ideas. These elements are important for program design. Creating a culture for learning and reflection was also important. This was done by creating a respectful, technical environment for discussion through facilitation and leadership.

### 3.2.3 Learning Must be Planned and Intentional

SMI design included budget and milestones related to learning. The program was committed to sharing successes and failures within and between countries and donors. Quality improvement provided a platform to use data and reflect on performance. Specific tools (quality and timely data, visualization, stories) and abilities (creating a learning environment, experimentation, translation, and brokering) were required to coordinate learning. In the case of SMI a dedicated team was created to carry out these activities.

## *3.3 Remaining Questions for Scale-Up, Sustainability, and Future Replications from a Complexity Perspective*

As SMI enters its third and final phase, many questions remain around sustainability, scale-up, and replication: (1) Is SMI sustainable in its current form; (2) Can it be scaled-up nationally; and (3) Can it be adapted and replicated in other programs?

We find that a coordinated learning system can take on many forms. In the case of SMI and in the newly launched Regional Malaria Elimination Initiative based on SMI, this system was created and managed by a small, dedicated unit within the managing organization, IDB. Regarding the sustainability and replication of SMI, these insights could help create new rules, policies, or best practices using exploitation mechanisms. For example, one recommendation is that future programs working in complex and adaptive systems should have a coordinated learning system with the four critical objectives mentioned. This system must be intentionally created and monitored, requiring both time and resources. One way to think about scale-up is by ensuring that actors outside of the those managing the learning system (in SMI's case, the coordination unit) acquire adaptive coordination abilities. This could be achieved by creating a focused mentoring program to key actors within the system, improving the ability of the system to experiment, translate, and broker.

## The Transformative Aspects of This Study

We found that to manage complex adaptive systems and mediate the tension between exploitation and exploration, it is necessary to create coordinated learning system with four critical objectives: creating a learning environment, experimentation, translation, and brokering. However, it is critical for programs considering working in complex adaptive systems to design a system that fits their context. Some programs may require dedicated teams, while others may intentionally assign these functions to existing stakeholders. To effectively design these systems, it is necessary to understand and map out the rules within the exploitation system of interest. Likewise, it is critical to understand the actors and to permit and detect emergent practices within their exploration system. Finally, it will require intentionally coordinating tension between these systems through learning with the right combination of data, actors and abilities to achieve meaningful change.

**Take Home Message**

- Conceptualizing the dynamic nature of a system through the coordinated tension model is important when innovation is a priority. It makes explicit how the micro, meso, and macro levels interact to create value.
- The bridge between exploitation and exploration is navigated through a process of coordination.
- Coordinating a system of learning requires dedicated resources (time, people, and money) to enable the mechanisms of (1) creating a learning environment, (2) experimentation, (3) translation, and (4) brokering.
- Using the coordinated tension model allows leaders to make explicit the priority they are placing on learning for the primary purpose of co-creating value with their stakeholders.

## References

1. Holland JH. Genetic algorithms and the optimal allocation of trials. SIAM J Comput. 1973;2(2):88–105.
2. Thietart RA, Forgues B. Chaos theory and organization. Organ Sci. 1995;6(1):19
3. Dooley KJ. A complex adaptive systems model of organization change. Nonlinear Dyn Psychol Life Sci. 1997;1(1):69–97.
4. Anderson P. Complexity theory and organization science. Organ Sci. 1999;10(3):216–32.
5. Plesk PE, Wilson T. Complexity, leadership, and management in healthcare organizations. BMJ. 2001;323(7315):746–9.
6. Braithwaite J, Churruca K, Long JC, Ellis LA, Herkes J. When complexity science meets implementation science: a theoretical and empirical analysis of systems change. BMC Med. 2018;218;16(1):63.

7. Buckley W. Society as a complex adaptive system. Modern systems research for the behavioral scientist. Chicago: Aldine; 1968. p. 490–513.
8. Plowman DA, Solansky S, Beck TE, Baker LK Kulkarni M, Travis DV. The role of leadership in emergent, self-organization. Leadersh Q. 2007;18(4):341–56.
9. Hausmann RC. Organizing ecosystems for social innovation: the relationality of contexts and mechanisms in a social entrepreneurship network. Unpublished manuscript. George Washington University; 2015.
10. Giddens A. The constitution of society: outline of the theory of structuration (reprint ed.). Berkley: University of California Press; 1984.
11. Barley SR, Tolbert PS. Institutionalization and structuration: studying the links between action and institution. Organ Stud. 1997;18(1):93–117
12. Stones R. Structuration theory. London: Palgrave Macmillan; 2005.
13. Axelrod RM, Cohen MD. Harnessing complexity: organizational implications of a scientific frontier. New York: Basic Books; 2001.
14. Uhl-Bien M, Marion R, McKelvey B. Complexity leadership theory: shifting leadership from the industrial age to the knowledge era. Leadersh Q. 2007;18(4):298–318.
15. Goldstein J, Hazy JK, Silberstang J. A complexity science model of social innovation in social enterprise. J Soc. Entrep. 2010;1(1):101–25.
16. Lewis MW, Andriopoulos C, Smith WK. Paradoxical leadership to enable strategic agility. Calif. Manag. Rev. 2014:56(3):58–77.
17. Hazy JK. Parsing the 'influential increment' in the language of complexity: uncovering the systemic mechanisms of leadership influence. Int J Complex Leadersh Manag. 2011;1(2): 164–91.
18. Maturana HR, Varela FJ. The tree of knowledge: the biological roots of human understanding, Paolucci R. (Trans.). Boston: Shambhala; 1998.
19. Weick KE. Sensemaking in organizations. Los Angeles: Sage Publications; 1995.
20. Hazy JK, Backström, T. Complexity and human interaction dynamics. Complexity. 2014;15(4). http://sm2015.org/es/iniciativa-salud-mesoamerica/iniciativa-salud-mesoamerica-inicio, 1904.html
21. Eichler R, Nelson J, Iriarte E, Gigli S, Zúñiga Brenes P, Ríos-Zertuche D. The initial prize in the Salud Mesoamérica Initiative results-based aid initiative (Technical Report No. 1314). Inter-American Development Bank; 2017. https://publications.iadb.org/handle/11319/8566
22. Mokdad AH, Colson KE, Zúñiga-Brenes P, Ríos-Zertuche D, Palmisano EB, Alfaro-Porras E, et al. Salud Mesoamérica 2015 Initiative: design, implementation, and baseline findings. Popul Health Metr. 2015;13(1):3.
23. El Bcheraoui C, Palmisano EB, Dansereau E, Schaefer A, Woldeab A, Moradi-Lakeh M, Salvatierra B, Hernandez-Prado B, Mokdad AH. Healthy competition drives success in results-based aid: lessons from the Salud Mesoamérica Initiative. PLoS One. 2017;12(10):e0187107.
24. Boisot M, Mckelvey B. Integrating modernist and postmodernist perspectives on organizations: a complexity science bridge. Acad Manag Rev. 2010;35(3):415–33.
25. Shirky C. Here comes everybody: the power of organizing without organizations. New York: Penguin Press; 2008.

# A Systems Perspective for Measuring Features of Transdisciplinary Knowledge Producing Teams (TDKPTs)

**Gaetano R. Lotrecchiano and Shalini Misra**

## 1 What Are Transdisciplinary (TD) Knowledge Producing Teams (KPTs)?

The first use of the term transdisciplinarity is credited to the Swiss psychologist Jean Piaget. In his treatise on the subject, he framed transdisciplinarity as a "*higher stage of succeeding interdisciplinary relationships … which would not cover interactions or reciprocities between specialized research projects, but would place these relationships within a total system without any firm boundaries between disciplines*" [1]. Hence, from its inception systems thinking grounded transdisciplinary economies of knowledge production. Systems thinking aimed to understand entire multilevel networks of individuals, organizations, and knowledge. Numerous scholars have continued to refine and expand upon the theoretical and applied properties of transdisciplinarity in an attempt to bridge this definition to applied problem-solving [2–6]. However, the application of the term as an applied model of problem solving is credited to the Romanian physicist, Basarab Nicolescu, who advanced the applicability of the term to contemporary problem solving by emphasizing how transdisciplinary perspectives aided in understanding the world beyond the frameworks of any one discipline [7]. A number of lines of inquiry have focused on the conceptual work of defining transdisciplinarity and have contributed to our understanding of the nature of knowledge integration—complex and adaptive systems perspectives [8]; humanities discourses [9]; socially

G. R. Lotrecchiano (✉)
Department of Clinical Research and Leadership, George Washington University School of Medicine and Health Sciences, Washington, DC, USA
e-mail: glotrecc@gwu.edu

S. Misra
Virginia Tech School of Public and International Affairs, Alexandria, VA, USA
e-mail: shalini@vt.edu



J. P. Sturmberg (ed.), *Embracing Complexity in Health*,
https://doi.org/10.1007/978-3-030-10940-0_12

responsible science [10, 11]; defining and dealing with "wicked problems" [12]; reimagining disciplinary silos and boundaries [13]; and the multiplicity of realities in science [7, 14].

This conceptual research over the past two decades has permeated the research agendas of many sectors. Reference to the TD paradigm has shown up in documentation about learning, education, and science by organizations such as the United States National Science Foundation (NSF), National Institutes of Health (NIH), National Academy of Sciences (NAS), the United Nations Education, Scientific and Cultural Organization (UNESCO), and the International Center for Transdisciplinary Research (CIRET). Each has invited conversation about the tensions and complexities in interchange across knowledge systems [15–18]. This process of engaging in "boundary crossing" [3], "boundary blurring" [19], and identifying "zones of interdependence" between boundaries is fraught with barriers and challenges. Strategies and approaches to overcome some of these barriers and manage the challenges of cross-disciplinary collaboration are critical for solving global problems. As well, emphasis on the differences and fundamental limitations of certain types of knowledge economies and methodologies are important topics to address to facilitate knowledge integration and solve contemporary societal problems.

Transdisciplinary knowledge producing teams (TDKPTs) explicitly aim to integrate knowledge and address wicked problems. Transdisciplinary teams are distinct from unidisciplinary, interdisciplinary, and multidisciplinary teams. While each of these teams strive to produce knowledge and address a scientific problem, there are several distinctions between these economies of knowledge and the level of collaboration that occurs within each type of team. One set of differences concerns the representation of distinct disciplines, the diversity of knowledge systems, and attitudes toward other disciplinary worldviews and methodologies. Unidisciplinary teams work within the confines of the traditions or expectations of a single disciplinary history and scope. Sometimes, these teams have negative biases toward other disciplines and deny the validity, rigor, and usefulness of certain disciplines, approaches, ontological assumptions, epistemic foundations, and methods [20]. For the purpose of comparison to other more cross-disciplinary interactive modalities, unidisciplinary teams typically adopt the oneness of a disciplinary approach with little consideration of parallel or adjacent disciplines.

Multidisciplinary teams involve individuals from two or more disciplines working together on a common problem [21]. This economy is employed in many cross-disciplinary teams throughout many sectors that require professional expertise to interface with scientific and scholarly expertise. Each participant brings to the discourse their own theories, methods, and techniques and provides insights within the confines of their own discipline. Multidisciplinary teams though extremely effective in incorporating multiple perspectives to understand or address a problem often lack the inventiveness to put forth new techniques or models, modify mainstream approaches, or construct new frameworks that integrate or transcend the confines of any one discipline. They are effective in solving problems that are less complex than those attempted by other more interactive cross-disciplinary teams. These teams often attempt to achieve greater understanding and knowledge through the multiplication of methods and not through hybridization of approaches [22].

Moving further along the continuum of cross-disciplinary collaboration, when teams made up of individuals from distinct disciplines modify (or synthesize) existing methods or theories stemming from the cross-pollination of two or more disciplines, they are interdisciplinary in nature [22]. However, interdisciplinary teams, though more intent on integrating knowledge are less focused on generating new knowledge that might result in new methods or frameworks that are the result of collaborative efforts. In both cases (multi- and interdisciplinary teams), a new level of discourse does emerge which ultimately leads to a further integration of knowledge [21, 22]. Klein suggests that interdisciplinarity is a paradox, generating productive tensions that supplement, complement, and critique existing structures [23]. This is in line with contemporary complexity thinking on adaptation in groups and organizations where tension and conflict can breed change and innovation [24–26]. The tensions promote the expansion of individual worldviews and the creation of new frameworks to manage knowledge. Without the development of new frameworks to manage such new knowledge, exchanges cannot have a lasting impact on problems requiring new theoretical or constitutive lenses [3].

Interdisciplinarity offers new ways of working in teams. New styles of thought begin to emerge and upend traditional methodologies and analytical enterprises to generate new frames of knowledge [27]. This sentiment echoes that of earlier theorists, who also focused on the shifts that occur between disciplinary boundaries resulting in novel perspectives and paradigm shifts, but highlighted different mechanisms like scientific paradigm shifts, differentiation and integration of scientific knowledge, and interdependences [28–30].

Multi- and interdisciplinary team approaches both fall short of knowledge integration in a manner unique to TDKPTs. Transdisciplinarity is a departure from mere considerations of hybridization and synthesis of disciplinary perspectives, methods, or frameworks. While multidisciplinary and interdisciplinary teams focus on exchange between disciplines, TDKPT teams operate from a fundamentally different paradigm that endeavors to work across disciplines and non-disciplinary knowledge systems with the goal of engaging in participatory knowledge creation across epistemic and methodological boundaries [31, 32]. Maasen and Lieven describe transdisciplinarity as a new mode of governing science where "*… practices are directed toward solving complex policy issues and address scientific knowledge production proper. It promises to circumvent the schism between scientific expertise and policy-making by … the involvement of stakeholders [that] make sure the 'right problem' gets addressed 'in the right way'*" [33]. Transdisciplinarity, therefore, moves us from a consideration of science as bound by disciplines and gravitates to a more holistic and systemic schema that considers the dynamics of entire systems of actors and concepts [22, 34–36]. Maasen and Lieven [33] characterize TDKPTs as "extending expertise," and "legitimation through participation" rather than "legitimation through knowledge."

In TDKPTs, participants are challenged to relate to and reconcile with different levels of reality [37] thus challenging the very core of their beliefs and assumptions about knowledge. Furthermore, the transfer of power, reinterpretations of service delivery, training and education requirements, and questions of legitimacy all contribute to a general resistance to transdisciplinarity [38]. These tensions become real as traditional roles and disciplines are challenged to change and evolve in

TD collaborations. TD team interactions are subject to unfavorable conditions that make it difficult to transition from an interdisciplinary mode to this more novel and integrative one. TDKPTs therefore require a reappraisal and a reconsideration of the systemic features and properties if integration and synthesis are to truly occur. Figure 1 provides a graphical representation of the distinctions between uni-, multi-, inter-, and transdisciplinarity. We now turn our focus to a systems analysis of the features of TDKPTs.

## 2 Features of Transdisciplinary Knowledge Producing Teams (TDKPTs)

To describe the overlapping themes in transdisciplinary knowledge economies and TDKPTs, we look at complexity science to understand how one might strive toward defining and developing the skills necessary to work within these teams. In the sections below, we introduce a typology of TD features under two categories—*structural system complexities* and *interactive system complexities* and elucidate the complexity factors they parallel and skills required to work within these environments. Underlying these features are several *key assumptions* about TDKPTs that are important to consider as we articulate the shared elements of TDKPTs with complex adaptive systems.

**Assumptions About TDKPTs**

TDKPTs operate within evolving environmental conditions as they strive to create new frameworks for managing novel knowledge outputs [40]. This evolving environment is recognizable through the dynamic interactions of teams [41].

TDKPTs by nature express adaptive qualities (those required for change) that are often manifested during moments of conflict and tension that are byproducts of evolution and change [42]. These conflicts are moments of knowledge awareness and exchange and not necessarily barriers to teaming [43, 44].

TDKPT mechanisms are not bound to any one feature. There is an enormous amount of overlap between different TDPKT features. To consider otherwise would be contrary to the systems approach being adopted here.

TDKPT features are found on the individual, group, and organizational levels of any system affecting individuals and teams as they interface with their environment [45]. Any description of features needs to be cognizant of the individual, team, and environmental factors that contribute to any knowledge economy.

TDKPTs are complex and adaptive environments (complex adaptive systems) that utilize techniques for communication and exchange that ascribe to principles found in systems theory like adaptation, nonlinearity, openness, and self-organization [8].

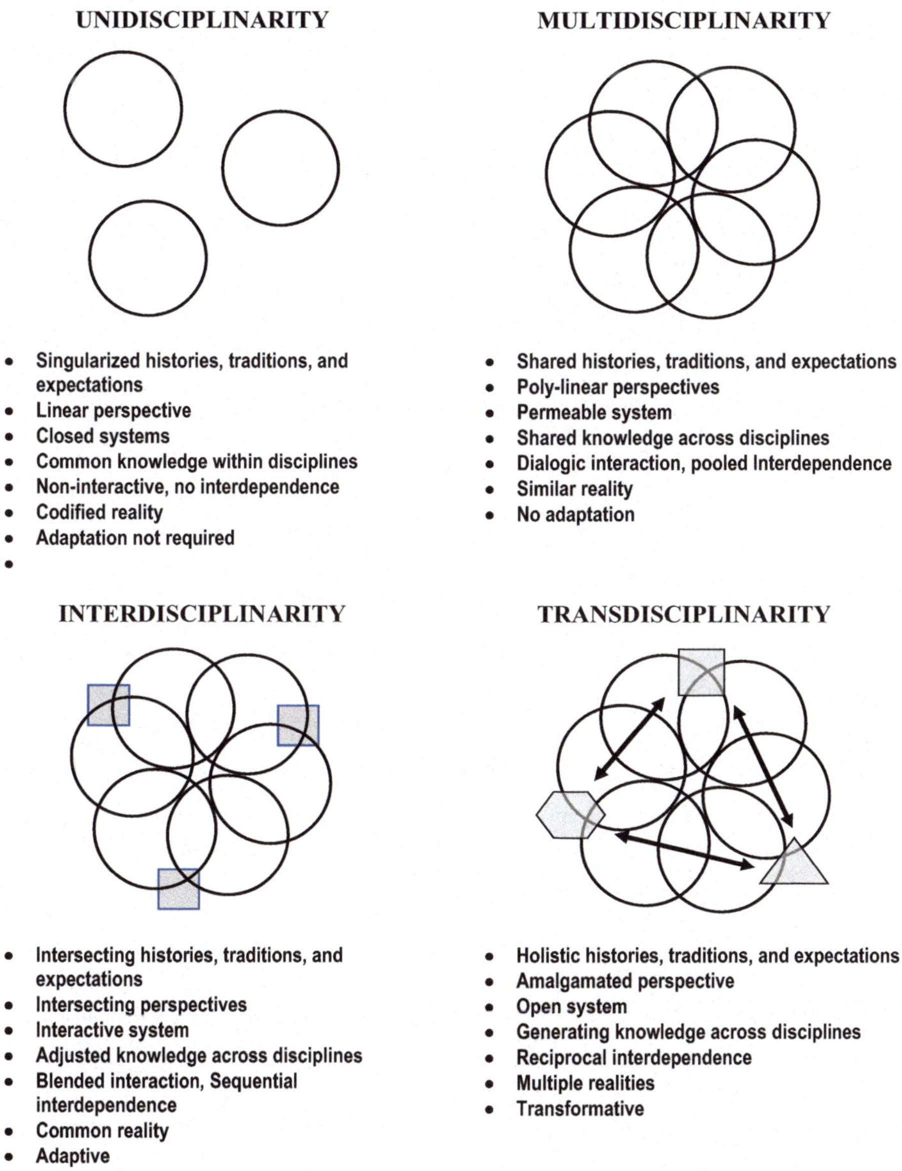


**Fig. 1** Complexity perspectives of cross-disciplinary knowledge economies (adapted from [39])

Having delineated the basic assumptions for a systems understanding of the features of TDKPTs, we present key features of TDKPTs, complexity factors at play, and areas of skill development that respond to challenge areas within structural system and interactive system complexities. Table 1 summarizes this information. We follow with an explanation of these concepts.

**Table 1** Features of TD knowledge producing teams categorized by the type of system complexity

**Structural system complexities**

*Challenges:*

- Perceived inequitable contributions to the project [46]
- Unbalanced problem ownership, discontinuous participation, and fear of failure [47]
- Variability in communication types and skills, overall lack of participant satisfaction with the project processes and outcomes [48]

| Feature | Complexity factor/ *Measurement of effectiveness* | Skill development foci |
|---|---|---|
| Complex problem solving | Information exchange occurs through the interactions of multiple elements<br>*The measure of sameness and difference in TDKPTs is dynamic as it relates to end goals and outcomes* | • A heightened focus on anticipated future states [10, 49]<br>• Goal alignment with conditions of a changing world [50]<br>• Focus on dealing with interpersonal team challenges<br>• Co-developed shared mental models within KPTs [51]<br>• Social learning as part of team engagement [52] |
| Stakeholder involvement | CAS are open systems with feedback loops, both enhancing, stimulating (positive), or detracting, inhibiting (negative). Both kinds are necessary<br>*Interconnective relationships in TDKPTs are measured by external relationships as much as internal team relationships* | • Translation of knowledge across disciplines [53]<br>• Development and sustainability of scientific and nonscientific partnerships [33]<br>• Establishing interdependence between knowledge partners [29] |
| Methodological pluralism | Change is a continual steady state in CAS where equilibrium is equated with death of the system<br>*The ability to approach problems with different methods of inquiry is the ability to adapt and assume new orientations* | • Boundary spanning over boundary forming [54]<br>• Shifting awareness of problems [55]<br>• Pluralism as a normative reality [56]<br>• Translation of knowledge [57] |

(continued)

**Table 1** (continued)

| | | |
|---|---|---|
| Praxis | Interactions between systems components is a foundational feature of CAS<br>*Effective knowledge production is as much a matter of producing process knowledge as much as it is a matter of outcome knowledge* | • Experience-based learning is necessary for impact-based solutions [58]<br>• Combining formal and informal knowledge [59]<br>• Reintegrating co-created knowledge [47] |

**Interactive system complexity**

*Challenges:*

- Differences in foundational training among team members, diverse and changing career paths, geographic dispersion, a lack of awareness of the breadth and complexity of the problem, perceived insufficient legitimacy of a team to solve the problem, conflicting methodological standards, and conflicting epistemological and ontological orientations [47]
- Differing levels of transdisciplinary orientation among team members [60]

| **Feature** | **Complexity factor/ *measurement of effectiveness*** | **Skill development foci** |
|---|---|---|
| Open systems capacity | Nonlinearity in CAS is the result of a lack of any one dominant framework bounding the flow of information<br>*Nondirectional and noncongruent thought and actions may be measured through confluence and conflict* | • Reception to knowledge from outside of one's system of knowledge [34]<br>• Conflict and power struggles can breed innovative thought [61]<br>• Interdependent relationships between actors need to contribute to shared goals [62] |
| Different (shifting) levels of reality | CAS are open systems where feedback loops serve as entropy in the system stimulating and inhibiting flow at any given time<br>*The degree of ability for simple components in TDKPTs to connect with the entire system is an emergent state that TDKPTs require to be effective* | • Navigation of multiple realities related to a single problem [63, 64]<br>• Mastering the consideration of diversity over different timescales, landscapes, and experiential episodes [8]<br>• Adaptation through self-organization [65] |
| Collaborative construction and reconstruction | The depth and history of a complex adaptive system is common<br>*Effectiveness in TDKPTs is dependent on the ability to self-organize amidst change in the systems* | • Openness to rearranging collaborative and knowledge arrangements [66]<br>• Direct contact with those affected by the problem attempting to be solved [54] |

# 3 Structural System Complexities

## 3.1 *Stakeholder Involvement*

While it can be easily surmised that multiple stakeholders representing different interests are needed to attempt complex problem solving, it is in the details of this sort of engagement where unique challenges emerge within TDKPTs. Interacting in ways that challenge unidisciplinary viewpoints requires an expansion of perspectives about the breadth of knowledge required in a process of inquiry and problem solving. Conflicts arise usually as a result of the lack of facility in translating knowledge to ensure accessibility across a team of stakeholders [67]. Maasen and Lieven find that these stifling dynamics can be observed when stakeholders representing both scientific and applied concerns interact and highlight "*the separation between scientific expertise and policy making*" [33, p. 401].

The emphasis here is not on conflict, but rather the barriers that are the result of singularizing perspectives around a problem. It reminds us to consider the reasons for multistakeholder interaction. Multistakeholder engagement is key to complex problems solving [68]. In TDKPTs, multistakeholder involvement arises from the need for task interdependence between actors to achieve a transdisciplinary end goal. If there is no interdependence between stakeholders within the system, there is no need for coordination across the system [29, 30]. Cohesion and interdependency among stakeholders stemming from their unique investments and agendas can be an opportunity for psychosocial investment in addressing a problem.

Differences in stakeholder understanding of problems in TDKPTs are not just a matter of the degree of involvement but also the ability to embrace the totality of the problem. The ability to integrate stakeholders with highly diverse perspectives including those who personally experience the problem is markedly different than that of other knowledge economies where knowledge production is left to those identified as knowledge specialists [33]. While the integration and synthesis of knowledge is of primary concern in these instances, such teaming engagements might lack the breadth of experiential knowledge to adequately engage all stakeholder perspectives. Translation between these factions requires an openness to seeking solutions across disciplines [53] establishing interdependent relationships as the core basis of teaming [29]. It is through the engagement of those who typically solve problems with those who typically are burdened with real-world problems where a unique stakeholder engagement specific to TDKPTs can be identified.

## 3.2 *Methodological Pluralism*

Complex problem-solving depends on the freedom to employ multiple approaches toward understanding and resolving the problem, with no single methodological approach dominating problem solving providing only a narrowly constructed solution [37]. If complex problem solving relies on a series of systematically and contextually related real-world factors, then solutions to these problems are just as complex. For this reason, no one method can adequately supply potential solutions. Constellations of methods are often employed in TDKPTs and they coexist as do the multiple realities that emerge as part of the problems seeking to be solved [57]. The logic behind this construction of problem solving processes is antithetical to many traditional unidisciplinary means to problem solving that rely on "risk reduction" over "risk production." Similarly, conflict becomes an opportunity for knowledge production and boundary spanning. Increasing risk in problem solving can be a means to expanding the scope of the problem and seeking greater input from different actors toward the resolution of the problem [33]. This multimethod approach to problem solving shows that more than one legitimate description of a problem exists and more than one potential solution is possible within a complex and adaptive system [8]. Different descriptions will decompose the system in different ways and are not reducible to one another. Different descriptions may also have different degrees of complexity [69].

Environments that adopt multiple methods toward problem solving are inherently complex. The adaptive nature of these environments will require the consideration of converging and diverging methodological practices and conflict may lead to both tension and creativity within the same teaming environment. When team members interface with different stakeholders and consider the ways in which they might utilize standardized methodologies from a host discipline in their quest to contribute to the solution of a problem, others will provide for complementary and possibly even contradictory ways of knowing and solving problems. As stated, this is a normative dynamic in a teaming environment where trust in methodological pluralism [56] shifts in reality perceptions [57], and boundary spanning [54] is a constant state. Translation therefore becomes the dominant behavior in TDKPTs, where individuals and the team are continually challenged to show the relational characteristics between different methods and how through selection and hybridization they can provide novel approaches to complex problems [70].

## *3.3 Praxis*

The term praxis is an often-used word with many contextual underpinnings. Here, we draw on the Aristotelian definition that emphasizes the relationship between thinking, making, and doing or transdisciplinary practice, knowledge, process, and application. The term was a key cornerstone in Marxist philosophy that challenged philosophical criticism to focus on the goals of philosophy to interpret the world for the sake of change and not just for the sake of critical analysis [71].

For the purposes of the consideration of praxis as a feature of TDKPTs, one should think about praxis as a process unique to the TD form of inquiry that takes action, considers impact, analyzes through reflection, alters and revises plans, and then implements plans for future actions. The praxical orientation of

TDKPTs is not unlike what Kolb [58] refers to as the experiential learning cycle, one grounded in experiential learning as a cyclical process of concrete learning, reflective observation, abstract conceptualization, and active experimentation. Here, new experiences give way to personal reflection on how the experience affects the individual, and ultimately, abstraction and the application of new ideas into practice. This is an interplay between what some would refer to as the intersection of formal and informal knowledge, or that which is practiced and that which is experienced [59]. This process is one where different forms of knowledge from divergent sources are related and reintegrated so as to represent a co-created knowledge form that is the result of the interactions between different components within a complex system [8]. This reintegration results in evidence-based practical applications incorporated into scientific discourse. All the while this process also provides a means by which new ways of knowing and decision-making can be observed as the byproduct of a praxical approach [47]. This process can contradict implementation science that is based on linear planning processes like those often found in scientific management [72] that emphasize the product orientation of scientific inquiry for a more knowledge-based purpose for inquiry. Praxis provides the vehicle for moving beyond system knowledge [10]. It is the summation of the relationships and dimensionality of systems, target, and transformational knowledge states.

In many ways, praxis underpins how individuals and teams might embrace the transition from unidisciplinary knowledge to action-oriented transformational and applied knowledge that results in structural change. In light of the coexistent multiple perspectives that make up the transdisciplinary environment, praxis becomes the normative model for integrating multiplicity. Praxis assumes that theory and practice are related, and each should inform each other in reciprocal relationship. In itself the achievement of a praxical orientation to knowledge building is a type of transdisciplinary endeavor. Wickson et al. [37] state that transdisciplinary praxis "*should co-evolve to a point where they are integrated and/or resonant. How this process proceeds in practice is one of the integrative challenges*" (p. 1053) yet to be fully understood. However, it suggests that application and conceptualization are unified entities in the transdisciplinary process [73].

## 4 Interactive Systemic Complexities

### *4.1 Open Systems Capacity*

The wicked problem solving ability of teams rests on their capacity to operate as part of an open system [74] allowing for knowledge from sources outside system to permeate within the system and be considered alongside other types of knowledge. An open system presumes interactions with entities from outside of a group of bounded actors, ideas, and/or entities with the intended result of recirculating knowledge through outputs back into the greater environment. Open systems are receptive to the input of tangible elements like resources and materials as well as the actors and ideas that are part of the input–output relationship between bounded systems (disciplines, teams, organizations, knowledge sets, etc.) and its interactions with other entities outside of it [34]. The capacity to learn from this permeable environment and adapt behavior for better fit can enhance knowledge integration. Under these conditions, TDKPTs can integrate and synthesize disciplines by providing "*synthetic reconfiguration of available knowledge regarding the social, economic, and ecological conditions*" [75].

In an open system environment, team members must expand the range of considerations beyond traditional outlets one is accustomed to. As input into a system occurs, conflict, and power struggles between discipline-defined team members can emerge as traditional ways of knowing are challenged by the integration of approaches from outside system. Ideas and information are key environmental inputs in this kind of open system. When ideas and information are exchanged in a TD team, individuals' internal knowledge frameworks are challenged. This destabilizes the system and can lead to conflict. Engaging with the information, questioning one's own assumptions, reconciling with the limitations of the discipline, and finding ways to synthesize ideas toward the common problem, results in TD integration. These moments of tension and conflict are exchanges of information which represent "triggers" of new awareness [43, 44] that have the potential to bring about novel awareness related to knowledge development [61]. These energetic input–output boundary-spanning events highlight that TDKPTs "*consist of patterned activities of a number of individuals and the activities are complementary or interdependent with respect to some common output or outcome*" [62] even though they may seem to be unrelated to a common goal as they are being played out. This exchanging of energy between individuals (interdependencies) within the system leads us to be able to identify the exchanges occurring within and without a system [30].

A TDKPT working under these conditions deals with the challenge of including all necessary inputs. Such inclusion may foster and breed conflict, as the multiple inputs might require a team to behave in transparent and freely uninhibited ways. This feature draws our attention to the input–output mechanisms associated with all groups and organizations that must include knowledge from alternative sources and provide outputs that are targeted to multiple audiences. Here, input–output interactions strive to develop a new integrated perspective [62]. This is a highly nonlinear pattern as outputs of these interactions are a function of future inputs. wicked problem [69]. The state of the system is determined by the values of the inputs and outputs over time and in relation to the evolution of new problems within the same.

## 4.2 Different (Shifting) Levels of Reality

One of the trademarks of scientific inquiry is the ability to frame and identify problems in light of their context within an agreed upon conceptual lens and analytic strategy [76]. TDKPTs engage in inquiry that challenges this trademark based on the possibility that in doing so a series of divergent realities can be considered alongside one another. Nicolescu [64] describes the intersection of these sometimes oppositional or conflicting realities as a zone of nonresistance where human-based considerations like political, social, and individual realities intersect with natural realities like the environment, the cosmos, and physical law. This intersection is where exchanges in knowledge can flow freely [63, 64]. A systems perspective to complex problems includes experiences of multiple actors and approaches from a range of lenses that may suggest that multiple realities exist in problem solving depending on one's proximity to it. In addition, reality itself can be skewed based on one's disciplinary lens or even the level of comfort one has with the complexity of a problem. Complex systems display reality over a diverse range of timescales, environmental landscapes, and experiential episodes [8].

As adaptive complex systems themselves, the network of actors involved in TDKPTs will display change as different stakeholders interface with one another, adjust their own disciplinary perspective, and contribute to new and emergent realities as part of their problem-solving efforts. Simultaneously, shifts occur within these complex systems as they adapt to a changing environment and self-organize themselves [65]. This is necessary in order for the system to cope with its environment and in TDKPTs this adaptation brings teams closer to considering problems with a more holistic viewpoint. Change is at the heart of such systemic emergence and it is a constant state that requires adaptation as a constant function. TDKPTs must adapt to changes to their environment quickly, as they can only sustain themselves if at least part of the system changes at a slower rate than changes in the environment [8, 77, 78].

Complex systems like those represented in TDKPTs display behaviors that are a direct result of interactions between actors and the knowledge being generated. In other words, the goal of generating new knowledge is more dependent on processes of creating knowledge, even if measured using different or divergent realities, than solely the synthesis of existing knowledge. Emergence is key to this feature as the goal of TDKPTs is to develop holistic approaches that are not subject to the parts of disciplines that make them up but rather are the culmination of including multiple states of reality related to a problem. As such, the environment of these teams can be one of disorientation where the environment is a constantly changing reality requiring individuals to develop skills that are multidimensional and access multiple states of reality as perceived through different stakeholders.

### 4.3 Collaborative Deconstruction and Reconstruction

As teams work toward affecting new arrangements of knowledge in their problem-solving activities, new arrangements of collaborators and stakeholders emerge [37]. This is partly due to inclusiveness and partly due to the creation of novel approaches and insights that may not lie within the perceived boundaries of a given problem. This process of boundary spanning in the interpretation of the complexity of problems invites new relationships between stakeholders that may be unusual or novel either because of their novel disciplinary arrangement or because of the viewpoint they may bring to solving the problem [66]. Often, these unexpected relational arrangements are the result of involving those who are directly affected by problems to work along those who merely work to solve problems [54]. Such construction of relationships can often deconstruct others and create strong ties out of loosely constructed ones [79].

Active exchanges between professionals of different disciplines or even from the same traditions can develop into novel interdependencies [30]. As coordination and collaboration develop into new interdependencies between actors of the system, increasing complexity of these relationships can support a reordering of the collaborative functions between those who work together in the same team [33]. These relationships may become more asymmetric than equal as team construction becomes a reflection of the complex environment in which the team works adapting to complex arrangements of relationships through an internal dynamic process. Overall team structure is maintained even through the components themselves are exchanged or renewed [8].

Groups, where changes in relationships and the strengthening and weakening of ties is a normative activity, can make for a challenging team environment. The consequences of these dynamics in parallel with the shifting landscape of problems and their solution seeking processes can cause emotional strain to existing relationships as disciplinary communal ties are tested and reshaped. There may even be emotional stresses requiring stakeholders to reevaluate their dedication to a strain of thought and the relationships with stakeholders that constitute one's loyalty. Such shifts can result in dissension from one's previously espoused epistemological commitments and require mediation and reflective skills as team members adapt through recombination. Recombination is the process of taking existing compositions and breaking them down into constituent elements and recombining them to form new ones [80]. Such reorganization of one's placement in the system of knowledge often results in reevaluating team values and can result in modifying behaviors to better navigate these relational changes.

**Acknowledgements** Parts of this chapter were originally presented at the 2017 Systems and Complexity Science in Health for Healthcare Conference, *Embracing Complexity and Health: The Transformation of Science, Practice and Policy*, at the George Washington University, Washington D.C. This paper was published in July 2018 in *Informing Science: The International Journal of an Emerging Transdiscipline in a Special Issue dedicated to Communication in Transdisciplinary*

*Teams*, edited by the authors of this paper. The present chapter is a reprint of the original paper published in Informing Science.

Lotrecchiano G and Misra S (2018). Transdisciplinary knowledge producing teams: Toward a complex systems perspective. Informing Science: the International Journal of an Emerging Transdiscipline; 21, 51–74.

## The Transformative Aspects of This Study

The paper bridges the gap between theories of transdisciplinarity, theories of knowledge producing teams, and the practice of transdisciplinarity. Defining transdisciplinarity in real-life cross-disciplinary team settings is challenging. This is coupled with a dearth of in-depth longitudinal field research on these types of teams, widening the gap between theory and application. This paper brings us one step closer to closing the gaps between theory and practice by identifying the characteristics of TD knowledge producing teams using a complex adaptive systems lens. In doing so, it distinguishes between different types of skills needed for transdisciplinary knowledge production. The proposed constructs are highly relevant to several sectors including health sciences and medicine, where knowledge production is interlinked with collaborative behaviors and performance. Behaviors and skills necessary for effective team science are system issues and fall into the realm of complexity science as understood in this collection. The transformational aspect of the work therefore is one of bridging the contributions of different sciences to arrive at a more holistic systems perspective on knowledge production and identifying indicators of transdisciplinarity that can serve as variables in research on science teams.

**Take Home Message**

- Transdisciplinary knowledge economies are by nature interactive and functional team environments.
- TDKPTs are evolving environments that are adaptive and generate knowledge through adaptation and change.
- Features of TDKPTs are overlapping yet can also be the source of specific inquiry and measurement of team effectiveness and the target of skills development.
- TDKPTs possess features of complex problem solving, stakeholder involvement, methodological pluralism, praxis, open systems capacity, different levels of reality, and collaborative construction and deconstruction.

## References


1. Piaget J. The epistemology of interdisciplinary relationships. In: Centre for Educational Research and Innovation (CERI), Interdisciplinarity: Problems of teaching and research in universities. Paris: Organisation for Economic Co-operation and Development; 1972. p. 127–39
2. Gibbons M, Limoges C, Nowotney H, Schwartzman S, Scott P, Trow M. The new production of knowledge: the dynamics of science and research in contemporary societies. London: SAGE; 1994.
3. Klein J. Crossing boundaries: knowledge, disciplinarities, and interdisciplinarities. Charlottesville: University Press of Virginia; 1996.
4. Kockelmans J. Why interdisciplinarity? In: Kockelmans J, editor. Interdisciplinarity in higher education. University Park: Pennsylvania State University Press; 1979. p. 123–60.
5. Jantsch E. Inter- and transdisciplinary university: a system approach to education and innovation. High Educ. 1972;1(1):7–37.
6. Jantsch E. Toward interdisciplinarity and transdisciplinarity in education and innovation. In: Center for Education Research and Innovation (CERI). Paris; 1972.
7. Nicolescu B. Manifesto of transdisciplinarity. Albany: State University of New York Press; 2002.
8. Cilliers P. Complexity and postmodernism. Understanding complex systems. In: Sturmberg J, Martin C, editors. Handbook of systems and complexity in health. New York: Springer; 2013.
9. Klein J. Inter- and trans-disciplinary boundary work in collaboration science and translational medicine. J Transl Med Epidemiol. 2014;2:1024–30.
10. Hadorn GH, Biber-Klemm S, Grossenbacher-Mansuy W, Hoffmann-Riem H, Joye D, Pohl C, Wiesmann U, Zemp E, editors. Handbook of transdisciplinary research. Heidelberg: Springer; 2007.
11. Maxwell JA. Qualitative research design. Thousand Oaks: SAGE; 2005.
12. Brown V, Harris J, Russell J. Tackling wicked problems: through the transdisciplinary imagination. London: Earthscan; 2010.
13. Choi BCK, Pak AWP. Multidisciplinarity, interdisciplinarity, and transdisciplinarity in health research, services, education and policy: 2. Promotors, barriers, and strategies of enhancement. Clin Invest Med. 2007;30(6):E224–32.
14. Nicolescu B. Transdisciplinarity: the hidden third, between the subject and the object. Hum Soc Stud. 2012;1(2):13–28.
15. National Science Foundation. Convergence research at NSF 2018 [cited 2018 May 1]. Available from: https://www.nsf.gov/od/oia/convergence/index.jsp.
16. International Center for Transdisciplinary Research. CIRET 2018 [cited 2018 May 1]. Available from: http://ciret-transdisciplinarity.org/index_en.php.
17. UNESCO–Division of Philosophy and Ethics. Transdisciplinarity: stimulating synergies, integrating knowledge. Symposium on Transdisciplinarity in Royaumont Abbey. Geneva; 1998. Available from: unesdoc.unesco.org/images/0011/001146/114694eo.pdf.
18. Cooke N, Hilton M. Enhancing the effectiveness of team science. Washington, DC: National Academies Press; 2015.
19. Becher T. The counter culture of specialization. Eur J Educ. 1990;25(2):333–46.
20. Allan K. The social lens: an invitation to the social and sociological theory. Thousand Oaks: Pine Forge Press; 2007.
21. Graybill J, Dooling S, Vivek S, John W. A rough guide to interdisciplinarity: graduate student perspectives. Bioscience. 2006;56(9):757.
22. Klein J. Interdisciplinarity: history, theory, and practice. Detroit: Wayne State University Press; 1990.
23. Klein J. The discourse of interdisciplinarity. Lib Educ. 1998;84(3):4.
24. Burnes B. Complexity theories and organizational change. Int J Manag Rev. 2005;7(2):72–90.

25. Plsek P, Wilson T. Complexity science: complexity, leadership, and management in healthcare organizations. Br Med J. 2001;323(7315):746–9.
26. Wheatley M. Leadership and the new science. San Francisco: Berrett-Koehler; 1999.
27. Pirrie A, Wilson V, Elsewood J, Hall J, Hamilton S, Harden R, Lee D, Stead J. Evaluating multidisciplinary education in health care. Edinburgh: The Scottish Council for Research in Education. Edinburgh: The SCRE Centre; 1998.
28. Kuhn T. The structure of scientific revolutions. 2nd ed. Chicago: University of Chicago Press; 1970.
29. Lawrence P, Lorsch J. Organization and environment; managing differentiation and integration. Division of Research, Graduate School of Business Administration, Harvard University. Boston: Harvard Business School Press; 1967.
30. Thompson J. Organizations in action: social science bases of administrative theory. New York: McGraw Hill; 1967.
31. Dillon P. A pedagogy of connection and boundary crossings: methodological and epistemological transactions in working across and between disciplines. Innov Educ. 2008;45(3):255–62.
32. Huutoniemi K, Klein J, Bruun H, Hukkinen J. Analyzing interdisciplinarity: typology and indicators. Res Policy. 2010;39(1):79–88.
33. Maasen S, Lieven O. Transdisciplinarity: a new mode of governing science? Sci Public Policy. 2006;33(6):399–410.
34. Tress M, Tress G, Fry G. Potential and limitations of interdisciplinary and transdisciplinary landscape studies. Tress M, Tress G, Fry G, editors. Wageningen: Delta Program; 2003.
35. Lotrecchiano G. Complexity leadership in transdisciplinary (TD) learning environments: a knowledge feedback loop. Int J Transdiscipl Res. 2010;5(1):29–63.
36. Hammond R, Dubé L. A systems science perspective and transdisciplinary models for food and nutrition security. PNAS. 2012;109(31):12356–63.
37. Wickson F, Carew A, Russell A. Transdisciplinary research: characteristics, quandaries and quality. Futures. 2006;38:1046–59.
38. Fine H. Transdisciplinarity: trying to cross boundaries. Tamara J Crit Org Inq. 2007;6(3/4):16.
39. Lotrecchiano G. Leadership is as simple as a game of marbles: transdisciplinary, learning and complexity in fairies, keepsies and mibs. Integral Leadersh Rev. 2011;11(4): http://integralleadershipreview.com/3261-leadership-is-as-simple-as-a-childs-game-of-marbles/.
40. Morgan N. Notions of transdisciplinarity. In: Somerville M, Rapport D, editors. Transdisciplinarity: recreating integrated knowledge. Oxford: EOLSS Publishers; 2002.
41. Stokols D, Fuqua J, Gress J, Harvey R, Phillips K, Baezconde-Garbanati L, Unger J, Palmer P, Clark MA, Colby SM, Morgan G, Trochim W. Evaluating transdisciplinary science. Nicotine Tob Res. 2003;5(S1):S21–39.
42. Hagemeier-Klose M, Beichler S, Davidse B, Deppisch S. The dynamic knowledge loop: inter- and transdisciplinary cooperation and adaptation of climate change knowledge. Int J Disaster Risk Sci. 2004;5(1):21–32.
43. Blau P. Exchange and power in social life. New York: Wiley; 1964.
44. Buckley W. Society: a complex adaptive system. Essays in social theory. Amsterdam: Gordon and Breach Publishers; 1998.
45. Börner K, Contractor N, Falk-Krzesinski HJ, Fiore S, Hall K, Keyton J, Spring B, Stokols D, Trochim W, Uzzi B. A multi-level systems perspective for the science or team science. Sci Transl Med. 2010;2(49):1–5.
46. Lotrecchiano G. Social mechanisms of team science: a descriptive case study using a multilevel systems perspective employing reciprocating struturation theory. Washington DC: George Washington University; 2012.
47. Lang D, Wiek A, Bergmann M, Stauffacher M, Martens P, Moll P, Swilling M, Thomas CJ. Transdisciplinary research in sustainability science: practice, principles, and challenges. Sustain Sci. 2012;7(1):25–43.
48. Crowston K, Specht A, Hoover C, Chudoba K, Watson-Manheime M. Perceived discontinuities and continuities in transdisciplinary scientific working groups. Sci Total Environ. 2015;534:159–72.

49. Weisbord M. Productive workplaces revisited: dignity, meaning, and community in the 21st century. San Francisco: Jossey-Bass; 2004.
50. Entin E, Serfaty D. Adaptive team coordination. Hum Factors 1999;41(2):312–25.
51. Cannon-Bowers J, Salas E, Converse S. Shared mental models in expert team decision making. In: Castellan N, editor. Current issues in individual and group decision making. Mahwah: Erlbaum; 1993. p. 221–46.
52. Schwandt D. Individual and collective coevolution. In: Uhl-Bein M, Marion R, editors. Complexity leadership, part 1: conceptual foundations. Charlotte: IAP Publications; 2008.
53. Colditz G, Wolin K, Gehlert S. Applying what we know to accelerate cancer prevention. Sci Transl Med. 2012;4(127):127rv4.
54. Klein J. A platform for a shared discourse of interdisciplinary education. In: Fenner Conference on the Environment; September; Guadalajara, Mexico; 2004.
55. Nicolescu B. Towards transdisciplinary education and learning. Science & Religion: Global Perspectives—Conference. June 4–8, 2005; Philadelphia, 2005. Available from: www.metanexus.net/archive/conference2005/pdf/nicolescu.pdf.
56. Lamont M, Swidler A. Methodological pluralism and the possibilities and limits of interviewing. Qual Sociol. 2014;37(2):153–71.
57. Nicolescu B. Towards a transdisciplinary education. J Transdiscipl Res S Afr. 2005;1(1):5–16.
58. Kolb D. Experiential learning: experience as the source of learning and development. Upper Saddle River: Prentice Hall; 1984.
59. Horlick-Jones T, Sime J. Living on the border: knowledge, risk and transdisciplinarity. Futures. 2004;36(4):441–56.
60. Misra S, Stokols D, Cheng L. The transdisciplinary orientation scale: factor structure and relation to the integrative quality and scope of scientific publications. J Transl Med Epidemiol. 2016;3(2):1042.
61. Eldridge J, Crombie A. A sociology of organisations. New York: International Publications Service; 1975.
62. Katz D, Kahn R. The social psychology of organizations. New York: Wiley; 1966.
63. McGregor S. Demystifying transdisciplinary ontology: multiple levels of reality and the hidden third 2011 [cited 2018 May]. Available from: http://integralleadershipreview.com/1746-demystifying-transdisciplinary-ontology-multiple-levels-of-reality-and-the-hiddenthird.
64. Nicolescu B. Hidden third theory. In: Haverkott B, Reijntjes C, editors. Moving Worldviews Conference Proceedings. Leusden: ETC/Compas; 2006.
65. Heylighen F. Complexity and self-organization. In: Bates M, Maack M, editors. Encyclopedia of library and information sciences. New York: Taylor and Francis; 2008.
66. Balsiger P. Supradisciplinary research practices: history, objectives and rationale. Futures. 2004;36(4):407–21.
67. Bennett L, Gadlin H. Collaboration and team science. J Investig Med. 2012;60(5):768.
68. Roloff J. A life cycle model of multi-stakeholder networks. Bus Ethics Eur Rev. 2008;17(3):311–25.
69. Cilliers P. Complexity and postmodernism. Understanding complex systems. London: Routledge; 1998.
70. Larson E, Landers T, Begg M. Building interdisciplinary research models: a didactic course to prepare interdisciplinary scholars and faculty. Clin Transl Sci. 2011;4(1):38–41.
71. Engels F. Marx/Engels selected works. Moscow: Progress Publishers; 1886.
72. Taylor FW. The principles of scientific management. New York and London: Harper & Brothers; 1911.
73. Lotrecchiano G. A dynamical approach toward understanding mechanisms of team science: change, kinship, tension, and heritage in a transdisciplinary team. Clin Transl Sci. 2013;6(4):267–78.
74. von Bertalanffy L. General systems theory. Gen Syst. 1956;1:1–10.
75. Pregernig M. Transdisciplinarity viewed from afar: science-policy assessments as forums for the creation of transdisciplinary knowledge. Sci Public Policy. 2006;33(6):445–55.

76. Burrell G, Morgan G. Sociological paradigms and organisational analysis: elements of the sociology of corporate life. London: Heinemann; 1979.
77. Barnes M, Matka E, Sullivan H. Evience, understanding and complexity. Evaluation. 2003;9(3):265–84.
78. Nicolescu B. Methods of transdisciplinarity–levels of reality, logic of the included middle and complexity. Transdiscipl. J Eng Sci. 2010;1(1):19–38.
79. Simmel G. Conflict. New York: Free Press; 1955.
80. Kerne A. Doing interface ecology: the practice of metadisciplinary. International Conference on Computer Graphics and Interactive Techniques. Los Angeles: ACM; 2005.

# How and Why Effective Leaders Construct and Evolve Structural Attractors to Overcome Spatial, Temporal, and Social Complexity

**James K. Hazy**

## 1 Introduction

Understanding how to succeed in an organization and to lead when needed are two interrelated skills that are especially salient for healthcare professionals during times of uncertainty. This article describes how individuals guide the emergence of efficacious organizing structures that facilitate coordinated action. By doing this, individuals enact organizational leadership that furthers the organization's purpose in ways that also further their own individual purposes.

### *1.1 Structural Attraction*

This chapter contributes the conceptualization of a new analytical framework called *structural attraction*. It uses a mean-field approach to describe how structures that have information and knowledge embedded in them bias and coordinate the choices and actions of individuals within population. They do this even as individuals pursue their own perceived self-interest in the context of efficacious cooperation with others who are like them. In a manner analogous to gravitation in general relativity, the information and knowledge embedded in physical and social structures are the "mass" that draws human activities toward the attractor. This bias creates order by making relevant events more predictable. In this way, *structural attractors* distort the spatial and temporal field of human interaction [1]. Observers see this as correlation patterns among individuals as they are drawn to the use of these structures: hospitals,

J. K. Hazy (✉)
Robert B. Willumstad School of Business Management, Adelphi University, Garden City, NY, USA
e-mail: hazy@adelphi.edu



J. P. Sturmberg (ed.), *Embracing Complexity in Health*,
https://doi.org/10.1007/978-3-030-10940-0_13

healthcare clinics, or firms, for example. "Structural attraction" as a social force arises in populations from the value of the information embedded in structure to those individuals who have access to it [2].

### *1.2 Value Potential as a Driver of Attraction*

The value potential of knowledge comes from its ability to make relevant events more predictable. By acting on this information, individuals expect to achieve greater benefit while also taking less risk. When the predictive value of an information signal encoded in the structure decreases, the distribution of individual choice across the organization become increasingly random and noisy. This background noise further exacerbates the confused and distracted conditions experienced by individuals who seek to decode the structural signals.

More precisely, we define *value* with respect to an outcome as an increase in the probability or expected value of that outcome (this benefit, called alpha, arises from the first statistical moment) or a decrease in variance (this benefit, called beta, arises from the second statistical moment) that the event will occur. Combined, these moments quantify the value of the attractor's signal as a predictor of a given outcome. Individuals make their choices in the context of the perceived value in this signal; structural attraction force flows from this value potential.

### *1.3 Overview of the Argument*

The chapter unfolds in four main sections. The first section shows how individuals experience more success (alpha) and lower risk (beta) by constructing models that take into account the implications of complexity. The second section identifies three types of complexity and describes the nature of structural attractors that individual leaders can construct to "simplify" choice and action in organizations. The third section describes how leaders use structural attractors to form communities and organizations and offers some caveats. The last section highlights key implication of this framework for research and practice.

## 2 Leaders Guide the Emergence of Structural Attractors

One of the key discoveries of complexity science is that in very complex environments, even ones that are apparently unpredictable in the fine-grain details, the observed outcomes that are relevant often continue to be predictable at the coarse-grain level. One simply has to peer through the complexity of the moment to see this. A river is a river, for example, and somewhere one has to cross. When viewed up close and only for an instant, the flow of water during a storm can be confusing and unpredictable, but this distracting fluctuation does not change the fact that a river is a river, until, that is, it no longer has the properties that define it as a river. Physical objects with a predictable benefit, such as a river, or a mountain pass, a freshwater spring, a highly visible landmark, or the Pole Star, make relevant aspects of lived experience predictable, at least in the short term. As a result, they "attract" activities toward them. These artifacts are "structural attractors" [3].

## 2.1 Human Agency and Structural Attractors

This article argues that life often seems simple because human beings have actively constructed structural attractors over the millennia to create collective experiences that are purposefully predictable. According to Goldstein [4], self-transcendent construction (STC) is the process of conceiving the bigger picture and actualizing that vision in the world. Managers do this by encoding the information from an abstract model into a locally experienced physical version of reality that can be accessed by those who possess the algorithms to decode it.

The notion of STC identifies the unique relevance of artifacts that past generations constructed over the millennia [5]: Today's human communities largely live in a constructed world of their own making. These constructions are prototype models that contain stored knowledge that at one time enabled effective short-term action in the world [2]. Human beings build and live in the safety and comfort of these interconnected and intermingled über-nests that were built by those who came before [6]. However, as robust and ubiquitous as they appear, these artifacts still exist within a more complex and uncertain physical world.

### 2.1.1 The Map (Model) Is Not the Territory (Reality): Three Types of Complexity

Complexity is ubiquitous because individuals cannot predict events as they unfold along three dimensions of complexity. First, they cannot predict where expected or surprise events will happen (spatial complexity). Second, they cannot predict when certain expected or surprise events will happen (temporal complexity). Third, they cannot predict who will take what action, follow or imitate which actions of others, or will believe whom about what (social complexity).

To act under complexity conditions, one needs a simplified "map" of the spatial territory, whether physical or conceptual, a forecast of temporal expectations about how events might unfold, and a playbook that clarifies how social interactions are expected to develop over time. All of these simplified "models" guide one's choices and actions over time—and influence the actions of others—even in the context of complexity. However, the map is not the territory. The next three sections describe how leaders construct distinct types of structural attractors that resonate with aspects of simplicity on the other side of these types of complexity.

## 2.2 *Physical Structural Attractors (PSA) Simplify Spatial Complexity*

The most straightforward type of complexity is spatial. This means that surprising events can occur anywhere in an abstract space of multiple dimensions. This is not limited to physical space, but can also be associated with a mathematical space that supports an abstract economic or some other type of model. To illustrate, it is useful to consider the simple example of clearing and paving a highway to make travel by automobile easier, which is to say more predictable. One might observe that by constructing relatively straight and smooth roads one transforms the experience of travel into one that approximates a proportional cause and effect relationship between time and distance. Thus, although variations in terrain and uncertainty with respect to temporal events are complex, this basic human experience is simple in the abstract, as simple as getting into a car, driving an hour at 50 km/h, and ending up 50 or so kilometers down the road. Human beings have constructed an environment that makes this thinking rational.

By clearing and paving roads and highways—and engineering efficient machines—one creates conditions where inputs of work or resources imply proportional levels of specific outcomes. One can therefore compare approaches and select the most efficient one. Thus, when one paves the road, builds a bridge, or bores a tunnel one is creating a predictable one-dimensional path through complexity from one point in space to another (at the coarse-grain scale of human activity). If one ignores traffic congestion and irrelevant details or "noise," then paving the road makes the travel experience very much the same at each point along the path. When an individual is sensing the environment, an object in the visual field is recognized because the observer is able to ignore details, implicitly assuming a type of native equivalence that is objectively present in the physical world. Similarly, in the context of the relevant outcome—a random variable intended to predict "travel time," for example—once a paved road is identified, on the human scale, one can safely assume that each point along it is "equivalent." By doing this, one is implicitly assuming translational symmetry along this path and, by Noether's theorem [7], that relevant coarse-grained properties are conserved everywhere along the path regardless of "noisy" local fine-grain events. This symmetry implies that within an acceptable range of error, one can assume away a good deal of spatial complexity at least along this one-dimensional path.

By paving more roads in a fractal pattern, starting from one's position, the entire space can eventually become "covered" with paths, and this fractal space can eventually be "closed" in the abstract so that travel experiences along a two-dimensional surface also become predictable. Crossroads become cities; these become metropolitan areas, and so on, as human imposed simplicity is scaled [8]. Average velocity connects distance and time in a proportional relationship that reduces temporal complexity for the "travel time" random variable.

Thus, although a model is not the territory, the territory can begin to act like the model if human beings export their simplified models into the territory for use by others. This STC results in structural attraction if a value potential field arises from improved predictability of specific relevant outcomes. This actionable simplicity objectively exists in the environment behind or on the other side of real-world complexity. The next section extends these ideas to another type of complexity and a distinct type of symmetry.

## 2.3 Dynamic Structural Attractors (DSAs) Simplify Temporal Complexity

The highway example demonstrates that human beings simplify their environment by developing conceptual models of the world that resonate with real-work symmetries and then build these abstract models into physical structures, like a road or a bridge that withstand local fluctuations. In this way, individuals transform and simplify their own experience and that of others. What had once involved living in an unpredictable and complex environment—with its surprising pitfalls, obstacles, twists, and predators—is transformed into a lived experience that is more predictable when connecting inputs to outputs. Predictability creates value and attracts individuals to them in order to participate in their use [2]. This idea of externalizing structural attractors also extends into other areas of experience and other types of complexity.

Temporal complexity relates to predicting exactly when events will happen. Uncertainty results because relevant aspects of unfolding time are not consistent with translational symmetry alone. Although to a certain extent, time passes with translational symmetry as the moments tick by, one like the next, in addition, many relevant temporal events unfold in cycles: periodicity drives daylight cycles, annual seasonal cycles, and lunar tidal cycles, and many related phenomena. Thus, although events unfold with temporal complexity, one can model time in the abstract under the dual assumptions that beneath some of this complexity there is localized translational symmetry that operates in resonance with longer-term periodicity described by rotational symmetry groups.

Humans who make use of rotational symmetry do so by developing models that help to make certain events more predictable. When an individual is physically sensing the environment, the auditory system recognizes when periodicity in air compression is recognized, the observer can ignore ambient noise, implicitly assuming a type of equivalence in the cyclic pattern in the temporal environment. Similarly, in dynamic environments generally, predictability exploits periodicity in the environment. Just as human beings construct translational symmetry into a physical highway system to simplify experience, in the dynamic case, human beings construct rotational symmetry into a dynamic structural "model" in the physical world—for example, the workday or work week—to make events more predictable over time. These self-transcendent constructions are dynamic structural attractors (DSAs).

To illustrate, consider those who live on a farm. If one individual works a little harder or uses extra seed (an increased input), a little more of a particular type of food (output) will result, within a probability distribution, in a proportional output level at a predictable point in time. Dynamic models of farms are constructed to provide signals about when, where, and how to plant, tend, harvest, gather, and safely store seed for the next season. The location and temporal availability of various crops are predictable because the growing cycle has the predictable simplicity of periodicity (the growing season) on the other side of temporal complexity. In contrast, as one forages in the wild, absent a DSA, even if one works a little longer, that person may or may not find more food. Furthermore, if one does find food, one cannot predict what and how much one will find. The constructed environment of the "farm model" makes human experience, including human needs and wants, predictable over time so that planning the timing and location of work can be coordinated with more precision. As long as those participating in the dynamic structure called a "farm" stay within the abstract dimensions of its construction, proportional cause and effect remains easier to predict. As in the case of highways, like the force of gravity, these simplifying constructions "attract" individuals to their use because they provide value potential for them: They make the achievement of their goals more predictable within the spatial and temporal environment.

More generally, dynamic structural attractors (DSAs) take into account periodicity in the physical world. They amplify and sustain an approximation of abstract rotational symmetry and by doing so they offer promised value as long as the "model" accurately reflects *and resonates with* the objective periodicity on the other side of real-world complexities, which is to say, the model only works if the underlying symmetry that it assumes is actually present in the environment. Thus, because some real-world events repeat themselves (e.g., sunrise, the seasons, flooding and weather cycles) in a certain sense, one can find this simplicity by focusing on the inherent rotational symmetry and ignoring details that might distract or perturb this discovered underlying simplicity on the other side of complexity.

To maintain this constructed simplicity, however, periodic forcing by individuals (i.e., knowledge-driven work) within the system-model is required to sustain resonance with actual rotational symmetries in the ecosystem. Individual must develop, share, and use algorithms to implement recursive operations that reinforce the cyclic simplicity in the models in resonance with periodicity in the environment. These self-transcendent constructions (STCs)—including iterative recursive operations that demand resources and work as inputs—result in dynamic structural attractors. The next section conjectures about a way to extend these ideas to potential symmetries within social network interactions.

## 2.4 *Social Structural Attractors (SSAs) Simplify Social Interaction Complexity*

Structural attraction would also seem to be relevant when individuals seek to predict the social interaction patterns of others. This article hypothesizes that norms are social structures that allow patterns of collective behavior to seem predictable. This predictability suggests potential value that might support the formation of social structural attractors (SSAs). To find simplicity on the other side of social complexity that would enable prediction, one must identify an analytical framework that suggests some symmetry group operation across some categories of social interaction—analogous to translational or rotational symmetry—that exhibits long-range correlation across a subset domain of the population over time.

In analogy with paving a road (PSA) or constructing and running a farm (DSA), an SSA would involve defining a subspace within social interaction space that, for some relevant random variable, has recognizable spatial and temporal symmetry across the population. In particular, one must identify a symmetry group operation on a particular domain associated with individual choices that supports an abstract model that predicts—that is, it provides a "path" through—the anticipated choices of others across a social network. The challenge is to identify the particular partition of the population that can serve as this beneficial domain. By analogy, when an individual is using smell or taste to scan the ambient surroundings for beneficial chemical agents versus toxic or innocuous ones, one must classify molecules as beneficial or not. Once classified into a category of beneficial agents, the observer can ignore other details, implicitly assuming a type of equivalence is present within the domain of beneficial agents. This article conjectures that symmetry in social choice may be based on an equivalence relationship among individuals who share a social identity [9, 10] and experience "generalized trust" [11]. This social choice symmetry holds due to an assumed equivalence across individual choices within a particular domain, but the domain itself may be specific to individual norms.

A potential mechanism that might enable this equivalence in the social interaction equivalence is an endogenously determined parameter called *social sensitivity* [12]. This parameter reflects each individual's tendency to "go along with what their neighbors are doing." Researchers [13] have shown that under certain conditions, a long-range correlation in the value of this parameter (that is, the tendency to, "just go along") can emerge across individuals in a social network and stabilize into two distinct phases. In one phase, which this chapter is calling the "social identity phase," there is a high probability that individuals will choose to cooperate with like others. In the other phase, which this chapter is calling the "autonomy phase," individuals choose to act independently across the population. During the social identity phase, there is a context for members to assume an equivalence across the domain of the organization's members with respect to the choice to go along with what others are doing. This would seem to imply that when an organization is in the social identity phase, each individual can effectively "trust" that an arbitrary "like-other" will "go along," i.e., cooperate, with and support him or her in pursuit of organizational purposes [14]. This opens the door to generalized trust [11].

The benefits that accrue from belonging to a community with a shared identity suggest that individuals would be attracted to participate in these communities. This attraction is conceptually similar to the well-documented tendency called homophily [15–17]. Individuals experience this "social structural attraction" as a sense of "belonging" to a "community" that is essentially an equivalence class of like-others who are aligned to provide mutual support. This implicit heuristic, what one might call a "norm of assumed interdependence" offers potential value to its members who believe that they can predict the behavior of others within such a community.

Individuals recognize the benefits of belonging to communities. In the abstract, they model SSAs as abstract organizations composed of an equivalence class of like-others along one or more normative dimensions. They then actualize these abstract models by constructing economic firms and institutions that encompass various types of PSAs and DSAs in the physical world. These firms and institutions provide benefit to their members by encouraging cooperative choices, coordinating action, and synchronizing iterative and recursive algorithms in ways that create value potential (both alpha and beta) for them in the world. The social identity phase tends to dominate the "autonomy phase" when "we" are in a better position to benefit from an opportunity than "I" am by acting alone. In other words, social identity dominates when potential value is available for those who participate and is the mechanism of social structural attraction.

## 3 Leaders Construct Structural Attractors

Individuals facilitate self-transcendent construction through actions that test one's expectations about the environment. Action is at root a search for predictability, a search for causal connection [2]. To find causal connections that are consistent across space and time, prototypical actions of a certain type must be comparable to one another along at least one dimension. This means that one must discover an underlying symmetry in the environment that implies equivalence between objects and events.

Individuals, "leaders," pave a more predictable pathway through an uncertain ecosystem by simplifying complexity across space, time, and social interactions. Once a "leader" has discovered and shared the better pathway, those who "follow" share in the opportunity to exploit the identified symmetry. Thus, leadership that "leads from the front" begins with potentially risky—but thoughtful—preemptive actions that probe the environment to identify cause and effect relationships. The generative process of iterative probing, reflection, and experimentation, followed by the construction of a physical prototype, gradually builds a structural attractor [18]. Once constructed, followers can exploit these structures and leaders can exploit their attractive force to organize others as well as themselves.

Structural attractors contain the embedded knowledge that comes from thoughtful experience. This information is stored for the use of others and is available for use by members of the collective for their own advantage [2, 5]. This structural knowledge, developed though the reinforcing feedback of collective experience, influences individual choice and action as they become norms within the organization. This occurs through what Hazy [19, 20] calls "influence process structural learning." The norms that express this learning require generalized trust that the benefits to individuals that accrue from these facilitating structures outweigh their costs [15]. Generalized trust in like-others clarifies the predictability of social choice as individuals navigate the ecosystem such that, by acting in their own self-interest, they also serve the organization's purposes.

### *3.1 While Structural Attractors Are Fragile, Dissipative Structures Are Emergent*

Finally, some cautionary observations are appropriate for individuals who would use structural attractors to organize the activity of others. Even though some aspects of experience appear to have underlying dynamic stability, the environment itself always holds the possibility of surprises along all three dimensions of complexity. Furthermore, any given organizing state can appear to be stable in a relatively certain or "fixed point" way, in a more complex or "periodic" way, and even in a very complex or "strange" way that is sometimes called "chaos." As systems switch among various states, some stable some not, a given system does not necessarily cross a clear boundary between stability regimes nor does it necessarily remain in a stable region. The boundary is not smooth and transitions can involve critical points such that change can be catastrophic: There can be a tipping point, a sudden change from one type of stability to the next. Change can be abrupt and unpredictable [21].

Furthermore, when a bounded system, like an organization, is under pressure from the outside, the system may respond by spontaneously changing its structure in ways that no one can anticipate or drive. The changes occur simply to alleviate pressure [22, 23]. These emergent "dissipative structures" release local tension, but do not necessarily serve the goals of the organization. In fact, these spontaneously forming structural attractors can channel choice and behavior in ways that run counter to overarching organizational purposes. An example of this would be the formation of corrupt subsystems within organizations [24].

## 4 Concluding Thoughts and Implications

Individuals can have a lasting impact on the direction of their organizations by identifying opportunities for simplicity on the other side of complexity, and through self-transcending construction, making their abstract model real in their organizations. Leaders can use structural attractors intentionally to clarify and amplify native simplicity in the environment. By doing so, they support the activities of other players in their organizations as they pursue their objectives. To summarize:

1. Individuals encounter spatial, temporal, and social interaction complexity that makes specific events difficult to predict.
2. To cope, individuals construct physical, dynamic, or social structural attractors that guide individual choice and action in order to achieve organizational purposes and by doing so, their own.
3. Structural attractors of three types, physical, dynamic, and social, exert a social attraction force due to the value potential they offer by making prediction more accurate for agents who choose to participate in the organization.
4. Just because a model enables prediction it does not imply there will be no surprises.
5. The model is not reality. Leaders must reinforce the models that work, and erase models that no longer work.
6. Sometimes structural attractors form to resolve local tensions and the attractive force of these structural attractors can run counter to organizational and individual purposes.
7. This process is iterative and never ending ... Return to (1) and repeat.

## The Transformative Aspects of This Study

This chapter suggests an analytical framework that allows researchers and practitioners to construct and use the emergent coarse-grain properties of human organizations to achieve individual and organizational objectives. It introduces a putative force called *structural attraction* that describes how coarse-grain organizational properties influence the choice and action of individuals in ways that result in consistent behavior patterns within populations. The chapter proposes that as individuals decode and use information signals encoded as the order in structures, a mean-field structural attraction force emerges that reflects a consistent biasing that affects the behavior of individuals. It describes three distinct types of structural attractors, each exploiting a different symmetry in the environment. Physical structural attractors exploit translational symmetry to reduce spatial complexity. By doing so, these attractors make physical action more efficient and predictable. Dynamic structural attractors exploit periodic, rotational symmetries that reduce temporal complexity and make iterative dynamic processes more effective and adaptive by improving their temporal predictability. Finally, social structural attractors exploit symmetry within social groups that share a social identity. This reduces social complexity by sorting people into formal categories as a means to make social interactions and task coordination within and among groups more understandable and predictable. Leaders can guide the construction of each of these attractor types from the fine-grain to the coarse-grain as a means to serve various individual and organizational purposes.

**Take Home Message**

- Individuals encounter spatial, temporal, and social interaction complexity that makes specific events difficult to predict. Leadership enables action by simplifying prediction.
- Structural attractors simplify prediction and by doing so create value potential that exerts a social attraction force that draws individuals to participate in the organization.
- Leaders construct physical, dynamic, or social structural attractors that guide the choice and action of followers toward achieving organizational purposes and by doing so, their own.
- The model is not reality and must evolve. Just because a model enables prediction does not imply there will be no surprises.
- Sometimes structural attractors form spontaneously through suboptimal fine-grain interactions that emerge to resolve local tensions; the attraction of these structural attractors can run counter to organizational purposes.

## References

1. Hazy JK, Backström, T. Human interaction dynamics (HID): foundations, definitions, and directions. Emerg Complex Org. 2013:15(4).https://doi.org/10.emerg/10.17357.b49794f57f1d3721cb1c501f05344d05
2. Sloman S, Fernbach P. The knowledge illusion: why we never think alone. New York: Riverhead Books; 2017.
3. Allen PM, Strathern M. Evolution, emergence, and learning in complex systems. Emergence. 2003;5(4):8–33.
4. Goldstein J. Emergence, creative process, and self-transcending constructions. In: Richardson KA, editor. Managing organizational complexity: philosophy, theory, and application. Greenwich: Information Age Publishing; 2006. p. 63–78.
5. Thomasello M. A natural history of human thinking. Cambridge: Harvard University Press; 2014.
6. Nowak M, Tarnita CE, Wilson EO. The evolution of eusociality. Nature 2010; 466(7310):1057–62.
7. Rehmeyer, J. Insights into symmetry. Science News Online, May 4, 2008. https://www.sciencenews.org/article/insights-symmetry?mode=topic&context=43. Accessed 14 Jul 2018.
8. West G. Scale: the universal laws of growth, innovation, sustainability, and the pace of life in organizations, and companies. New York: Penguin Press; 2017.
9. Fukuyama F. Trust: the social virtues and the creation of prosperity. New York: The Free Press; 1995.
10. Hazy JK, Silberstang J. The emergence of collective identity as a means for creating and sustaining social value. In: Goldstein JA, Hazy JK, Silberstang J, editors. Complexity science and social entrepreneurship. Litchfield Park: ISCE Publishing; 2009. p. 447–70.
11. Glaeser EL, Laibson D, Scheinkman J, Soutter C. Measuring trust. Q J Econ. 2000;115(3):811–46.

12. Mahmoodi K, West BJ, Grigolini P. Self-organizing complex networks: individual versus global rules. Front Physiol. 2017;8:478
13. Mahmoodi K, Grigolini P, West BJ. On social sensitivity to either zealot or independent minorities. Chaos Solitons Fractals. 2018;110:185–90.
14. Wang Y, Wang X, Zuo W-L. Research on trust prediction from a sociological perspective. J Comp Sci Technol. 2015;30(4):843–858.
15. Mcpherson M, Smith-Lovin L, Cook JM. Birds of a feather: homophily in social networks. Annu Rev Sociol. 2001;27:41544.
16. Zak PJ, Knack S. Trust and growth. Econ J. 2001;111:295–321.
17. Kossinets G, Watts DJ. The origins of homophily in and evolving social network. Am J Sociol. 2009;115(2):40550.
18. Surie G, Hazy JK. Generative leadership: nurturing innovation in complex systems. Emerg Complex Organ. 2006;8(4):13–26.
19. Hazy JK. Leading large organizations: adaptation by changing scale-free influence process structures in social networks. Int J Complex Leadersh Manag. 2012;2(1/2):52–73.
20. Hazy JK, Cürüklü B. Influence process structural learning and the emergence of collective intelligence. Collective intelligence. Boston: MIT; 2014. arXiv preprint arXiv:1406.7547.
21. Bak P. How nature works. New York: Springer; 1996.
22. Prigogine I. The end of certainty: time, chaos, and the new laws of nature. New York: The Free Press; 1995.
23. MacIntosh R, MacLean D. Conditioned emergence: a dissipative structures approach to transformation. Strateg Manag J. 1999;20(4):297–316.
24. Hazy JK, Lichtenstein B, Demetis D, Dooley K, Backstrom T. Notes on the complexity of corruption. Paper presented at the Academy of Management Annual Meeting in Atlanta on August 7, 2017.

# Physician Burnout: A U.S. Public Health Crisis in Need of a Socio-Ecological Solution

**Suzie Carmack**

> *We tell physicians to get more sleep, eat more granola, do yoga, and take better care of yourself. These efforts are well intentioned. The message to physicians however is that you are the problem, and you need to toughen up . . . We need to stop blaming individuals and treat physician burnout as a system issue. It affects half of our physicians, so it is indirectly affecting half of our patients.*
>
> Dr. Tait Shanafelt [1]
>
> *Chief Wellness Officer for Stanford Medicine*
> *Director of the Stanford WellMD Center and*
> *Associate Dean for Stanford School of Medicine*

## 1 Why I Care (My Personal Burnout Story)

Late one night, after I had taught two yoga classes, after I had put my children to bed, after I had written payroll checks to the instructors in my yoga studio, I sat down to work on finalizing a paper on well-being for the doctoral program I was in. My instructor was so disappointed in my prior draft that he made a point to call me to discuss the paper—saying that I really needed to learn more about well-being measurement tools if I was to call myself a well-being researcher. "*If we can't measure it, it doesn't exist*," he told me.

I had mixed thoughts about his assessment of my work. On the one hand, I knew I had a lot to learn from him. As the academic equivalent of a walk-on player

S. Carmack (✉)
George Mason University, Washington, DC, USA

Adjunct Faculty School of Integrative Studies, George Mason University, Fairfax, VA, USA
e-mail: Scarmac2@gmu.edu



J. P. Sturmberg (ed.), *Embracing Complexity in Health*,
https://doi.org/10.1007/978-3-030-10940-0_14

in my PhD program—a researcher who was not published—I was just beginning to discover what was expected in scholarship. On the other hand, I had over 20 years of experience in the field of well-being promotion—what I now know is called "grounded experience" in the qualitative research community. I had not yet connected all of the dots between my real-world experience working with clients as a yoga and movement therapist and integrative health coach, with my scholarship in health communication and well-being promotion. All I knew is that I had worked with a lot of people to solve their real-world stress, burnout, and work/life balance challenges—to help them to improve their well-being—and that I was being told by my professor (who was 10 years younger than me) that I better figure out how to define and measure well-being if I was going to hang my professional hat as a well-being promotion scholar.

So, knowing I had a lot to learn, and wanting to do this whole PhD thing the right way not the easy way, I sat down at 11 pm at night, after my regular responsibilities were concluded for the day, and got to work on the paper.

At the time, I had no idea how ironic this moment was. I was in the doctoral program in the first place because I wanted to learn how to promote well-being more effectively—through the science of health communication—and yet here I was jeopardizing my own well-being by pushing myself too hard with unrealistic demands on my time (i.e., pursuing a PhD as a single mom of three teenagers; owning and running a yoga studio; teaching classes and clients in my yoga therapy practice; presenting yoga teacher training workshops; and teaching courses at the university where I was earning my PhD as part of my graduate assistantship). At the time, I saw this all as quite normal and necessary for the mosaic of my life—I was trying to turn myself around professionally and personally after an unexpected divorce, and I had to support my family. I was also driven to excel, as a self-made geek who put herself through school to survive.

In the months prior to this night, I had spent the past several months trying to find, understand, and evaluate well-being assessment tools as per my professor's request. I unearthed an underworld of what I now call the "*Beauty and the Beast*" sides of well-being assessment. On the one hand, well-being assessment tools can measure the beautiful aspects of our lives and our well-being, such as thriving, flourishing, happiness, resilience, grit, hope, meaning/purpose, and joy. On the other hand, well-being assessment tools can measure the not-so-beautiful aspects of our lives and well-being, such as burnout, compassion fatigue, depression, and suicidal ideation. The more I looked at them and their respective questions, the more I realized that these constructs were not mutually exclusive—e.g., one can be depressed with suicidal ideation and still experience joy. One can have high meaning and purpose and still be burned out.

So, when I sat down at 11 pm to finish this paper—with the added heat of knowing it was due the next day—I decided to pull back and take an aerial view of all of these well-being assessment tools, and categorize them by their subjective or objective approach. Subjective well-being assessment tools are self-rated; they are completed by the individual to rate themselves. They are inherently vulnerable to subjective bias—our inability to see ourselves holistically and/or realistically. As humans we have innate tendencies to either over-criticize or over-glamorize our self-assessments; so, asking us to subjectively self-rate ourselves is complicated; where is the reality in the midst of our own perception of truth?

Objective well-being assessment tools are completed by some type of other—at the individual, local, regional, or national level. Our friend tells us "we look great today" or "we don't look so good"—informal and qualitative assessments to be sure, but objective well-being assessments nonetheless. A public health specialist analyzes our water to tell if it is safe or not safe for us to drink.

Together, these subjective and objective appraisals—whether qualitative or quantitative—form the full 360 degree view of our well-being. Here we can hopefully blend the best of both rating (assessment) worlds—we know ourselves well enough to know when we are and are not doing well (experiencing and/or having well-being) through our own subjective self-appraisals, and we pay attention to the people and organizations and agencies that are looking out for our well-being objectively—so that we know how well we are doing with respect to national trends, health guidance, and public safety.

After grouping these subjective and objective assessments, I realized how biased the well-being assessment world is to subjective analysis. There are many validated subjective well-being assessment tools; there are very few objective ones. This makes it interesting from a well-being promotion perspective: How was I to start taking a systemic approach to promoting well-being, when everyone is using different tools, everyone is defining it differently, and not everyone has the ability to be fully candid with themselves in their subjective appraisal and/or is open to candid appraisals from "others"? As a well-accepted axiom in the mental health community states, "the people who need the most mental health support are usually the last to know."

**All of this begs the question, if we are going to promote well-being, who gets to measure how well we are or are not doing that, and how do we measure our success?**

At that point, I realized I had the central premise for my paper—what would end up becoming a key chapter in my doctoral dissertation [2].

After I finished the draft, around 3 am, I felt pretty good about my ability to meet the professor's call to action for my paper. I had stepped up my social science game, and although I knew I had a long way to go, I felt like I could see a place where I could do what many of my more academically thoroughbred colleagues thought was functionally and phenomenologically impossible—that I could actually contribute to the health communication literature. This was what we think of as a good professional day in academia.

But then, as I got into bed, ready to get exactly 2.5 h in of sleep before I needed to get up to start another demanding day, I had a personal moment that was not pretty. It was a really, really bad day.

**I realized that I might be that very person I was writing about—that person that had a mental health issue who was the last to know.**

I decided to pull out one of the assessment tools on well-being that I had been avoiding looking at more closely in my analysis. It was an assessment of worker engagement and burnout. I knew that self-diagnosis does not yield "valid" results, and that it is never a great idea, but I was sitting there with the publicly available instrument and I figured it could not hurt.

"Why not fill it out myself?," I thought.

So I did.

And in that moment, at 4 am, I realized the irony.

I had burnout.

Yep, me, the well-being promotion scholar/practitioner.

Do you see the irony? If not, I will explain.

In the act of researching burnout, so I could teach people not to have it (i.e., promote their work/life balance and well-being through health education, promotion, and communication), I realized that I had it.

I had become my own subject.

After this moment, I had a lot of shame about the fact that I had committed my entire professional life to helping people to "optimize their work/life balance," and be more "happy peaceful and centered" as a yoga teacher ... and that I was burning myself out in the process of doing that. What was painfully true, and equally painful to accept, was that I really knew better about the importance of "*self-care*" and "*health behaviors*" that could mitigate and even prevent burnout.

Here is the really scary, ironic, and hard-to-admit part:

I was not engaging in the very healthy activities and habits that I knew from my grounded, empirical, and formative research to be preventative to burnout—because I was so committed to protecting other people from burnout and promoting those solutions to them.

This discussion leads me to the central point of this introduction—how I became fascinated with the idea that healers (people who help other people to be happier and/or healthier) can easily hurt themselves if they do not balance their desire to be of healing service with their own self-care needs. This fascination fuels my desire to promote well-being, but also challenges me to take a much different approach to it than I did prior to my doctoral work researching the beauty and the beast sides of well-being. Today I realize that there is great complexity in promoting well-being to populations that are in healing fields in general, and healthcare professions in particular. In their (our) desire to be of service, our work often asks a lot of us: sleepless nights to complete a shift, respond to an emergency, complete a continuing education activity, finish a paper, prepare a lecture, and analyze data. And, as part of our giving, healing role, we are expected to be of service without fail—to ensure the safety and well-being of those we are serving. We can't afford to fail those who we are helping; but at what point, in our accomplishment of the demands of our work, do we fail ourselves by ignoring own personal and quite physiological needs for self-care?

Now that you know why I care so much about the issue of burnout in general, and how it applies in healthcare settings in particular, I would like to walk you through a very specific discussion of physician burnout in the USA. I hope that the reader does not misconstrue my choice to discuss physician burnout as implying that this is the only healthcare provider role in need of burnout intervention. Instead, think of this discussion as one that begins a host of other discussions I feel we all need to have about other professionals in other healing fields—in traditional healthcare settings and in complementary and alternative healthcare settings, too.

This chapter will limit its discussion to physicians in the USA due to space demands, but this real-world discussion should not be limited solely to the USA. When I originally presented the content in this essay (in Fall 2017 at the 3rd International Conference for Systems and Complexity Sciences for Health at George Washington University), I was originally focused on data researched of U.S. physicians because I had only 5 min to present my findings within the confines of the conference's "TED-style" format. After delivering that presentation, I had many colleagues come up to me on breaks to share with me that this issue of physician burnout is also burgeoning in their respective host countries. Although I was personally glad to make some new professional acquaintances based on my talk, I am neither professionally nor personally glad to know that the problem is bigger than I imagined—and that, globally, it is getting bigger every year.

## 2 Defining the Problem: What Is Burnout, Really?

Before we review the rising prevalence of physician burnout in the USA, and before I offer a few possible solutions for addressing it from a socio-ecological point of view, I would like to first articulate what I/we mean by "*burnout*". Burnout is a term that is often used loosely in everyday speech, in everyday conversation but is much less known as an ideological construct. Making its study more complicated is the fact that like well-being, burnout is very complicated from a scholarly and investigative point-of-view: like well-being, burnout is defined and measured differently by different scholars. All of these scholars define burnout differently, and therefore measure it differently—which makes tracking it from an epidemiological point-of-view quite difficult both domestically and internationally.

Burnout is considered a life management disorder [3], but it is also closely related to work engagement. However, engagement and burnout are not mutually exclusive—similar to the ways that depression and happiness are not mutually exclusive. In other words, a person can be depressed and still experience happiness; a person can be highly engaged and still experience burnout.

Despite these complexities, the most popular definitions of burnout that are cited in the literature include the following. Burnout has been defined as a "*progressive loss of idealism, energy, and purpose experienced by people in the helping professions as a result of the conditions of their work*" [4] and there are three key characteristics of burnout: *physical and emotional exhaustion, cynicism, and inefficacy* [5]. Burnout is listed as a problem condition (Z-73) and life management difficulty but not as a psychiatric disorder in the International Classification of Diseases (ICD-10) [3].

Burnout is not to be confused with compassion fatigue, a separate construct that is measured differently and stems from different fundamental issues—but is experienced symptomatically in ways that present to the individual experiencing them in ways almost identical to burnout (i.e., exhaustion, feelings of distress, mood disorders, feelings of hopelessness, and overwhelm). Unlike burnout, compassion fatigue is considered a secondary post-traumatic stress disorder—it stems from a caregiver or clinician "taking on" the biopsychosocial effects of the stress of caregiving and/or the stress of those they are caring for, it is therefore considered a psychiatric disorder. One way to conceptualize the distinctions between burnout and compassion fatigue is to consider burnout as being grounded in professional identity questions such as "Why am I here?" Compassion fatigue is grounded in the body's inability to adapt to interpersonal demands of caregiver-related stress and/or prolonged bouts of caregiving.

Since they are not well-recognized by the general public as illnesses per se, and because "*no diagnostic criteria for burnout have been developed*" [6], it is quite possible that the alarming trends we see with regards to burnout are actually misinformed if not inaccurate. In other words, if we have not trained providers or the public in standard practices for diagnosis or self-disclosure, it is safe to assume that the prevalence rates we do see are at least inaccurate and at most woefully underreported. Moreover, in the cases of burnout we do know about and have measured, we have differences of scholarly opinion with regards to burnouts sub-constructs and their measurement, which only further dilutes our ability to track burnout epidemiologically at a public health level. And, since compassion fatigue and burnout present so similarly, we may not be seeing the whole compassion fatigue/burnout picture; we may be misdiagnosing one as the other and/or we may not realize both issues are present because we are only measuring for one of them (if at all).

## *2.1 Conceptualizations*

Asking the reader to at very least accept that there is great confusion surrounding what exactly it is we are or are not talking about when we refer to, discuss, or measure burnout, I will now highlight two measures of burnout which I feel are both pertinent and important for the reader's understanding of this chapter's overarching discussion of physician burnout. Although other measures (beyond those in this discussion) are also quite capable of helping to illuminate the prevalence of physician burnout, I have chosen to focus on the following two instruments for simplicity's sake. I also will admit both for the transparency that is needed for autoethnographic essays such as this and to alert the reader to the inherent bias I have with regards to these instruments that I have a personal connection and bias with regards to both of these instruments. The first was the instrument that helped me to discover I had burnout (as described earlier in this essay), while the second instrument was conceptualized by my colleague, friend, and former boss Dr. Anne Nicotera of George Mason University.

With full acknowledgement of these personal biases with regards to these measurements, I can now share why I have chosen to highlight these two measures for this discussion. First, as mentioned earlier there is a well-established notion in research that states "*if we can't measure it, it doesn't exist*." By understanding how something is conceptualized and measured, we can better understand the thing itself—because it tells us more about what that thing really is like and by default, what it is not. Second, I highlight these two measures of well-being to give the reader a small insight into the complexities of not only conceptualizing and measuring burnout, but to ensure that the reader can feel the full weight of what it means to say that approximately half of U.S. physicians are burned out today.

### 2.1.1 Maslach Burnout Inventory

The first measure of burnout pertinent to this discussion is the Maslach Burnout Inventory, selected both because of the rigor used to develop it and because of the ground-breaking work of its namesake Christina Maslach, who was instrumental (pun intended) in both giving "burnout" its name and in finding ways to actually measure it. In 1976, Maslach discovered in the process of conducting exploratory research into the ways that workers in healthcare and human service occupations coped with strong emotional arousal on the job that several workers were using a term that was also used to refer to drug use at the time—"burnout." Soon thereafter, other scientists as well as the public shortened the term, to what we now know is "burnout."

In an intriguing retrospective of the history of burnout, Maslach and her colleagues describe burnout as being more than an individual's issue, but one that emerges based on workplace relationships. She and her co-authors state that "*from the beginning, burnout was studied not simply as an individual stress response, but in terms of an individual's relational transactions in the workplace*" [7]. In Maslach's pioneering work, she discovered during exploratory interviews (qualitative research) that three common themes evolved which correlated with what participants were calling burnout:

- Exhaustion or feelings of low energy,
- Depersonalization or feelings of inappropriate professional cynicism,
- Inefficacy or feelings of low self-competence for work performance.

She then developed an instrument to measure for these themes, the Maslach Burnout Inventory (MBI) which is now well-recognized as being statistically valid. The MBI has been adapted over the years to the needs of several professions—including physicians most recently.[1]

[1]Because the MBI is proprietary, its questions cannot be included here.

### 2.1.2 Structurational Divergence Instrument

An alternate instrument that is publicly available and that offers a more holistic view of burnout is the structurational divergence (SD) instrument conceptualized and initially validated by Nicotera, Mahon, and Zhao [8]. As its name might imply, this measure does not examine burnout per se, but does describe the experience of structurational divergence—i.e., the experience of becoming caught in "*negative communication cycles resulting from the interpenetration of incompatible meaning structures*" [9]. Because structurational divergence is highly correlated with (predictive of) burnout, and because there are also strong statistical correlations between SD and role conflict, bullying, depression, and intention to leave (the occupation), as well as a negative correlation between SD and job satisfaction [8], structurational divergence offers anyone interested in conducting burnout investigations (for themselves, for physicians, or for anyone in or outside of the healthcare system) a more comprehensive and systemic view of the entire "burnout problem."

So, what is structurational divergence exactly? In layman's term, structurational divergence is one way to describe those moments that you are "caught between a rock and a hard place" and "feel damned if you and damned if you don't." (The reader may smile upon learning that these are actually two of the questions on the SD self-report scale). To understand structurational divergence as a construct it helps to put it into a real-world context. Imagine that your boss tells you that it is imperative that you are present for an important meeting, and you tell him you will be there (because you want to maintain the performance expectations of your role as well as your professional relationship with your boss and your colleagues). Then 5 min later you receive a phone call that you are requested by a family member to accompany them on an important and unexpected medical visit that has been scheduled at the same time as your important meeting. Your role as worker is at direct odds with your role as mother, sister, daughter, and/or caregiver, and you have a "structurationally divergent" moment on your hands.

Although the example above illustrates my own theoretical understanding and interpretation of this construct, and I have situated this example in a somewhat cliché'd "work vs. life" scenario, I feel it is important to emphasize here that structurational divergence can be experienced WITHIN either work and/or our lives: we often have multiple roles we play at "work" and at "home." And it is also important to emphasize that structurational divergence is not just about being overloaded by the multitude of demands these roles ask of us, it is the social norms that surround each of these roles and the cultural norms and expectations embedded within them that cause the trouble (i.e., incompatible meaning structures). When the expectations of our roles are at odds, we find ourselves stuck in the middle in that rock and hard space of structurational divergence.

Because the structurational divergence (SD) instrument was developed through a study designed for nurses, the instrument measuring SD has a clearly healthcare-oriented tone as shown in the following partial sample of questions from the SD instrument (survey). Participants are asked to rate the degree to which they agree with statements such as:

- Administrative procedures get in the way of what is best for the patient.
- I feel like I am "between a rock and a hard place."
- I am "damned if I do and damned if I don't."
- I feel like I am fighting "unnecessary fires at work."
- The concerns of the hospital/organization surpass the needs of the patient.

The reader is invited to see the full instrument as well as its rating scale in Nicotera, Mahon, and Zhao's article [8].

### *2.2 Glimpses into the Complexities of Burnout*

These two measures give you a small glimpse into the complexities of burnout. It is clear that there is real need for more comprehensive solutions for conceptualizing it, understanding it, and measuring it, so that we can more effectively track it and eventually address it. Still, we cannot let the messiness of its measurement get in the way of our pursuing clearer understandings of it as a construct in general, or its impact on physicians in particular. As we will see in the next section, physician burnout is an epidemic in the USA—one that calls for socio-ecological solutions.

## 3 The Crisis of Physician Burnout in the U.S. Healthcare System

As of 2018, U.S. doctors are more burned out and less satisfied with their work than the general U.S. working population. Both burnout and depression develop cumulatively and burnout peaks during residency [10]. According to Medscape's 2018 national study of over 15,000 physicians from 29 specialties, the highest rates of burnout occurred amongst critical care (48%), neurology (48%), family physicians (47%), and ob/gyns (46%) and internists (46%) (see Fig. 1). Interestingly, 40% of all physicians surveyed reported that they are both depressed and burned out, as indicated on Fig. 2 [11].

When viewed from a systems-perspective, physician burnout affects the individual, the organization, the community, and the healthcare system as a whole. Some scholars describe burnout not as an individual's problem, but as a systems-level issue. The individual experiences it, but it is caused by systems-level challenges that impact the individual.

For the individual physician, burnout can be experienced as job dissatisfaction, less altruistic values, broken relationships, and problematic alcohol use. Burnout also threatens providers' ability to improve patient outcomes, because burnout and medical errors are positively correlated. Physicians who are burned out have

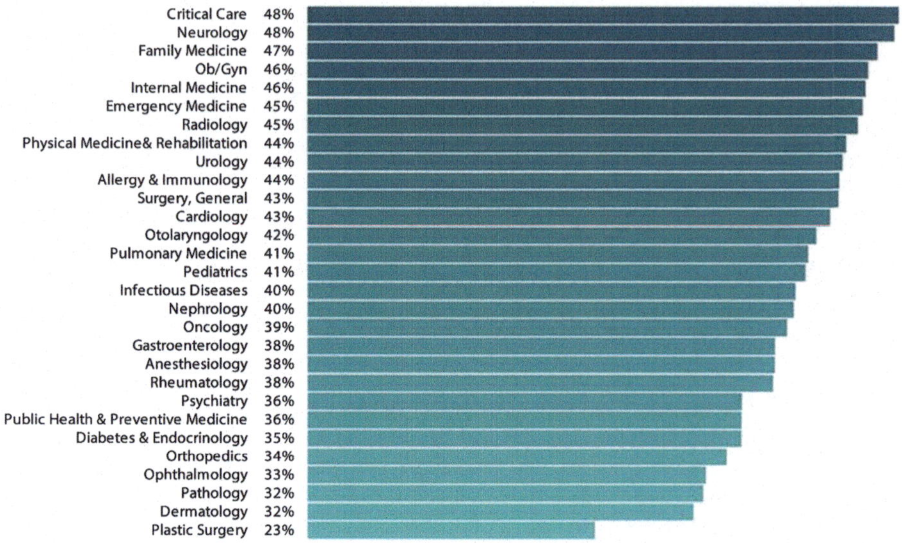


**Fig. 1** Physician burnout by specialty, 2018.
Source: Medscape (2018): National Physician Burnout and Depression Report

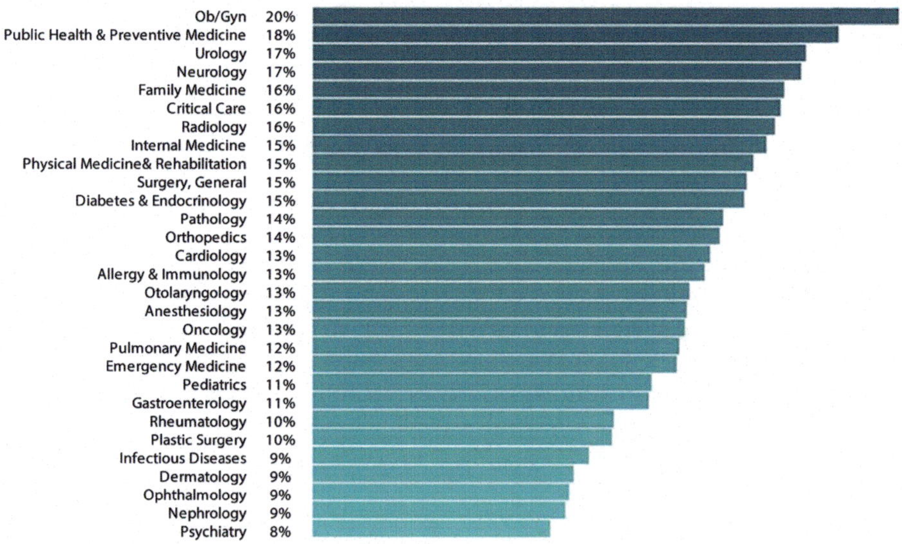


**Fig. 2** Physicians with both burnout and depression by specialty, 2018.
Source: Medscape (2018): National Physician Burnout and Depression Report

decreased physician empathy and increased physician unprofessional conduct. Not surprisingly, patients who are cared for by burned out physicians report lower patient satisfaction and have reduced patient adherence to their treatment plans [10, 12].

Like depression, burnout is also associated with suicidal ideation.[2] In the USA, approximately 1 doctor commits suicide every day—approximately 40,000 Americans commit suicide annually. Physicians have the highest prevalence rate for suicide relative to any other professional group in the general U.S. population—including the U.S. military—at a rate of approximately 28–40 per 100,000. Male physician trainees commit suicide at a rate that is 40% higher than that of U.S. men, while female physician trainees commit suicide at a rate that is 130% higher than that of U.S. women [13].

While these prevalence rates at the individual (physician) and interpersonal (patient–provider) levels are enough to qualify burnout as a U.S. healthcare crisis, physician burnout also makes a crisis-level impact at other levels of the socio-ecological model, namely, organizational, community, and policy levels.

At the organizational/healthcare delivery and practice level, burned out providers are less professional in their conduct [14]. They have decreased productivity, make more medical mistakes, and are more likely to engage in unprofessional conduct and disruptive behaviors [10].

At the policy and U.S. healthcare systems-level, physician burnout today causes a shortage of physicians tomorrow: the U.S. Department of Health and Human Services estimates a shortage of over 50,000 physicians in the USA by 2020 [10]. Recruitment costs to replace a physician are estimated to be $ 250,000 per physician [14].

## 4 Solving the Problem: Proposed Socio-Ecological Solutions

When considering solutions for the future, it is helpful to look at how solutions posed in the past have or have not worked. Interestingly, a recent study examined burnout in primary care settings, with 422 primary care physicians in 119 practices and 1785 of their patients [15]. The study showed that there are four key variables that predict burnout, and these are closely linked to the socio-ecological model [16], as shown in Table 1.

This same study made recommendations for ways that practices can address burnout, which the authors call "making primary practices safer." They recommended three key solutions: "(1) Emphasizing information systems; (2) Promoting a culture of quality; and (3) Improving the hectic environment" [15].

While today (13 years later), the notion that information systems can improve burnout is being challenged (since many physicians and providers today blame electronic health information systems as a major source for their burnout [17]), the idea that improving the hectic environment and promoting a culture of quality are still relevant. Based on my grounded experience working with individuals and

[2] Author's note: depression and burnout are separate illnesses, and as with compassion fatigue, are not mutually exclusive.

**Table 1** Socio-ecological analysis of burnout predictors

| Socio-ecological model | Predictor of Burnout as per MEMO study |
|---|---|
| Individual level | Work control |
| Interpersonal level | Time pressure (time w/patients needed vs. available) |
| Organizational level | Organizational culture |
| Societal/Policy level | Work pace (including productivity demands) |

Adapted from: Krugg EG et al. Violence—a global public health approach. World Report on Violence and Health [16]

organizations (ironically, the same work that burned me out in ways described at the beginning of this chapter), I can personally see several ways that public health promotion and well-being intervention design can help address this physician burnout crisis—at least domestically (within the USA) and potentially internationally.

First, at the individual, interpersonal, and organizational levels, awareness campaigns in occupational settings—such as burnout and compassion fatigue awareness campaigns—can address the workplace organizational culture and work control variables that increase the likelihood of burnout. These types of campaigns can help physicians to be aware of their vulnerability to these health risks and help to prevent the likelihood that they fall prey to them and/or know how to treat their conditions adaptively if they discover they have them. These trainings can also include training in health communication practices, since there are seven pathways through which communication can lead to better health:

1. Increased access to care,
2. Greater patient knowledge and shared understanding,
3. Higher quality medical decisions,
4. Enhanced therapeutic alliances,
5. Increased social support,
6. Patient agency and empowerment, and
7. Better management of emotions [18].

Additionally, these trainings can include self-care and self-compassion education to help providers to not only express compassion to their patients more effectively but to also protect themselves from compassion fatigue [19].

## *4.1 Principles of Preventing Burnout*

Inspired by my own lived experience with burnout as well as the stories of my yoga and integrative health coaching clients, I have conceptualized, designed, developed, and disseminated two well-being promotion interventions aimed at helping individuals to both prevent them and/or manage them should the need arise. *Well-Being Ultimatum* [21] is a meta-intervention that empowers individuals to take a strategic and holistic strategy approach to the many dimensions of their daily lives and well-being: physical, financial, social, mental, purpose, and emotional. Participants are taught that through their commitment to daily self-care, weekly social support, and monthly services (help-seeking) they will be able to optimize their well-being strategically through the full continuum of surviving through thriving. Participants of the intervention are taught to be "strategic healers"—who recognize that in order to best care for others we must first care for ourselves and treat ourselves with self-compassion.

The second intervention, *Genius Breaks* [19], teaches participants to take mini-breaks of mindfulness, movement, and meaning (self-compassionate self-talk) throughout the work or school day. Whereas *Well-being Ultimatum* [20] is strategic in its approach to empowering individuals to transform their well-being over a 6- or 12-month period, *Genius Breaks* offers participants the ability to take mini-breaks throughout the work or school day in as little as 10 min. The intervention is inspired by research that indicates that both movement and mindfulness can improve physical, mental, and emotional well-being, while promoting and protecting longevity. The intervention teaches participants to engage in a "mindful movement vitamin" [19]—a kinesiology protocol which helps participants to know which movements to engage in daily in order to fight sitting disease while ensuring they have engaged in all three planes of motion.

The mindfulness and meaning dimensions of the Genius Breaks' "3M" Method add two other somatic dimensions to the experience of taking a regular stretch break. The mindfulness theme is practiced through simple breath strategies, so that participants do not have to feel as though they have to "go to a beach" in order to practice mindfulness. (Closing one's eyes and taking 10 deep breaths is a less indulgent but still beneficial alternative.)

The third "M" in the Genius Break Method (framework) is "Meaning." Participants are taught to take time during their Genius Break of mindfulness and movement to consider the meaning of the day's events, and to decide if and how they would like to reframe the meaning surround them. For example, a leader may feel overwhelmed by the difficulties of the day's demands, but upon reflection, reframe the difficulties as an opportunity for her team to rally their collective expertise and evolve. Participants in the intervention are taught to link their movement and mindfulness to a meaning framework, which I call the *Chakras of Communication* [19]. The framework includes 8 communication meaning themes, that are inspired by and adapted from the chakra system. Participants are taught to link movement to these themes in a form of stylized gesture, so that they are communicating non-verbally with themselves. When they put movement, mindfulness and these meaning things together, they have a system for moving through the blocks within their day and inside of themselves, and for reframing the stressors of the day into a new (and less stressful) narrative. I have seen their utility work both inside the yoga study (as a structure for cueing classes) and in the board room (as a way to redirect energy when I am facilitating an important discussion).

When practicing their Genius Breaks, participants learn the 8 Chakra of Communication themes—Respect, Gratitude, Commitment, Courage, Kindness, Insight, Community, and Consciousness—and how to link them to their body. This somatic approach enables each Genius Break to be more than just a mindfulness or movement break; it becomes an opportunity for each participant to feel as though they are in control of the way that they see their day—an important mechanism for either preventing and/or managing burnout and as a way to reconnect with themselves, their colleagues and their loved ones.

I designed both interventions—*Well-Being Ultimatum* (2015) and *Genius Breaks* (2017)—to make them easy-to-implement for the busy folks they are designed to help and easy-to-integrate for the organizations in which they work. Although neither intervention offers a turn-key solution for the physician burnout epidemic, anecdotal evidence (from my individual and organizational clients) indicates that both interventions hold great potential for helping to prevent physician burnout.

In addition to these individual-centric approaches to addressing the epidemic of burnout, workplace well-being campaigns at the organizational, community, and societal levels can also help to address organizational and professional culture issues, and help to raise awareness for needed policy changes for physician occupational expectations. Although residency hours have been addressed in previous policy mandates by the American Medical Association [21], these required changes have not completely solved the physician burnout problem. Additional changes can be made to occupational policies for physicians, similar to expectations in the aerospace (pilot) and emergency response (lifeguard) communities where breaks and "crew rests" are mandated to help these workers to sustain the high stress demands of their work.

## 5 Limitations

This discussion is by no means intended to have all of the answers for solving this healthcare crisis—domestically or internationally—but it is meant to stimulate a discussion that can hopefully lead to viable solutions generated in both the healthcare and public health contexts.

There are several limitations in this discussion that I feel the need to call out into the open. As mentioned previously, physicians are only one type of healthcare provider in the U.S. healthcare system who are burned out today; it is well-established that there is rising prevalence in other healthcare roles, especially in the field of nursing [22].

I also recognize the inherent limitation of taking on this discussion from an autoethnographic point of view; it is my own personal reflections on the causes of and potential solutions for an admittedly very complex systems-level crisis. Though the use of autoethnographic structure [23], I attempted to use narrative and personal experience to (hopefully) compel the reader to see beyond the numbers into the real world of its complexity—from its diagnosis to its intervention design to its prevention, treatment, and management. And while I admit freely that I am not a physician, I am a provider in the integrative health community dedicated to promoting well-being at all levels of the socio-ecological framework. I therefore know both through my own lived experience navigating through burnout and through my work helping individuals and organizations to do the same that it will take a concerted, collaborative, and calibrated approach to raising the public awareness about the complexities and impact of burnout if we are to be successful in treating it nationally and globally.

## 6 Conclusion

This discussion has provided the reader with both an individual- and systems-level understandings of the rapid rise of physician burnout prevalence in the USA, as well as an expanded understanding of how intervention and policy design might address it. Ultimately, I hope that my personal experience and narrative has helped the reader to see that burnout is not just an individual's problem it is a systems-level problem in need of socio-ecological approaches to its solution—through intervention designed to recognize its complexities through the continuum of formative research, conceptualization, design, delivery, message testing, and dissemination.

With the prevalence rates of burnout rising rapidly, it is important that we continue a systems-level awareness discussion that this chapter has hopefully contributed to. If we now know that one out of every two physicians has been identified as being burned out, and we also know that burnout is very difficult to identify, diagnose, and discuss—then perhaps the problem is even larger than we currently imagine. The time is now for us to look to socio-ecological solutions that address the crisis as a public health systems-issue that negatively impacts individual providers and patients.

## The Transformative Aspects of This Study

Since physicians have the highest burnout and suicide prevalence rates of any U.S. profession, it is important that we raise public awareness about its prevalence and start discussing systemic solutions. If we are to address this U.S. public health crisis of physician burnout appropriately, it is important that we understand the issue through the lens of the individual, the community, the organization, and the national healthcare landscape. This therefore challenges traditional thinking surrounding this often undiscussed yet systemically pervasive national issue, and begins with an overview of the complexities surrounding conceptualizing and measuring burnout, presented through the lens of my own lived experience discovering that I had burnout while researching it. After illuminating for the reader the difficulties of being inside of burnout, I then examine the impact of physician burnout at other levels on the socio-ecological framework: organizational, community, and societal. After examining the problem with this socio-ecological approach to systems-thinking, I then wrap up the discussion with possible solutions. I share two frameworks that I designed to prevent burnout and promote well-being that are informed both by my lived experience realizing I had them and inspired by my work as an integrative health (yoga and movement therapy) provider. Ultimately, I hope that through my open and candid discussion that I will raise the awareness of the public, patients, and providers of the prevalence of burnout and the importance of burnout prevention and treatment.

TAKE HOME MESSAGE

- Burnout 101
  - Burnout is not to be confused with compassion fatigue, although it is experienced symptomatically in similar ways by the individual.
  - Burnout is a systems-level issue, felt and experienced by the individual.
  - Compassion fatigue is a post-secondary stress disorder, caused by the repeated experience of "taking on" the stress of the people we care for.
  - Most scholars agree that burnout is a combination of exhaustion, cynicism/depersonalization, and inefficacy (low perception of professional self-competency).
  - It is difficult to know if you have burnout, compassion fatigue, or both, making its identification, diagnosis, epidemiology, and treatment difficult.
- Physician Burnout Today (2018)—A Public Health Crisis
  - According to Medscape's 2018 national study of over 15,000 physicians from 29 specialties:
    - U.S. doctors are more burned out than the general U.S. working population.
    - 40% of all physicians surveyed reported that they are both depressed and burned out.
    - Physicians have the highest prevalence rate for suicide relative to any other professional group in the general U.S. population—including the U.S. military.
  - When viewed as a public health epidemic through the lens of the socio-ecological framework, the impact of physician burnout is felt at all levels:
    - Individual: Job dissatisfaction, less altruism, less work/life balance, less empathy, higher depression, higher anxiety, and higher suicidal ideation.
    - Interpersonal Patient–Provider Level: Worse patient outcomes, lower patient satisfaction scores, and decreased patient adherence.

(continued)

  - Organization/Practice Level: Decreased productivity and increased medical mistakes, increased unprofessional conduct, and disruptive behaviors.
  - Societal/Healthcare System Level: Reduced patient adherence to treatment plans (means lower patient engagement and compliance), a predicted shortage of over 50,000 physicians nationally by 2020, and rising costs of replacing physicians who leave the field ($250,000 per replacement).

- Potential Socio-ecological solutions
  - Individual Level: Burnout and compassion fatigue awareness trainings, as well as self-care and self-compassion based interventions can help individuals to raise their health literacy with regards to burnout and its solutions.
  - Interpersonal Level: Burnout and compassion fatigue are both "quiet challenges" that can be difficult to talk about; however, social support has been positively correlated with well-being.
  - Organizational, Community, and Societal Levels: Workplace well-being campaigns can also help to address organizational and professional culture issues, and help to raise awareness for needed policy changes for physician occupational expectations.
  - Societal/Healthcare Systems Issue: Policy changes can be made to support and protect physicians, similar to expectations in the aerospace (pilot) and emergency response (lifeguard) communities where breaks and "crew rests" are mandated to help these workers to perform well despite high stress demands of their work.

## References

1. Shanafelt T. Physician burnout: Stop blaming the individual. NEJM Catalyst. 2017. https://catalyst.nejm.org/videos/physician-burnout-stop-blaming-the-individual/. Retrieved: 08/02/2018.
2. Carmack S. Making Sense of Well-Being: A Mixed methods study applying sense-making theory to explore the role of communication competence and social support in physical, emotional, mental and comprehensive well-being. Dissertation; 2014. http://mars.gmu.edu/xmlui/handle/1920/8841.
3. Ninnivaggi FJ. "Burnout": The indelicate reality of job exhaustion. Am Psychol Today. 2016. https://www.psychologytoday.com/blog/envy/201609/burnout-the-indelicate-reality-job-exhaustion. Retrieved: 08/02/2018.
4. Sanchez-Reilly S, Morrison LJ, Carey E, Bernacki R, O'Neill L, Kapo J, Periyakoil VS, Thomas Jde L. Caring for oneself to care for others: physicians and their self-care. J Support Oncol. 2013;11(2):75–81.

5. Maslach C, Schaufeli WB, Leiter MP. Job burnout. Annu Rev Psychol. 2001;52:397–422.
6. Bianchi R, Schonfeld IS. Defining physician burnout, and differentiating between burnout and depression-I. Mayo Clin Proc. 2017;92(9):1455.
7. Maslach C, Leiter MP, Schaufeli W. Measuring burnout. In: Cartwright S, Cooper CL. The Oxford handbook of organizational well being. Oxford, UK: Oxford University Press; 2008.
8. Nicotera AM, Mahon MM, Zhao X. Conceptualization and measurement of structurational divergence in the healthcare setting. J Appl Commun Res. 2010;38(4):362–85.
9. Nicotera AM, Clinkscales MJ. Nurses at the nexus: A case study in structurational divergence. Health Commun. 2010;25(1):32–49.
10. American College of Physicians Wellness Champion Report (2017). Physician wellness: Promotion and prevention. https://www.acponline.org/system/files/documents/about_acp/chapters/ut/16mtg/lopez.pdf. Retrieved: 08/02/2018.
11. Peckham C. Medscape national physician burnout & depression report 2018. https://www.medscape.com/slideshow/2018-lifestyle-burnout-depression-6009235. Retrieved: 08/02/2018.
12. Dyrbye LN, Massie FS Jr, Eacker A, Harper W, Power D, Durning SJ, Thomas MR, Moutier C, Satele D, Sloan J, Shanafelt TD. Burnout and suicidal ideation among US medical students medical student burnout and suicidal ideation. Ann Intern Med. 2008;149(5):334–41.
13. Goldman ML, Shah RN, Bernstein CA. Depression and suicide among physician trainees: recommendations for a national response. JAMA Psychiat. 2015;72(5):411–2.
14. Dyrbye LN, Massie FS Jr, Eacker A, Harper W, Power D, Durning SJ, Thomas MR, Moutier C, Satele D, Sloan J, Shanafelt TD. Relationship between burnout and professional conduct and attitudes among US medical students. JAMA. 2010;304(11):1173–80.
15. Linzer M, Manwell LB, Mundt M, Williams E, Maguire A, McMurray J, Plane MB. Organizational climate, stress, and error in primary care: the MEMO study. In: Henriksen K, Battles JB, Marks ES, Lewin DI, editoes. Advances in patient safety: From research to implementation (Volume 1: Research Findings). Rockville, MD: Agency for Healthcare Research and Quality (US); 2005.
16. Krugg EG, Dahlberg ZL, Mercy JA, Zwi A, Lozano R. Violence—a global public health approach. World report on violence and health. Geneva: World Health Organization; 2002.
17. Shanafelt TD, Dyrbye LN, Sinsky C, Hasan O, Satele D, Sloan J, West CP. Relationship between clerical burden and characteristics of the electronic environment with physician burnout and professional satisfaction. Mayo Clin Proc. 2016;91(7):836–48.
18. Street Jr RL, Makoul G, Arora NK, Epstein RM. How does communication heal? Pathways linking clinician-patient communication to health outcomes. Patient Educ Couns. 2009;74(3):295–301.
19. Carmack S. Genius breaks: Optimize your workday performance and well-being. Fairfax, VA: Body Doctrine Press: 2017.
20. Carmack S. Well-being ultimatum: A self-care guide for strategic healers—those who live in the service, leadership and healing of others. Fairfax, VA: Body Doctrine Press: 2015.
21. Gopal R, Glasheen JJ, Miyoshi TJ, Prochazka AV. Burnout and internal medicine resident work-hour restrictions. Arch Intern Med. 2005;165(22):2595–2600.
22. Nicotera AM, Mahon MM. Between rocks and hard places: Exploring the impact of structurational divergence in the nursing workplace. Manag Commun Q. 2013;27(1):90–120.
23. Vryan KD. Expanding analytic autoethnography and enhancing its potential. J Contemp Ethnogr. 2006;35(4):405–9.

# Part V
# Health Systems and Policy

# Organisational Relativity—Changing Our Perspective on Health and Health Care

**John Watkins**

## 1 Introduction

On the 24th of November 1859, Darwin's 'On the Origin of Species' [1] was published. This was the culmination of ideas that had been fermenting in Darwin's mind since he travelled on the Beagle as a Naturalist some 25 years earlier. By the late 1830s Darwin had formulated the basis of his theory of evolution but it would be a quarter of a century before it was formally released to the world. Nearing the 160th anniversary of this event it is important to reflect that Darwin himself made two observations, firstly he noted, 'survival of the fittest' and equated this to the well-known practice of selective breeding, whereby environmental change led to changes in survival potential and hence 'natural selection' of individuals with traits that gave them an advantage. His second, often overlooked, observation was the concept of a 'tangled bank'. During his long voyages in the Southern Hemisphere and particularly the Galapagos Islands, he noted not only the biodiversity of the fauna and wildlife compared to his home but also the variation between islands. Despite this biodiversity on land, the thing that caught his attention was the comparative paucity of species diversity and abundance of wildlife compared to the fertile Pacific waters lapping on the shores. Underwater, despite what one may interpret as a nutritionally impoverished environment, there existed a 'tangled bank' comprised of hundreds of species, each interdependent on the other, an ecosystem in secular equilibrium, the ebb and flow of populations dependent on each other—a food web, not a food chain.

J. Watkins (✉)
Centre for Population Medicine, Cardiff University and Public Health Wales, Cardiff, UK
e-mail: john.watkins@wales.nhs.uk; watkinsj8@cardiff.ac.uk



J. P. Sturmberg (ed.), *Embracing Complexity in Health*,
https://doi.org/10.1007/978-3-030-10940-0_15

## 2 Challenges to Darwin's Original Ideas

Despite a turbulent and often difficult birth, Darwin's concept of natural selection has remained a central theme through successive iterations. As time passed into the early twentieth century it was clear that the original Darwinian concepts needed to be modified. His theory, as first conceived, could not explain adequately inheritance of quantitative variation, such as eye colour, which is not driven by selection bias [2]. In addition, Darwin and Wallace knew nothing of the extent of genetic variation that existed within species [2]. In an attempt to accommodate Darwin and explain these emerging 'difficulties', the Modern Synthesis was developed, bonding together ideas from biology, the emerging field of genetics and palaeontology, the modern synthesis sort to blend Darwin's ideas of natural selection with Mendelian inheritance accepting that genetic variation was giving rise to quantitative variation [2].

The Modern Synthesis, despite its undoubted success in addressing issues of evolutionary origins and variation, was, in it's turn, unable to explain the unfolding knowledge of the latter decades of the twentieth century.

Findings flowing from the new science of molecular biology demonstrated that the genome was anything but what scientists at the time imagined, for example, the most developed species on the planet, us humans, had less definable genes, around 20,000, than some very lowly creatures, e.g., nematode worms, and much of our DNA did not appear to code for proteins, as Crick would contest in his central dogma. In contrast, we now know that the genome itself is an historical collection of DNA, partly made up of genes that code for proteins, a large proportion involved in functions of control and expression of genes and some parts that have viral origins, amongst others, from antiquity [3].

Rather than Darwin and Wallace's concept of survival of the fittest,[1] in relation to species, many genes have been conserved over billions of years and inherited independent of species survival, e.g., pax6 genes that code for proteins in the eye [4].

[1]On the origin of 'Survival of the Fittest', the origin of the expression 'survival of the fittest is probably not Darwin's, in that, he did not use this term in the first 5 editions of *On the Origin of Species*. There are only two sentences that relate to the notion:

*... the wolves inhabiting a mountainous district, and those frequenting the lowlands, would naturally be forced to hunt different prey; and from the continued preservation of the individuals best fitted for the two sites, two varieties might slowly be formed* (p. 86). and *But the utter extinction of a whole group of species may often be a very slow process, from the survival of a few descendants, lingering in protected and isolated situations* (p. 300). It was Herbert Spencer—philosopher, biologist, anthropologist, sociologist and prominent classical liberal political theorist—who first used the term: *This survival of the fittest, which I have here sought to express in mechanical terms, is that which Mr. Darwin has called 'natural selection', or the preservation of favoured races in the struggle for life* (Principles of Biology of 1864, vol. 1, p. 444).

Possibly the greatest discovery in biology, since Watson and Crick worked out the structure of the double helix of DNA and it's role in the genetic code, has been the increased understanding of the role of epigenetic changes in gene regulation. Epigenetic changes occur and accumulate throughout life and are transmitted beyond a single generation. These changes arise due to host environment interactions and are heavily influenced by individual behaviours [5], e.g., during the Second World War, as the war-torn Netherlands were annexed by the Germans, famine set in—'the Dutch hunger winter'—when much of the population starved to death. Interestingly, those pregnant women who survived this ordeal gave birth to children who themselves had problems with obesity in later life, this trait passing on in turn to their children. This is an example of how environmental/personal behaviour can have lasting phenotypical consequences for inheritance outside of classical Darwinian control.

## 3 Innovation, Variation, the Adjacent Possible and Complex Adaptive Systems

We now know that rather than the genome being the book of life it would appear to be more like a library, with individuals parts being defined as 'genes' and non-coding regions. These non-coding regions, rather than being 'junk', as first thought, now appear to have a role in gene expression and are the origin of some inherited diseases [3]. We are therefore drawn to the conclusion that DNA rather than being the all controlling centre defining a species, it is but a part of a complex adaptive system, a point to which we shall return.

Andreas Wagner in his wonderful book, *Arrival of the Species* [2], poses the question:

> ... where do innovations come from? ... where do the new variants come from that selection needs?

Wagner sets about answering his rhetorical questions by suggesting that '*life can innovate ... while preserving what works through faithful inheritance*'. Wagner looks at the genome and the proteome for that matter, like the mythical '*Library of Babel*' [2] in which exists an infinite number of copies of the genetic code. Any single genome, or protein coding gene, in this library will have multiple near neighbours differing from the original by a single nucleic acid base, these new 'books', will in turn, have near neighbours that they themselves will differ from, by a further single nucleic acid change. Wagner suggests that it is possible to 'walk' across this library, near neighbour, to near neighbour, slowly changing the genetic code, without changing phenotypical characteristics, or biological function, arriving at a distant place in the genomic '*Library of Babel*', whereby the genetic code may be different and individual proteins made up of different amino acid sequences but in phenotypical terms have little, or no, impact on form, or function. This natural variation in the genome can give rise to phenotypical variation which is neutral in terms of survival, or variation in characteristics that have their origins in a large number of genes, e.g., human height, human propensity to develop disease, etc.

The cover of Steven Johnson's best-selling book '*Emergence*' [6] headlines a number of questions, answered within its pages:

> ... why do people cluster together in neighbourhoods? How do Internet communities spring up out of nowhere? Why is the brain conscious even though no single neuron is? What causes a media frenzy?

to this we can add what causes the variation of life on earth? How do adaptations arise to fit an ecologic niche?

Johnson brings together three themes to answer these questions [6]; the variation that exists at all levels in the universe, the concept of the 'adjacent possible' defined by Stuart Kauffman [7] and complex adaptive systems and what they mean for biology, society and our place within it [8].

At its simplest Kauffman's 'adjacent possible' [7] is eloquently defined by Johnson, as

> ... a kind of shadow future, hovering on the edges of the present state of things, a map of all the ways in which the present can reinvent itself. ... captures both the limits and the creative potential of change and innovation.

Another way to look at this, from both the biological and societal perspective, is that any system or set of systems are peppered with variation, most of which confers, at any given time, little, or no, advantage. However, now consider some change in the environment that redresses the balance and perhaps confers an advantage for some variants over others, or alternatively, a new innovation arising. In this circumstance, some of those 'shadow worlds' that existed beyond the closed door to the 'adjacent possible' now become available and redress the balance in favour of one variation/adaptation over another. In the 'real' world people have traded goods ever since societies have existed, but it was the invention of, first the telephone, then the Internet and then Amazon and PayPal, that has allowed books to be traded instantly from one continent to another.

The third of Johnson's strands in '*Emergence*' [6], complex adaptive systems, were initially explored by Stuart Kauffman and the Danish physicist Per Bak when they were at the Sante Fe Institute [8]. They worked together for a number of years trying to come up with a consistent theory as to how the origins of life could have started from a complex mixture of chemicals that self-organised to a point of criticality. Ideas Kauffman would expand on in his book '*The Origins of Order*' [7], meanwhile Bak and colleagues [8, 9] published their seminal paper on complex adaptive systems. What Bak and colleagues [8, 9] demonstrated, using a very simple sand pile model as a metaphor for many complex adaptive systems (e.g., earthquakes, economic fluctuations in market value, punctuated evolution, etc.), was that such systems undergo avalanches of all sizes and scales which occur with a power law frequency distribution. From this work they concluded that in many complex adaptive systems the natural evolution of the system is to a point of criticality, with regions of relative calm and other areas at the point of collapse into chaos. In the sand pile analogy they describe and experimentally demonstrated, that when the sand pile reaches this critical point, the addition of more sand causes avalanches across a broad spectrum of sizes and timescales—small avalanches more common that large ones, periods of great turmoil are interspersed with periods of relative calm.

## 4 Fitness Landscapes and Organisational Relativity

Both Kauffman and Bak built on the work of Sewall Wright [10], who, in 1932, introduced the concept of fitness landscapes. In this concept, evolution by selection will, within a particular environment, select out those traits that impart a survival benefit. This benefit will lead to change whereby, over time, a species will evolve upwards to an optimal survival/adaptive peak. In a static landscape, with multiple peaks, the newly evolved species will be trapped at the top of its own local peak, unable to travel to higher, more suitable, vistas without travelling down into the adjoining valley and relinquishing some survival advantage. Both Kauffman and Bak see such a landscape, both in biology and society, as being constantly changing, like the surface of the ocean thrashing around in three dimensions. In reality, this seascape will be multidimensional and hence always at a point continual change in some direction. Bak has shown us that rather than being unique and unlikely to arise by chance, complex adaptive systems evolve naturally to this point of criticality [9], a point from which the system can change quickly in response to small perturbations in the fitness landscape. Sergey Gavrilets has explored this concept of high dimensional fitness landscapes and their role in speciation [11], whereby the interplay between environmental change genotypical and phenotypical variation leads to evolutionary flow across multidimensional fitness landscapes.

Recently Denis Noble, Emeritus Professor of Cardiovascular Physiology at the University of Oxford in the UK, in acknowledgement of Einstein, has coined the phrase biological relativity to evoke the same liberating vision of there being no universal point of reference in the biology of life, just as Einstein disposed of the universal reference frame for space and time [12]. Noble contests that there is no privileged position from which biology and life flows, the genome, in and of itself, is neither the conductor of the orchestra, or the blind watchmaker. Noble sees life as a whole and not just the sum of its parts, a complex interaction of the organism with its cells, its intracellular environment and its genetic code. Life playing out a constant complex dance between the environment, social networks (in their broadest sense—be they colonies of bacteria, or humans), organisms, cells and intracellular machinery. It is the environment and the reaction and interaction, of a species to its changes, that brings out life in all its diversity. This co-evolutionary development is in fact the underlying engine room of Darwin's tangled bank.

Gavrilets, writing with Vose [13], explored the explosion of diversity, adaptive radiation, that arises in a species that is rapidly growing and inhabiting a new ecological niche. It was just such an ecological niche, the Galapagos islands, that led Darwin down the road to the Origin of Species. Darwin's finches have long been the 'pin-ups' for the Origin of the Species and it was their apparent adaptations to niche environments that led Darwin and the generations of evolutionary biologists that followed, to put this down to rapid evolutionary change. However, as Andreas Wagner points out [4], the rate of change achieved by random variation and selection is far too slow to drive this diversity. Noble [12] in '*Dance to the Tune of Life*' cites recent work by Skinner et al. from Washington State University in which they explore the interaction between the epigenome and the environment and the role it may have played in contributing to the diversity in beak morphology in Darwin's Finches [14]. Skinner et al. found that between closely related individual species of finches there were a far greater number of epigenetic changes detected compared to genomic variation. This led the authors to speculate that it is the environmental impact on the epigenome that is driving change and this change may eventually result in permanent genetic sequence differences and not the other way around [14].

## 5 Complexity—A Science for the Twenty-First Century

The nineteenth century was the period of time when man reached the pinnacle of his engineering prowess, using the then known laws of physics, we were able to harness hitherto unimaginable power and drive the industrial revolution. The twentieth century was the golden age of reductionism, where we brought nature itself under man's control, we 'split' the atom and worked out the very elements of how life is organised. However, the twenty-first century sees the dawn of a new realisation that reductionist ideology, as powerful as it is, will not lead to a deeper understanding of how the world, from atoms to academies, works. This realisation will fundamentally change the way we think of ourselves and our place in the world. With the discovery of the DNA by Watson and Crick in 1953, people felt that it was only a matter of time before we were to gain the understanding required to cure many diseases, but the promise of the human genome has come and gone and we now realise that we need a deeper understanding of how the pieces we have discovered fit together. Our molecular level understanding of many chronic diseases today is like a metaphorical box of body parts, we could not possibly predict the splendour of a Mozart symphony from examining his body, and by the same token we cannot, at present, work out the complexities at play in the origin of disease. For example, one of the greatest health challenges medicine faces today is dementia, a disease responsible for the deaths of millions annually, as each year goes by we discover another 'gene' implicated. The difficulty arises in knowing: How do these 'genes' interact? Which are important? Where do we target? What are the implications of this action? Small steps are being made in answering some of these questions, e.g., Zhang et al. [15] using network theory. However, the challenges in our fight for health and triumph over disease do not stop there, in that, once we identify a target we need to discover and test the new drugs and treatments. For example, breast cancer, once thought of as a single disease caused by a single cancer cell line, is now known to be a much more complex set of diseases, often treated by combination therapies, which, in turn, moves us well away from either certainty in outcome, or optimization.

## 6 Implications

So what does this mean for the way we think about ourselves, our interactions with each other, the organisation of civil society, the organisation and delivery of health care, the way we think about diseases, the way we diagnose and treat conditions and the robustness and type of evidence we use on which we base our decisions. From a young age we are taught to think in a hierarchical way, food chains with pyramid structures, organisations with CEO's and commanders in chief, reductionist science that places the gene at the centre of health and disease, but are these concepts wrong? Much of this chapter has concentrated on exploring and dispelling a number of scientific 'givens'; the gene is at the centre of the control of life that leads exclusively to proteins, which in turn lead to phenotype and not the other way around, evolution moves by a slow process of random variation, etc.

We now know that food chains/pyramids with a top predator are not how life works; in reality, both society and predator/prey interactions are complex networks with essential nodes that are vital for survival—it may be the loss of the bee and not the 'King of the Jungle' that leads to the trophic cascade of a food web. Noble [12] has directed us to the realisation that there are no privileged positions in biology and the same can be said for societies. Cities and human endeavour are just as much ecosystems as those of biology and are no more predictable. Just like any other complex adaptive system, societies and a sub-organisational structure, like health care, are akin to Per Bak's sand pile model [8, 9], there will be areas of relative calm and some areas of instability, most societies are in this inter-land poised on the edge of chaos. Kauffman [7] contests that this poised edge gives systems the potential for maximum adaptability able to take advantage of changes in the fitness landscape [7, 8, 10] that allow access to the adjacent possible [6, 7]. Does this way of thinking have any evidence to support it? One can draw on a number of events in the recent past that have resulted in rapid change occurring in very short timescales: the fall of the Berlin Wall and the reunification of Germany, the Arab spring driven by mass communication outside of normal news and governmental channels. At its heart huge social change is being driven, not by slow footed top down governments but by highly connected citizens using social media, run on the same smart devices that have spawned Google, Amazon and Twitter, to name but a few. These devices have allowed unprecedented access to information, on-line market places and social interaction. No one would have predicted, not even 10 years ago that 'High Streets' in the UK would struggle for shoppers, or that historical left wing socially deprived communities would vote for right wing policies and politicians—Brexit and Trump.

Equipped with a new way of thinking about the world and its connectedness, at all levels, we should embrace this knowledge and learn the lessons from biology.

Man is not distinct from the ecosystem and our destiny, in health and disease, is part of and determined by our environment. Our cities and civil societies are complex adaptive systems that will evolve and emerge into futures that, by and large, we cannot foresee, or control. We need to learn from life that we need to innovate, embrace variation and adapt to change readily. There is no central control on life, or society, it is all a collaborative endeavour, emerging out of simple rules which we need to discover and define for ourselves.

**Acknowledgements** I would like to thank the organisers of the *3rd International Conference for Systems and Complexity for Health*, Washington, DC—October 2017, for giving me the opportunity to present the content on which this chapter is based and to Joachim Sturmberg for his hard work, dedication and guidance in allowing my ideas to come to life in print.

## The Transformational Aspects of This Study

In this chapter we have set out to explode the myth that simple solutions can be found to complex problems and that disease aetiology can be solved by simple behaviour change. We have sort to demonstrate that, as a product of our western culture and education, we erroneously try to solve problems we face in life, particularly in health and health care, by breaking them down into simple manageable parts and seeking solutions to these. For example, to solve long delays in an emergency room we put in place waiting time targets for patients to be seen, this action, in the UK, has resulted in a shortage of availability of emergency ambulances, as they are forced to wait outside hospitals, delaying handover, while those with the most complex health needs are ignored as being too time consuming to ensure targets are met. In reality, to this problem, a more holistic approach is required that not only ensures the availability of front line services but also changes in the population's health seeking behaviour and greater collaboration across and between public services and health care.

In addition, it is commonly assumed that we are able to make predictions about the evolution of a system going forward, such as health care and the future demands placed on it—in management terms, we assume we can gear supply to this predicted demand, hence maximising efficiency. The fallacy we highlight is the assumption that an adaptive nonlinear network, such as a health system, is predictable, yet we accept uncertainty in other aspects of life, such as the weather and to some extent the performance of financial markets.

Society has many of the features of a complex adaptive system e.g., who just a few years ago would have predicted that the UK would seek to leave the EU, or that Donald Trump would be the incumbent in the White House!

On the issue of predicting future demand, in numerical terms and gearing supply to match, there is an underlying assumption that demand is predictable and can be calculated using simple parametric statistics, where we can specify, for any data set, mean values with confidence intervals. The assumption that healthcare demand, for example, over time, is normally distributed following some linear process, giving a fixed output for any particular input is clearly false. In reality, health seeking behaviour is highly sensitive to multiple related factors and is highly sensitive to small changes in the parameters, e.g. a media story that life-threatening influenza is spreading in the population, or that a local service is in threat of closure. In reality the decision to consult the healthcare system is a complex mix of social, psychological and physical factors, driven by norms and peer pressure.

We need to learn the lessons from biology, outlined in this article, that complex adaptive systems evolve in unpredictable ways, with emergent properties, in order to cope with this, biology builds in surge capacity and resilience and does not necessarily have efficiency as its sole guiding principle. In public services and health care we would do well to recognise this.

**Take Home Message**

- The whole is greater than the sum of its parts, this cliché applies to human health and society as much as it does to biology.
- Health and hence health seeking behaviour is a complex interplay of biological, physiological, psychological, social and environmental processes.
- Disease presentation is a result of all these agents at play with causal relationships moving up and down in scale. For example, adverse events in childhood lead to changes in brain structure and function, which in turn lead to changes in mental health later in life.
- Pressing public health issues of today, such as drug dependency in adolescents, need a whole system approach, addressing the whole ecology of the illicit drugs industry; production, trafficking, drugs culture, etc., and not just concentrating on those affected.
- Individuals and organisations need to awaken to the realisation we live in a complex world and there rarely exists simple solutions to a complex problem, failure to recognise this can have unforeseen and sometimes catastrophic consequences.

## References

1. Darwin C. On the origin of species by means of natural selection, or preservation of favoured races in the struggle for life. London: John Murray; 1859.
2. Wagner A. Arrival of the fittest - solving evolution's greatest puzzle. London: Oneworld; 2014.
3. Carey N. Junk DNA. London: Icon Books; 2015.
4. Kozmik Z. Pax genes in eye development and evolution. Curr Opin Genet Dev. 2005;15(4):430–8.
5. Carey N. The epigenetics revolution. London: Icon Books; 2012.
6. Johnson S. Emergence. New York: Scribner; 2001.
7. Kauffman S. The origins of order. New York: OUP; 1993.

8. Bak P. How life works. New York: Springer-Verlag; 1996.
9. Bak P, Tang C, Wiesenfeld K. Self-organized criticality. An explanation of 1/f noise. Phys Rev Lett. 1987;59(4):381–4.
10. Wright S. The roles of mutation, inbreeding, crossbreeding, and selection in evolution. Proc Sixth Int Congress Genet. 1932;1(8):355–66.
11. Gavrilets S. High dimensional fitness landscapes and speciation. In: Pigliucci M, Müller GB. Evolution—The extended synthesis. Cambridge MA: MIT Press; 2010.
12. Noble D. Dance to the tune of life. Cambridge: CUP; 2017.
13. Gavrilets S, Vose A. Dynamic patterns of adaptive radiation. PNAS. 2005;102(50):18040–5.
14. Skinner MK, Gurerrero-Bosagna C, Haque MM, Nilsson EE, Koop JA, Knutie SA, Clayton DH. Epigenetics and the evolution of Darwin's finches. Genome Biol Evol. 2014;6(8):1972–89.
15. Zhang B, Gaiteri C, Bodea L-G, McElwee J, Podtelezhnikov AA, Zhang C, Xie T, Tran L, Dobrin R, Fluder E, Clurman B, Melquist S, Narayanan M, Suver C, Shah H, Mahajan M, Gillis T, Mysore J, MacDonald ME, Lamb JR, Bennett DA, Molony C, Stone DJ, Gudnason V, Myers AJ, Schadt EE, Neumann H, Zhu J, Emilsson V. Integrated systems approach identifies genetic nodes and networks in late-onset Alzheimer's disease. Cell. 2013;153(3):707–720.

# A Systems Model of HIT-Induced Complexity

**Craig Kuziemsky and Andrea Ghazzawi**

## 1 Background

Health information technology (HIT) is playing a key role in transforming the healthcare system into a collaborative patient centered system. However, unintended consequences (UICs) such as workflow, communication, or information entry or retrieval issues commonly emerge post-HIT implementation [1, 2]. Healthcare delivery is a complex adaptive system [3] and UICs occur because of a complex array of interactions between technology, users, organizational policies, and other situational contexts [4, 5]. Understanding the nature of these interactions and the manner in which they occur is a necessary first step to understanding and managing UICs that arise from HIT implementation.

While there is a history of using complexity science to study healthcare delivery, a criticism is that it has been used as a fad or descriptor for different healthcare delivery issues and not as a robust method [6]. Addressing that issue requires us to design systematic approaches for studying the complexity of a healthcare system and why and how this complexity leads to UICs. Many of the existing HIT evaluation models are static and fail to properly illuminate the complexity of how users, processes, and technology interact [7]. Complex adaptive systems and complexity science have been advocated for understanding HIT-induced complexity [8–10]. However, there is still a need to understand how to use complexity science to study HIT usage and UICs that emerge from it. A particular need is to understand how HIT-induced complexity evolves over time. While UICs occur and may be measured in the moment, they often are the result of ongoing interactions between people, processes, and technology [11, 12]. While models of UICs exist [13, 14],

C. Kuziemsky (✉) · A. Ghazzawi
Telfer School of Management, University of Ottawa, Ottawa, ON, Canada
e-mail: Kuziemsky@telfer.uottawa.ca; aghaz091@uottawa.ca



J. P. Sturmberg (ed.), *Embracing Complexity in Health*,
https://doi.org/10.1007/978-3-030-10940-0_16

a shortcoming with them is that they tell us about the occurrence of issues but not about the development of them [15]. Counts of incidents of UICs need to be complemented by observational studies that provide insight into the complexities of clinical practice and how UICs emerge from it [15]. Others have described how HIT-induced complexity is varied and that we need to understand both the degree of HIT-induced complexity (e.g., simple vs. complex) and how complexity issues develop over time [10, 16].

To develop evidence on how UICs occur we need to view healthcare systems as complex adaptive systems rather than mechanistic systems [17] and study HIT implementation issues from an upstream–downstream continuum [18]. This paper addresses the above need and uses a case study of a perioperative information system to study UICs and then develop a systems model of HIT-induced complexity.

## 2 Methodology

We use a case study of a perioperative system called the surgical information management system (SIMS) to develop an upstream–downstream model of HIT-induced complexity. SIMS was implemented across all perioperative areas (pre-admit unit (PAU), same day admit (SDA), surgical day care (SDC), operating room (OR), and post-anesthesia care unit (PACU)), of a multi-campus hospital in a major Canadian city. Other analyses of the case have been described elsewhere [19, 20].

### *2.1 Data Sources*

Two data sources were collected during the case study. First, we conducted 150 h of non-participant observations across all the perioperative areas and campuses. Second, eight semi-structured interviews and three focus groups were also conducted with different categories of users including anesthetists, nurses, and managers. Interviews and focus groups were recorded and professionally transcribed.

### *2.2 Data Analysis*

Figure 1 shows our analytical framework. Ash, Berg, and Coiera provided a framing of UICs classifying them as errors of information entry and retrieval, and communication and coordination [1]. We first analyzed our case data looking for UICs according to this classification. Second, we further analyzed the identified UICs using complex adaptive system concepts such as non-linearity, emergent behavior, and requisite variety [21, 22] to understand the context of the complexity of UICs and how they evolved from the interaction of people, processes, and

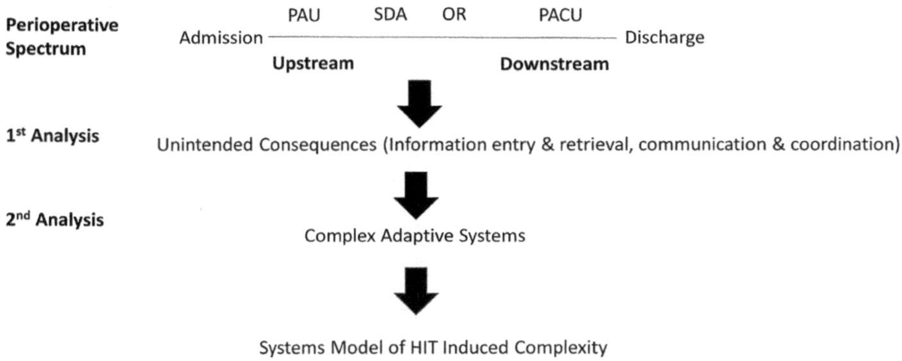


**Fig. 1** Analytical framework for UICs and complex adaptive systems

technology over time. Finally, we summarized our findings as a systems model for HIT-induced complexity that describes the upstream–downstream evolution of UICs and provides insight on how to manage them.

# 3 Results

## *3.1 Information Entry Issues*

Several examples of complexity in information entry tasks were observed. One example of information entry complexity was that although data entry tasks exist in all perioperative areas, the tasks were non-linear. After the SIMS implementation, users in some areas found the transition from paper to electronic to be quite manageable, while others struggled with the change and said the data entry workflow was much more difficult using SIMS. Further analysis identified that requisite variety was the primary reason for non-linear data entry issues. A specific example of requisite variety was the difference between a general patient assessment and data entry for a patient's specific case. Prior to surgery all patients receive a common assessment of overall health and other relevant data such as current medications and medical, surgical, and anesthesia history. Because this assessment was common to all patients a template could be built for it where data was entered category by category. In contrast, once a patient had their surgery, the data entry became tailored for a patient's specific case as surgeries could require data entry fields for drains, wounds, and external lines. While a post-surgical data entry template was created, anesthetists in the OR and nurses in PACU still needed to supplement the template with additional data to fit the patient's surgical context. Some users said adding the supplemental data added a lot of extra work as per the quote below:

*They're not really [patient] case-specific, they're more, you know, start the GA, for all cases. We tried to go generic, but they went middle of the road, not lowest common denominator, and, so that's ... You can get maybe sixty percent, and then the outliers, whatever, it's hard to Satisfy. You end up doing a lot of manual entry ...* Anesthetist

Other information entry issues were less predictable and arose due to emergent system behavior from both people and technology. An emergent issue nurses described was a change in the OR to PACU handover process. In the previous paper-based system, anesthetists provided nurses a written handover document, but post-SIMS implementation nurses described how some handovers were hybrid verbal-written handovers. Nurses described this as a substantial workflow change as the OR-PACU handover is busy and now they had to receive and manage the patient's IV's and other lines as well also having to process verbal handover data. Further analysis of the issue identified that the UIC was actually a data entry issue that originated downstream in the OR. One anesthetist described how he was not a good typist and could not type fast enough to fill in the discharge template during the short time transition between the end of surgery and transfer to PACU. Therefore, this anesthetist changed parts of his handover process to a verbal one.

Evolving technological complexity also led to data entry issues. One benefit of the SIMS system was that it supported direct interface and data uptake from some clinical machines such as heart rate and blood pressure monitors. Some anesthetists described this as a positive feature as it allowed them to focus on the wider array of clinical tasks rather than having to manually enter vital signs. However, automated data entry is not perfect and in the quote below by an anesthetist describes how over time they realized that automated entry was leading to artifactual data appearing in the patient record. Anesthetists had to adapt their data entry workflow to be cognizant of the issue to prevent artifactual data from becoming part of the patient's record. Deleting electronic data created additional workload as formal auditing purposes require a note made as to why the data was changed.

*But we know that that's an artifact. So, but there are mechanisms again to go in there and literally, physically, change the number that's presented to you with a little notation saying "That's an artifact." We have a screen, which is, again, a bunch of descriptors that just, you can put in there actually very quickly, saying "This number is artefactual." And it's not really the patient has become very, very hypertensive, or a very, very high heart rate, because there have been issues; it's a complete artifact. So, you know, I'm trying to prevent that sort of information from being captured, or not data mined, because it's artefactual* ... Anesthetist

## *3.2 Information Retrieval Issues*

Information retrieval issues were common as a patient's case data grow as the patient moves down the perioperative trajectory. Nurses downstream in the perioperative spectrum (e.g., PACU) were far more likely to encounter retrieval issues as there will just naturally be more data downstream in the spectrum. Some anesthetists recognized that nurses in PACU were having trouble finding the relevant data on a patient's case which could lead to important data being missed. To facilitate easier data retrieval some clinicians developed emergent solutions. In the quote below one anesthetist describes a workaround he uses to make sure the handover document from the OR to PACU was easier to read for the downstream users.

> *Well, that's what, when I deal with residents, I tell residents to put their preoperative assessment on the anesthesia record so that instead of just clicking off a bunch of anesthesia history and physical review, meds review, the allergy review, blah blah blah, they actually put in some meaningful information, like a little, like a little full of this, of pertinent medical issues, pertinent medications, pertinent—that we'll use. So in fact, in recovery, when the nurse it's the little note button, she can scan back and see a complete snapshot of that patient in two seconds ...* Anesthetist

However, in further analyzing the data retrieval issue we found that not all of the excessive patient data was necessary. Simple rules existed for how and when data should be entered on a patient but such rules were not always followed. Users found it very easy to just "click and enter" another data element and that led to more data entry points than were necessary. Further, when these simple rules are ignored early in the perioperative spectrum the excessive data ripples downstream to all subsequent data retrieval tasks. At one point a perioperative manager commented how she had to go to upstream users to remind them of the data entry rules.

> *I mean actually what we have to do with our staff in PAU is remind them that are standards for charting where this, because people just automatically chart everything. And it's like, you don't need to chart the patient's color every fifteen minutes if, unless there's a change. So, a few years back we were reminding people. Because it's all stuff that goes into the data, you know, so it actually clogs it, there's a lot of extra data ...* Nurse

## *3.3 Communication and Coordination Issues*

SIMS was implemented as a corporate system at all clinical sites and used across the entire perioperative spectrum. Thus, users assumed that data would pass seamlessly across the different perioperative areas. However, a UIC that emerged was that data transfer was non-linear and some data fields were not transferring across the different areas. This issue was not apparent right away but rather emerged over time as some clinicians began noticing inconsistencies in communication between areas.

> [In] *PACU, the nurses don't seem to have access to all the information in anesthesia manager that they could have access to. [...] Sometimes I've actually gone onto the PACU record and wanted to see if they could see what I was doing in the operating room and some of the things just aren't there. Some of the fields just aren't there. [...] The big key there is to know what you can and cannot see. That helps you out at least with the thinking process. 'Well they don't know that so it's not on there.' ...* Anesthetist

The same communication issue was also described when patients move from PAU to the OR. Patients would come into PAU on their day of surgery and disclose an allergy or some other data item relevant to their surgery. However, those data fields would not transfer into the OR system and thus nurses in the OR stated that they only found out about the issues when the patient arrived in the OR, resulting in a scramble to deal with the issue. In further analyzing the above communication issue, a number of emerging solutions were devised to deal with the issue. As described in the above quote, anesthetists in the OR began consciously tailoring their data entry based upon the fields that nurses in PACU would have access to. An emerging solution to the PAU-OR issue involved nurses in PAU phoning the OR to pass along relevant patient data.

The corporate design of SIMS was needed to standardize processes across the perioperative spectrum. However, one issue that emerged was between coordination at the individual and the unit level. At the individual level a common complaint was that SIMS added additional workflow to users and that it took longer to do clinical tasks than in the pre-SIMS paper-based system. Further analysis identified that not all of the workflow issues were technological issues but rather some were due to the corporate standardization imposed by SIMS. Despite its complexity, the basis for much of the perioperative workflow is simple rules by which a patient is assessed pre-surgery and then proceeds downstream for their surgery and recovery. One example is the recovery score that determines when a patient can be discharged from PACU. Pre-SIMS each campus had their own way of recording recovery scores but the corporate design created standards for these simple rules. While the rules for data entry of these concepts were straightforward and provide corporate coordination, individual users found it challenging in that they had to learn both a new IT system and a new process for doing recovery scores as described in the quote below.

> *So they weren't even all three using the same. And then the [] had a totally different recovery score that had been developed for them years ago in collaboration with anesthesia and a whole lot of other things. So that was a big learning curve for people, because it was one of the items that we had to take really corporate and redo. So that was something brand-new for some people. So if they're learning a new system, and now all of a sudden they have this new recovery score, so you're trying to teach them that at the same time …* Nurse

## 4 Systems Model of HIT-Induced Complexity

Figure 2 shows our systems model of HIT-induced complexity. The model summarizes the findings from this paper into an upstream–downstream model that defines four dimensions of HIT-induced complexity: temporal, policy, workflow, and connectivity complexity. The model emphasizes that we cannot think of HIT implementation as a static in-the-moment event. While specific tasks such as information retrieval or care coordination are done in the moment, these tasks will be impacted by downstream tasks and will impact upstream ones. Therefore, a first task in defining HIT complexity is to understand the upstream–downstream continuum where technology will be used. The more the clinical units and tasks that exist in the continuum, the higher the potential for complexity. The top part of the continuum

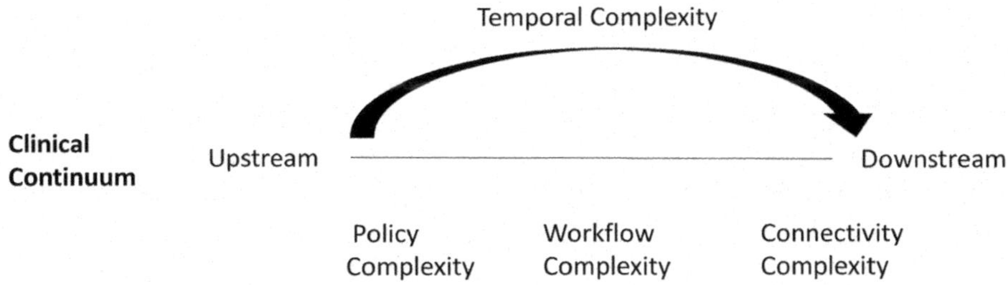


**Fig. 2** Systems model of HIT-induced complexity

highlights how there will always be temporal complexity any time that patient care is provided over time, as more patient data is collected over time it will lead to retrieval issues. Particular attention needs to be paid to information retrieval tasks that occur downstream as tailored solutions are required to support the increased complexity of downstream data retrieval tasks.

However, the natural course of time is not the only complexity factor from HIT implementation. Most of the UICs described in this paper were non-linear and resulted from the interaction or evolution of different components of the complex perioperative continuum. Policy complexity draws attention to the need to define the simple rules by which clinical processes are done and to ensure that people follow the simple rules when tasks are automated by HIT. We identified a UIC where users were having data retrieval issues due to excess data but complexity analysis identified that part of the excess data was due to people not following simple rules for when data points should be assessed and instead using the technical ease of "click and enter" to enter far more data on a patient than necessary. Policy complexity can also cause UICs due to the standardization of data across different care delivery units or settings. One example from our case study described how users had to learn both a new HIT system and a new way of doing recovery scores at the same time. While SIMS was blamed for having to learn a new recovery score approach, it was in fact a corporate policy issue and not a technological issue.

Workflow complexity refers the manner in which people's work practices will change because of HIT. Our case study identified numerous examples of workflow UICs including the change in handover from written to verbal and increased data entry burden because of the need to customize a data entry template for a patient's specific case. However, these issues are non-linear and only occurred for certain clinicians and patient cases. Workflow complexity raises the need to understand how work practices will change before technology is implemented so that appropriate training and data entry solutions can be developed. It also emphasizes that user training is more than just technical training on the system being implemented [19]. Training on supplemental skillsets such as typing or data retrieval must also be provided before HIT is implemented to minimize post-implementation disruptions due to issues such as typing deficiencies.

Connectivity complexity looks at the different ways in which people, processes, and technology connect as part of care delivery. Interoperability of healthcare systems is rarely linear and assuming that data will flow seamlessly through all areas can be a precursor to communication issues and medical errors. Our case study provided examples where key patient data was not being communicated across different perioperative areas. Worse, this issue was an evolving one that was only identified over time. Addressing this issue requires us to identify and conduct a hazard analysis prior to HIT implementation to define the requisite data that needs to be communicated across settings and to ensure that the data is able to be communicated appropriately.

We also need to consider specific contexts of the complexity dimensions and the UICs that arise from them. Some UICs are permanent such as clinical process changes due to standardization or data entry or retrieval issues caused by temporal complexity. While these issues cannot be eliminated, they can be managed proactively such as developing better data retrieval templates and dashboards to allow people to see relevant patient data in a concise summary form. Other UICs are temporary such as poor typing skills altering handover between units. But again, this issue requires proactive management such as training clinicians on ancillary skillsets such as typing prior to implementing HIT. Finally, complexity science also emphasizes the need to define the simple rules that define a particular context of clinical care delivery and to use these rules as the basis for establishing common ground across all users of HIT.

## 5 Implications

HIT implementation frequently causes a gap between users and technology. Complexity science helps us understand this gap by drawing attention to the interactions between people, processes, and technology and how these interactions evolve over time. It emphasizes that we cannot look at UICs in isolation but rather we need to look at both the upstream and downstream implications of them and how they evolve over time. Some UICs start upstream but evolve in complexity downstream due to the accumulation of data. Other issues emerged because users do not follow simple rules such as when certain assessments should be done.

Our paper confirms what others [23] have said in that implementing in health care cannot be done on a step-by-step basis because of the inherent complexity in healthcare systems. We also confirm what others have said in that complex health system issues must be studied using observational approaches and by eliciting details of clinical practice from the front line users [15]. However, our paper also addresses the call for more analytical approaches to applying complexity science approaches in health care [6]. Our systems model goes beyond just describing complex health system issues and provides a framing for how to study the occurrence of UICs along the dynamic upstream–downstream continuum where care delivery takes place. While the complexity of healthcare delivery prevents us from predicting the specific interactions that lead to UICs, our model enables us to make inferences about the likelihood of some interactions and the contextual circumstances of how they occur. Overall, complexity science provides an understanding of the nature of these complex interactions so we can proactively manage them.

## 6 Conclusion

Implementing HIT in complex healthcare settings is a significant challenge. While the complexity of healthcare delivery prevents us from predicting the specific interactions that lead to UICs, our systems model of HIT complexity enables us to make inferences about how certain interactions occur and the contexts where they occur. Our model helps us understand the complexity of HIT implementation and so we can proactively manage UICs.

**Acknowledgements** We acknowledge funding from a Discovery Grant from the Natural Sciences and Engineering Research Council of Canada and the Research Chair in Healthcare Innovation from the University of Ottawa.

## The Transformative Aspects of This Study

The research presented in this paper helps transform how we design and implement health information technology (HIT). It reminds us that health care is not delivered by technologies or models but rather by complex systems of people, processes, and technologies that are wrapped in unique contexts. Our ability to deliver healthcare outcomes such as safe, collaborative patient centered care will be dependent on our ability to account for this complexity in the policies, tools, and services we design to support healthcare delivery.

Complexity science enables us to look at the broader system where HIT is used and how it interacts with people, processes, and technology during healthcare delivery. HIT usage will not be equal across all providers or settings but rather it will be non-linear, perhaps even within the same organization, as was the situation in our case study. We also emphasize that HIT evaluation must go beyond simple models of technology adoption and include longitudinal evaluation of the emerging properties that will arise from the complex interactions between people, processes, and technology. Our research also transforms how we study HIT and its use in healthcare systems. We cannot just ask people about how they use technology or do a survey about what they like or dislike about a system. To understand the nature of complex system interactions we need to observe systems in their natural environment such as by using ethnographic approaches.

TAKE HOME MESSAGE

- Health information technology (HIT) implementation is a complex adaptive system.
- Unintended consequences arise because of a failure to account for the complex nature of interactions that occur between users, processes, and technology.
- We developed a systems model of HIT-induced complexity to help us understand the complexity of HIT implementation so we can proactively manage UICs.

## References

1. Ash JS, Berg M, Coiera E. Some unintended consequences of information technology in health care: the nature of patient care information system-related errors. J Am Med Inform Assoc. 2004;11(2):104–12.
2. Kuziemsky CE, Randell R, Borycki EM. Understanding unintended consequences and health information technology: Contribution from the IMIA organizational and social issues working group. Yearb Med Inform. 2016(1):53–60.
3. Sturmberg JP, O'Halloran DM, Martin CM. Understanding health system reform - a complex adaptive systems perspective. J Eval Clin Pract. 2012;18(1):202–8.
4. Coiera E. Interaction design theory. Int J Med Inform. 2003;69(2–3):205–22.
5. Kuziemsky CE, Andreev P, Benyoucef M, O'Sullivan T, Jamaly S. A connectivity framework for social information systems design in healthcare. AMIA Ann Symp Proc. 2016;2016:734–42.
6. Reid I. Complexity science. Let them eat complexity: the emperor's new toolkit. BMJ. 2002;324(7330):171.
7. Koppel R. The health information technology safety framework: building great structures on vast voids. BMJ Qual Saf. 2015.
8. Abbott PA, Foster J, Marin HDF, Dykes PC. Complexity and the science of implementation in health IT-knowledge gaps and future visions. Int J Med Inform. 2014;83(7):e12–e22.
9. Patrick Albert P, Lori TP, Miguel Noe Ramirez N. Health information technology: Anticipating, recognizing, and preventing disruptions in complex adaptive healthcare systems. In: Vaughan M, Deborah JR-L, Stephen RG, Wendy C, editors. Handbook of research on patient safety and quality care through health informatics. Hershey, PA, USA: IGI Global; 2014. p. 214–35.
10. Kannampallil TG, Schauer GF, Cohen T, Patel VL. Considering complexity in healthcare systems. J Biomed Inform. 2011;44(6):943–7.
11. Harrison MI, Koppel R, Bar-Lev S. Unintended consequences of information technologies in health care—An interactive sociotechnical analysis. J Am Med Inform Assoc. 2007;14(5):542–9.
12. Borycki E. Trends in health information technology safety: From technology-induced errors to current approaches for ensuring technology safety. Healthcare Inform Res. 2013;19(2):69–78.
13. Magrabi F, Baker M, Sinha I, Ong MS, Harrison S, Kidd MR, Runciman WB, Coiera E. Clinical safety of England's national programme for IT: a retrospective analysis of all reported safety events 2005 to 2011. Int J Med Inform. 2015;84(3):198–206.

14. Magrabi F, Ong MS, Runciman W, Coiera E. An analysis of computer-related patient safety incidents to inform the development of a classification. J Am Med Inform Assoc. 2010;17(6):663–70.
15. Coiera E, Ash J, Berg M. The unintended consequences of health information technology revisited. Yearb Med Inform. 2016(1):163–9.
16. Kuziemsky CE, Borycki EM, Kushniruk AW. Studying the HIT-complexity interchange. Stud Health Technol Inform. 2016;225:38–42.
17. Lipsitz LA. Understanding health care as a complex system: The foundation for unintended consequences. JAMA. 2012;308(3):243–4.
18. Kuziemsky CE. Review of social and organizational issues in health information technology. Healthcare Inform Res. 2015;21(3):152–60.
19. Kuziemsky CE. A model of tradeoffs for understanding health information technology implementation. Stud Health Technol Inform. 2015;215:116–28.
20. Kuziemsky CE, Bush P. Coordination considerations of healthcare information technology. Studies Health Technol Inform. 2013;194:133–8.
21. Widmer MA, Swanson RC, Zink BJ, Pines JM. Complex systems thinking in emergency medicine: A novel paradigm for a rapidly changing and interconnected health care landscape. J Eval Clin Pract. 2018;24(3):629–634.
22. Ellis B, Herbert SI. Complex adaptive systems (CAS): an overview of key elements, characteristics and application to management theory. Inform Prim Care. 2011;19(1):33–7.
23. Braithwaite J, Churruca K, Long JC, Ellis LA, Herkes J. When complexity science meets implementation science: a theoretical and empirical analysis of systems change. BMC Med. 2018;16:63.

# Salutogenesis Revisited

**Alonzo H. Jones**

## 1 Introduction

Some are looking for solutions to the complex problems with which we are all confronted, but most seem to get glassy eyed when more than two variables are discussed. Complexity is seen as impossible to understand so why bother. But we do live in a complex world and we need to try to understand it so that we can manage it better. We have written on the subject in the past: looking at how Craig Reynolds modeled flocking behavior we took his three rules and applied them to our society and our health [1]; looking further into health care and evolution we developed a nasal spray that optimizes our primary nasal defense system and when used regularly eliminates most upper respiratory problems [2]; and elaborating on the importance of evolutionary medicine we wrote of the paradigm shift from our current illness care model of medicine to the evolutionary model that supports our health by optimizing all of our evolutionary defenses [3].

### *1.1 Adaptation*

Others looking at complex systems continue to use our analytical model; they find help with big data and mathematical tools and models that help us find patterns in the attractors of our complex systems. It seems to me, however, that there is an added layer between the complex systems in the physical world and those of our own making. That added layer is adaptation. Adaptation is a characteristic of all living

A. H. Jones (✉)
Common Sense Medicine, Plainview, TX, USA
e-mail: drjones@commonsensemedicine.org



J. P. Sturmberg (ed.), *Embracing Complexity in Health*,
https://doi.org/10.1007/978-3-030-10940-0_17

organisms. It enables us, and every other living organism, to adapt to elements in our environments. Adaptation does not fit into our equations; it is emergent, novel, and unpredictable. It is on a different level. On a genetic level this adaptation is not purposive, but in the long-term natural selection gives it direction: survival and diversity.

Bacteria are the experts at adapting. If they are threatened they adapt to survive. If they are not threatened, but constrained in their spread so they cannot easily get to another host, they tend to adapt in a friendlier manner toward ways to live with their current host. This pattern permeates nature.

It also extends into areas other than genetics. Adaptation on a mental and social stage is purposive. Every animal constantly evaluates its environment and quickly decides whether an object is a threat or safe to approach. We do the same thing. These responses are a part of evolutionary psychology as described by Kahneman [4] and Haidt [5]—and it is, to some degree, predictable. These psychological researchers both point out that sensory input—which introduces our environment to us—goes first to the midbrain where threats are identified. The midbrain has a long history. In evolution it is first found in reptiles, which prompted MacLean [6] to call it the "reptilian brain." If a threat is identified here neural responses bypass the cortex and go directly to trigger what we call the fight or flight response. The fact that this response saved many lives in the days when our predators ate us has made it both strong and durable. Haidt uses the metaphor of the rider on the elephant, with the rider being the cortex and the elephant being the midbrain. It is a very accurate portrayal of their respective powers. But it also shows the limits, for while human responses to fear are more nuanced they are still mostly the tactical responses of fight, flight, or freeze. They all fit into the survival pathway of evolution. We need a way to open up the diversity pathway that adds strategy, novelty, resilience, emergence, increases both the health of the members and the system, and as the bacterial example suggests, helps us all get along better.

## *1.2 Evolutionary Perspective: Survival and Diversity*

Some are looking at complex problems from an evolutionary perspective. Darwin saw the two pathways: survival and diversity. But without understanding genes his explanations were cloudy. Diversity is best seen in the variety of organic life on the earth. The processes leading to it are seen on an evolutionary scale in the pattern of punctuated equilibrium. In genetic evolution periods of survival seem to oscillate with emergence. Cell walls, for example, got more defined in the archaebacteria, which enhanced their survival, and then organisms with these cell walls were able to protect and live with organisms—cyanobacteria—able to use light to create energy. The result of this symbiotic relationship was the plant kingdom and a boost to the oxygen in our life sustaining atmosphere.

A similar process occurred later when some bacteria learned to use the sugars and oxygen created by the cyanobacteria and the plants to make energy. In a similar symbiotic relationship with a larger bacterial cell they became what we know as the mitochondria—the energy producing part of every animal cell. This step, about 2 billion years ago, introduced the world of animals.

These two pathways—survival and diversity—are both necessary, but as anyone familiar with complex systems will tell you, the health of any living system is best seen in its diversity—much more than in the survival of its members. We know from bacterial behavior that a threat stimulates mutation rate. We know for human and animal behavior that threat and fear promote survival based resistance. It is entirely appropriate to ask how to stimulate diversity.

## 2 Salutogenesis

Salutogenesis is the study of what makes good health. Some people are just healthier than others and Aaron Antonovsky studied a group of them, mostly female Holocaust survivors, in Israel more than 40 years ago. He found that healthy survivors had what he called a sense of coherence, defined as:

> a global orientation that expresses the extent to which one has a pervasive, enduring though dynamic feeling of confidence that
>
> 1. the stimuli deriving from one's internal and external environments in the course of living are structured, predictable and explicable;
> 2. the resources are available to one to meet the demands posed by these stimuli; and
> 3. these demands are challenges, worthy of investment and engagement. p. 19 [7]

While the vagaries of life may be a bit more complex and unpredictable than Antonovsky's subjects thought it makes little difference. Salutogenesis is a sterling example of Thomas's theorem "*If men define situations as real, they are real in their consequences*" [8]. Antonovsky's three elements may be mostly mental advantages but salutogenesis has been validated in a questionnaire [9] which measures one's sense of coherence and is available for clinical practice.

A *sense of control* or *manageability* has some carry-over from understanding but is mostly related to how easily one is overcome by environmental stresses. It is closely related to one's financial ability to cope with these stresses. *Understanding* is related to how one sees the physical elements of one's world: as overwhelming and mysterious, or rational and understandable. *Meaningfulness* is how one relates to the environment and it is very much influenced by community support.

But with all due respect this is an analytical approach to a complex system and complex systems, by their very nature, defy analysis—especially when they are alive and able to adapt in totally novel ways. At the same time, however, the elements of salutogenesis point to conditions that are fundamental in evolution and thus of importance beyond the sociological perspective.

# 3 Bacterial Adaptation: Mastering Survival and Diversity

Bacteria clearly show the survival aspect of evolution as they ramp up their mutation rate in developing antimicrobial resistance when threatened with an antibiotic. But, as stated above and explained by Paul Ewald in the *Evolution of Infectious Disease* [10], if not threatened but constrained in their spreading—if the challenge is not life threatening—bacterial adaptation tends toward a friendlier commensalism. If they cannot spread to another host, as Ewald puts it, they must learn to live with the current one. An example of these processes has been demonstrated in the study of tooth decay and explored further in the next section. Other examples include cholera shifting to a less virulent strain when water is cleaned up and HIV morphing similarly when condoms are used regularly.

## *3.1 Tooth Decay*

Tooth decay begins from the action of bacteria that produce acids from their digestion of the sugars in our diets. The acids eat through the enamel surfaces of our teeth and a cavity forms. Many studies have been conducted to look at the effects of xylitol on this process. Xylitol is a five carbon sugar alcohol that is commonly used as a sugar substitute and has been well shown in the "Turku Sugar Studies" and others to decrease tooth decay when used regularly, and up to 80% when used five times a day [11].

One of the most interesting studies with xylitol was done in Belize where decay is rampant due to the plentiful sugar cane that is nice to chew on. The initial study was done on young elementary school children and consistent with others showed a xylitol benefit. However, the more interesting finding arose from a follow-up study—children had stopped xylitol and their teeth were re-examined 5 years later. Researchers found that the teeth that had erupted during the initial study had 90% less decay than their neighbors in the same mouth [12]. This long-term benefit shows the stability of the biofilm on our teeth and means that either the bacteria causing the decay are not there any longer or that they have changed to not make the tooth destroying acids. There are no other explanations. Consistent with this is a study done feeding xylitol to the predominant type of these acid producing bacteria that showed them to become "resistant" to xylitol in that they learned not to eat it [13]. But when they did they also stopped producing acids.

These are genetic adaptations in bacteria, and they are the experts in mutation. Individual microbes do not have a brain so the sociological notion of salutogenesis cannot be applied; however, they organize into biofilms, or communities of bacteria, and these communities behave just as do our human adaptive systems. We know microbes have a sense of control from their successes in adapting to our antibiotics, and a sense of understanding by selecting mutation sites. If meaning comes from community response the sharing of their successful mutations in plasmids with any other organism that needs it suggests that this element is present as well. They suggest that we really can, as Ewald argues, negotiate with bacteria by playing with their environment so that they are a challenge, but not a threat.

### *3.2 Cell Surface Adherence*

Nathan Sharon, an Israeli researcher who helped to show how bacteria attach to us, prosecutes the same argument. Attachment is a bacterium's first objective when it gets to a new host as if this fails it just gets washed out and there is no problem in the host. Attachment occurs to sugars and sugar complexes on our cell surfaces [14].

Sharon studied how *E. coli* attach. They are responsible for most urinary tract infections and they attach by holding on to mannose molecules which are plentiful in the genitourinary tract. Sharon argued, and he and his colleagues proved, that eating mannose regularly allowed the bacteria in the GI tract, which is the source of most infections, to bind with the dietary mannose and get washed out—they are no longer there to cause more infections [15].

Blocking adherence in this way applies the same pressure that Ewald sees in blocking transmission. In a very real way this negotiation is salutogenesis applied on a bacterial level. It is a win–win that enhances the health of both bacteria and host.

## 4 Salutogenesis Is Ubiquitous

While the survival aspect of evolution has been our focus for some time the things that make a system resilient—diversity, redundancy, and we add a sense of coherence—are equally important. They lead to better health. When living organisms are not confronted with an existential threat the challenges are those that fit into the salutogenic model (Fig. 1). They have time to play with their environment—a play that often leads to novelty and diversity, a play that often results in win–win outcomes. It is not just the door to good health for us; it is the doorway to the diverse, novel, and resilient adaptations that make all living systems healthier. We see this as the *simplicity on the other side of complexity*.

### *4.1 Salutogenesis on a Genetic Level*

Look at living organisms and see how they adapt. Bacteria are the simplest and one of the most studied. As Ewald points out, if they are not threatened, but constrained in their spread, and we add adherence, they adapt toward commensalism [10]—this is *salutogenesis on a genetic level*.

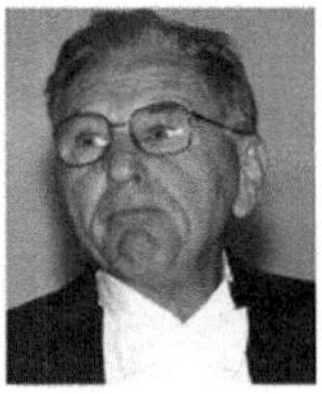

Aaron Antonowsky
1923-1994

**... is concerned with**
**the factors that support human health and well-being**
**the relationship between health, stress, and coping**

**... results from a *Sense of Coherence***
**# Comprehensibility**
**# Manageability**
**# Meaningfulness**

| **Adaptation - the Key for Survival** | |
|---|---|
| ***Salutogenesis at ...*** | |
| **# genetic level** | **bacterial become commencials** |
| **# memetic level** | **childhood development** |
| **# social level** | **addressing underlying causes of conflict** |
| **# business level** | **loose collaboration to develop radical innovation** |

**Fig. 1** Salutogenesis

### *4.2 Salutogenesis on a Memetic Level*

Memes have to do with the mental models we build to make sense of our world. It is what children, the archetype of adaptive systems, do as they grow, and it appears to have the same evolutionary pathways. No other organism adapts memetically into such a wide range of environments and cultures as a child. If they are threatened they can respond by fighting/biting, fleeing/copping out, and freezing, and even, as ignored orphans showed us, by dying. But if raised in a safe, caring, and enriched environment they tend to thrive—that is *salutogenesis on a memetic level.*

### *4.3 Salutogenesis on a Social Level*

Social evolution deals with mental memes rather than genes. It is much faster than genetic evolution but the evolutionary trends and the environmental conditions pushing them are similar. Memetic survival is akin to the existential survival seen with predator recognition and escape, but the memetic threat is to our ego or to our sense of self, which includes our belief systems. It leads to what Kahneman calls "System 1" or fast thinking [4]; threatening input is routed to the midbrain—Paul MacLean's "reptilian brain" [6]—and the responses are rapid. They saved our lives when we had predators that ate us, but they persist in us despite the lack of existential threats. Coming from the midbrain they are mostly those we see in reptiles: flight, fight, or freeze. They are tactical and reactionary; they are not strategic.

As such they have a military aspect. Kalev Sepp, who teaches Defense Analysis at the Naval Post Graduate School in Monterey, California, sees this pattern in our wars. In his historical study "*Best Practices in Counterinsurgency*" [15], he looks at insurgencies that have been fought over the past century and concludes that the empire tends to lose if the focus is only military—it becomes an existential threat that promotes resistance. But if the empire addresses the underlying issues they tend to win, and it is a win–win, it is not a zero sum game—it is *salutogenesis on an international social level.*

### *4.4 Salutogenesis on a Business Level*

When Lockheed-Martin needed more novel and creative solutions they created the skunkworks—that is *salutogenesis in business.*

## 5 Salutogenesis in Health Care

### *5.1 Infectious Disease*

Twenty years ago my wife Jerry and I played with xylitol to help prevent our granddaughter's recurrent ear infections. Xylitol draws water into the airway surface fluid that lays on top of the cells lining the nose and this added moisture optimizes our normal nasal defenses. It also, as discussed above, addresses bacterial adherence and brings into play the same constraints that Ewald shows come with preventing the spread of the infecting organism. It is negotiating with the bacteria in a war we cannot win. It is not threatening—it is *working with bacterial salutogenesis.*

### *5.2 Mental Health*

Tom Insel quit the National Institute of Mental Health (NIMH) 2 years ago because he saw the truth in a comment to his presentation on the work his institutes were doing: Dobbs [16], writing in The Atlantic (July/August 2017), tells the story:

> Around this time, Insel told me recently, he'd just finished a talk describing the wonderful things the NIMH was discovering about the brain when a man in the audience said, "You don't get it."
> "Excuse me?," Insel said. "I don't get what?"
> "Our house is on fire," the man said, "and you're telling us about the chemistry of the paint. We need someone to focus on the fire."
> "I heard that," Insel told me. "I went home and thought, There's truth to that. It's not just that we don't know enough. The gap between what we know and what we do is unacceptable."

Now he is fostering online communities of those with mental health problems using Google apps to predict crises and a professional who helps cope with them. That is *memetic salutogenesis.*

## 5.3 Hospital Practice

Curt Lindberg, beginning with the Plexus Institute and now at the Billings Clinic, uses positive deviance [17], a program that encourages employees to come up with novel solutions to company problems. As with skunkworks he creates a safe place to play, takes the experts who know the territory, and makes it meaningful with both colleagues and rewards—that is applying *salutogenesis to the business of health care and health care in itself.*

## 5.4 Salutogenesis in a Healthcare System

In any area where living adapting organisms are involved and we work to provide an environment that is safe and non-threatening—where we are in control, rich in elements with which to play—so we can understand them, and in a community of agents that share the challenge—and foster the sense of meaning—the outcome is much more likely to be creative, novel, diverse, and healthy for all adaptive organisms. This model is in practice in Singapore where everyone has control of their Central Provident Fund.

Paid for by individual and employer deductions, with other funds from government if needed, it can be used for health care, housing, and education, and it can be shared within the family. It goes a long way toward providing a sense of control. Putting these elements into the sandboxes of our lives helps us to understand them, and sharing the journey enhances meaning. Adding these elements to our healthcare systems makes for systemically healthy adaptations as we all continue to evolve (for more details see https://www.cpf.gov.sg/members).

# 6 Final Thoughts

Salutogenesis is working; it is part of what appears to be a universal law—we cannot stop it. But we can fail to give it support by focusing on survival and the profits to which it is so closely tied. Thomas Kuhn in his paradigm explaining monograph points out that the major hurdle to the acceptance of a new paradigm is a vested interest in the one it is replacing [18]. While we certainly are not against the dominant pathway of evolution we are confident that our collective survival is not at risk, except from our destructive abuse of nature—perhaps. But not from other agents and our translation of evolution into society and economy based only on self-interest and survival is misguided. The first step in supporting a new paradigm is to open our collective eyes and look.

**Acknowledgements** Much of this material and the ideas about children and their adaptations comes from my wife, Jerry Bozeman, a Registered Play Therapist Supervisor who has spent many years learning the language of a child's play so she can put it into words.

## The Transformative Aspects of This Study

We all live in a world with other living organisms, but the need to survive still dominates in our thinking. Existential threats abound, but they are existential largely because the amygdala of our reptilian brains makes them so. Sensory input to the amygdala is routed differently depending on its threat level. If the threat is serious our fight or flight response is triggered (to which should be added freeze). This response is powerful—it saved many lives when we had predators that ate us. This response center is akin to the elephant in Jonathan Haidt's metaphor, while our cortices—the parts of our brains that make us humans or *Homo sapiens*—are the rider on the elephant. It is an accurate portrayal of their respective powers. Shifting this emphasis on survival to the perspective that honors others and the resulting diversity is not easy, it requires us all to control the elephants in us, but it is the message of all the world's religious leaders. Salutogenesis tells us about the steps in the process:

- manageability—make the path (sandbox) safe for the elephant (the emotional midbrain);
- understanding—create the conditions for fruitful play, i.e., lots of familiar, and some new toys in our sandboxes;
- meaning—promote a rich social network and share the play.

**Take Home Message**
This is a paradigm shift in our thinking from survival (size, wealth, and power) to diversity (novelty, resilience, redundancy, and health). Like all paradigms it changes the way we see. But in this case we need both survival and diversity; they are both a part of evolution and they both have value. The problem today is that our focus has been on survival—we want to *Make America Great Again*. We don't see clearly the value of diversity—the pathway that goes through the human cortex—which can *Make America **Healthy** Again*.

## References


1. Jones AH, Bozeman J. The boids and the bees: guiding adaptation to improve our health, healthcare, schools and society. Phoenix: Emergence Press; 2009.
2. Jones AH. No more allergies, asthma, or sinus infections. Los Angeles: Freedom Press; 2010.
3. Jones AH. From microbes to models: how coping with ear infections led to a new paradigm. In: Sturmberg J, editor. Putting systems and complexity science into practice. Cham: Springer; 2018. A revised edition of this article is available online at http://commonsensemedicine.org/recent/defense-medicine-evolutionary-medicine-good-medicine/. Accessed 19 May 2018.
4. Kahneman D. Thinking, fast and slow. London: Penguin Books; 2011.
5. Haidt J. The righteous mind: why good people are divided by politics and religion. New York: Vintage Books; 2012.
6. MacLean PD. The triune brain in evolution: role in paleocerebral functions. New York: Plenum Press; 1990.
7. Antonovsky A. Unraveling the mystery of health - how people manage stress and stay well. San Francisco: Jossey-Bass Publishers; 1987.
8. Thomas WI, Thomas DS. The child in America: behavior problems and programs. New York: Knopf; 1928.
9. Antonovsky A. The structure and properties of the sense of coherence scale. Soc Sci Med. 1993;36(6):725–33.
10. Ewald E. The evolution of infectious disease. Oxford: University Press; 1994.
11. Peldyak J, Mäkinen KK. Xylitol for caries prevention. J Dent Hyg. Fall 2002;76(4):276–85.
12. Hujoel PP, Mäkinen KK, Bennett CA, et al. The optimum time to initiate habitual xylitol gum-chewing for obtaining long-term caries prevention. J Dent Res. 1999;78(3):797–803.
13. Trahan L, Bourgeau G, Breton R. Emergence of multiple xylitol-resistant (fructose PTS-) mutants from human isolates of mutans streptococci during growth on dietary sugars in the presence of xylitol. J Dent Res. 1996;75(11):1892–900.
14. Ofek I, Goldhar J, Zafriri D, Lis H, Adar R, Sharon N. Anti-Escherichia coli adhesin activity of cranberry and blueberry juices. N Engl J Med. 1991;324(22):1599.
15. Sepp KI. Best practices in counterinsurgency. Mil Rev. 2005;84(3):8–12.
16. Dobbs D. The smartphone psychiatrist. The Atlantic. 2017(June-July Issue)
17. Lindberg C. Guest Blogger: Curt Lindberg on Positive Deviance. Culture of Health Blog. Robert Wood Johnson Foundation. 20 Jul 2007. https://www.rwjf.org/en/culture-of-health/2007/07/guest-blogger-c.html
18. Kuhn T. The structure of scientific revolutions. Chicago: University of Chicago Press; 1970.

# Disappointment-Driven System Improvement in Health Care

**Kevin E. Nortrup**

> *The reasonable man adapts himself to the world; the unreasonable one persists in trying to adapt the world to himself. Therefore, all progress depends on the unreasonable man.*
>
> George Bernard Shaw

## 1 Introduction

There is growing recognition that the complexity of health care mandates systemic treatment. In May 2014, the President's Council of Advisors on Science and Technology (PCAST) issued a report to President Obama, *Better Health Care and Lower Costs: Accelerating Improvement through Systems Engineering*, whose cover letter recommended, "*Systems-engineering know-how must be propagated at all levels,*" and "*the United States* [must] *build a health-care workforce that is equipped with essential systems engineering competencies that will enable system redesign.*" In an ever more complex world, the systemic disciplines—including systems thinking, systems and complexity science, and systems engineering[1]—may be the "killer apps."

[1]Broadly distinguishing between these as examples of the range of systemic endeavors:

- Systems thinking = a fundamental, transdisciplinary understanding of the interrelated nature of everything; a vital, adjunct capability of modern knowledge-workers in a complex world;
- Systems and complexity science = a constellation of theoretical inquiries into the universal laws, patterns, and nature of systems of all types; and

K. E. Nortrup (✉)
Sugar Creek Solutions LLC, Fairland, IN, USA
e-mail: kevin@sugarcreeksolutions.com



J. P. Sturmberg (ed.), *Embracing Complexity in Health*,
https://doi.org/10.1007/978-3-030-10940-0_18

Yet this begs a vital question: how does an entire workforce acquire systemic capabilities to facilitate "system redesign"—or at least, to improve health care through a systems approach?

The journey begins by committing to a systemic perspective. It is counter-productive to proclaim health care to be a system, then to approach it through the traditional silos and lenses, such as management engineering, process improvement, and quality management; instead, the focus must be on systems engineering, systems improvement, and systems management.

Responsibility for the health of health care must be demystified and decentralized. Subject matter experts may coach and coordinate, but the monitoring and improvement of healthcare deliverables must be incorporated as a fundamental part of everyone's job-description.

Finally, the "sibling rivalry" between theory and practice must end. Practical theorists must equip theoretically sound practitioners with simple, accessible yet powerfully effective mindsets and methodologies to think and to act systemically in performance of everyday responsibilities.

This chapter explores one possible approach to accomplish such an ambitious agenda. It describes preliminary, in-progress work in emerging fields, born of reflection on what previously has not seemed to work and why—not the first word, nor the last, but a waypoint.

## 2 "The Quality Problem"

Quality management, process improvement, and similar disciplines have had unquestionable success in addressing emergent issues and increasing efficiency in mass-production systems. However, as those systems and their environments grow in complexity, the disciplines and supplemental systems that seek to manage and to improve them also become more complex—with growing risk of unintended consequences from such compounded complexity.

Furthermore, traditional quality-management and process-improvement efforts tend to center on individuals with extensively specialized skill sets, cloistered in separatist departments whose objectives and initiatives may not always align with those of other departments or the organization as a whole. This can create adversarial objectives and an "us-versus-them" atmosphere within the organization, further disenfranchising workers whose connectedness and motivation may already be limited by organizational silos and bureaucracy.

Finally, such efforts also run the risk of localized or irrelevant optimization. As Peter Drucker noted in T*he Effective Executive*, "*Efficiency is doing things right;*

---

- Systems engineering= the application of systems sciences to real-world problems and objectives.

*effectiveness is doing the right things.*" Such a critical distinction is often lost in the quest to quantify quality.

Presently, health care is transitioning from episodic intervention and management of illness to the cultivation and facilitation of healthy, preventative lifestyles that promote wellness. Shortfalls and setbacks would still require the temporary imposition of external remedial structures (such as casts and crutches on broken legs), but only until inherent, internal wholeness is restored. If the casts and crutches remain forever, then health care will fail to deliver fully its objective.

Perhaps quality management and process improvement similarly could seek to transition from episodic intervention and external imposition of structure to the cultivation and facilitation of inherent, internal wholeness throughout the hospitals and similar sociotechnical enterprise systems. The resulting focus would become continuous, organic system improvement, for which everyone throughout the organization would have contributory responsibility.

Such a transition requires a simpler, more efficient yet highly effective concept of quality.

## 3 Inherent Qualitative Quality

A comprehensive definition of "a system" enumerates many important characteristics. Perhaps two of the most fundamental characteristics of systems can be summarized simply as:

- A system has input, and a system has output.[2]
- Between the input and the output, something happens.

Particularly for man-made systems:

- The "something" that happens is the purpose of the system—typically, to add **value**:[3] how the world is better because of the system's behavior and operation.
- The inputs, outputs, purpose, requirements, and constraints—basically, all expectations—are explicitly documented as the specifications of the system.

[2]A closed system does not have input or output; it only has interactions among its internal elements (subsystems). Although some human conceptual models are abstracted as closed systems for simplicity, the fundamental "interconnectedness of everything" suggests that the only truly closed system is the entirety of the physical universe itself—and even that is dependent upon the absence of any metaphysical context or interconnection.

[3]Arguably, all value is instrumental value as efficacy toward one or more ends, which may be short-term or long-term, siloed or big-picture, concrete or abstract. The concept of the "triple bottom line" and similar holistic perspectives of results seek to enlarge the "scope of the system in question" and thereby to close the artificial gap between instrumental value and system/ethical/esthetic value.

For example, if the system under discussion is a single-serving coffee-maker:

- The system inputs are ground coffee beans, filter, water, electricity, and an empty cup.
- The system outputs are a cup full of coffee, used coffee grounds, and used filter.
- The system purpose is to produce a cup full of hot, freshly brewed coffee.
- The system specifications (expectations) are summarized in the owner's manual.

If the customer's expectations are met or exceeded by their experience (a cup of hot, freshly brewed coffee), then the customer is satisfied. If the expectations are not met by experience (cold coffee, or nothing), then the customer is disappointed.

This is a qualitative assessment of quality that applies easily and equally to any system:

**Quality is the degree to which Experience meets or exceeds Expectations.**
Experience < Expectations = Disappointment (low quality)
Experience >= Expectations = Satisfaction (high quality)

Accordingly, improving quality can be accomplished by increasing (improving) experience and/or by decreasing (managing) expectations (Fig. 1).

This applies not only to expectations and experience between the system and its environment, but also to expectations and experience between elemental subsystems within the system itself. Furthermore, it applies bi-directionally at every interface (external and internal): both the provider of output and the receiver of input have expectations of the interaction's unfolding.

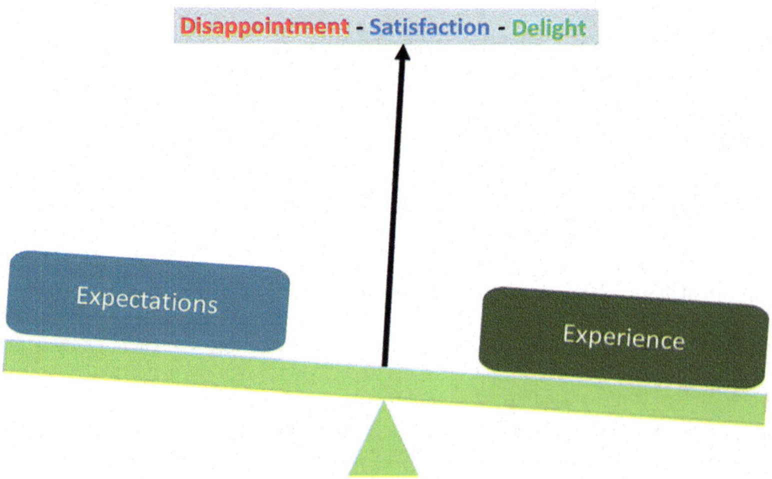


**Fig. 1** Qualitative quality. (*Courtesy of Kevin Nortrup / Sugar Creek Solutions*)

If a patient walks into a hospital and asks for a flu shot, yet no such flu shot is available, then that patient's experience falls short of expectations, the patient is disappointed, and poor quality is perceived. The possible location of the root cause(s) of the perceived poor quality includes:

- An intermediate task within the hospital, perhaps far in time and space from the patient: last week, inventory may have been miscounted, failing to trigger a re-order of vaccine.
- An entity in the larger supersystem outside of the hospital: over-caution by a regulatory agency may have delayed production or shipping of new vaccine by the manufacturer.
- The patient's own expectations: perhaps the hospital's emergency department does not advertise or have the resources to provide elective, walk-in vaccinations.

Therefore, patient experience of "poor quality" can originate anywhere within the health-and-wellness supersystem, within the hospital itself, or even within the patient's own expectations. Such an understanding both demands and facilitates a substantial shift in paradigm:

- "Quality" is not an esoteric alchemy with specialist wizards and separatist departments; instead, it is a cultural commitment that experience will meet or exceed expectations, for which everyone throughout the health-and-wellness supersystem is responsible!
- A "Quality system" is not a department, infrastructure, process, or other supplemental system whose purpose is to impose quality onto an otherwise deficient primary system (such as a hospital or a primary or community care clinic); instead, it is a primary system of inherently high quality!

## 4 Disappointment-Driven System Improvement

Wherever and whenever experience falls short of expectations, the resulting disappointment serves as a "check-engine" light, bringing attention to some part of the system whose proper operation is suddenly in question, and thereby inviting follow-up investigation into it. Harnessing disappointment can drive and fulfill the promise of continuous improvement, utilizing the eyes, ears, hands, feet, and minds of everyone throughout the system—not just a few select specialists—to be active, participatory agents of quality and performance improvement.

This requires a cultural climate of trust, safety, and unity of purpose. The entire system must value honest discussion, appreciative inquiry, root-cause analysis, ongoing improvement, and the restoration of collegial professional relationships. Everyone throughout the system must feel comfortable in expressing and addressing disappointment, confident in ground-rules and processes that acknowledge potential emotional implications but moderate potential drama.[4] Leaders must accept responsibility to facilitate organic growth and wellness in the system.

Investigating disappointment must be a holistic inquiry, with minimal assumptions and no agenda other than bridging the “disappointment gap” by reconciling expectations with experience in both directions of the interface, recognizing that one or both may need adjustment:

- Expectations: identifying and articulating initial expectations; revisiting, validating, and adjusting as appropriate; documenting (specifications/job-descriptions) when done.
- Experience: clarifying/validating/adjusting objectives; reviewing/verifying/improving design; reviewing/verifying/improving execution.

Many instances of disappointment will be resolved simply between the individuals involved—especially when handled early, before disappointment grows into frustration, anger, bitterness, or worse. Some instances will require mediation by a facilitator or escalation to higher authorities. Larger systemic issues may require more extensive troubleshooting by a supplemental team. However, no report of disappointment should go unaddressed.

All inquiry and investigation should be both systemic (holistic) and systematic (methodical), going through all three prioritized stages of troubleshooting and resisting the ever present temptation to conclude prematurely:

- Alleviate the symptoms that caused the disappointment.
- Find and fix the specific underlying problem(s) that caused the symptoms.
- Find and fix the general vulnerability(s) that facilitated the problem(s).

Metaphorically, fire-fighting always should transition into fire-investigation, which always should facilitate better fire-prevention. Organizations that “don’t have time” for post-firefighting follow-up, usually spend all their time fighting fires (many of which could have been prevented).

## 5 Managing Healthcare Expectations

The first stage of investigating the root cause of disappointment includes examining, validating, possibly adjusting, and then better documenting the expectations of both parties. The systemic disciplines can bring innovative and useful perspective to

[4]Such openness initially may be awkward, even painful, as typically there is minimal precedent or preparation for it. However, workplace morale will improve (and stress will decrease) when everyone feels heard and sees positive response to their concerns, and job-satisfaction will increase as everyone sees their contributions valued. Therefore, a better workplace environment is both a prerequisite and a by-product of harnessing disappointment productively, and disappointment-driven system improvement will become progressively easier over time.

such investigation, both in identifying where to examine and in performing such examination.

## 5.1 Purpose and Requirements Specification

Systems engineering emphasizes the need to identify, to clarify, and to document why an effort is being undertaken and what to expect from its successful completion before embarking on the actual design process. In the absence of a clear definition of the destination, a route can be highly problematic to establish and to travel.

Certainly, the expectations of patients are of critical importance. There is growing (and, arguably, long overdue) awareness within health care of "customer service" and "user experience." However, patient expectations are not just of "quality of service" but also of "quality of life": what does it mean to be healthy or well, despite or amidst various conditions?

There are also expectations from providers, payors, and others—sometimes consistent, sometimes in conflict, with patient expectations. Expectations in both directions, at every interface, need to be discussed holistically, then validated or adjusted, and documented as specified requirements.

There remains much divergence in thought—and little public discussion—about the full expectations and specifications for health care, particularly at national levels. There may be unspoken assumptions or contentious assertions by various groups and individuals, but these must be collected, reconciled, and ratified authoritatively before effective reform is possible.

This is especially problematic in pluralistic democracies with conflicting or polarized, deeply held ideologies among their citizens. For example, the equilibrium between individualism and collectivism must discuss and develop consensus on enormously sensitive and difficult yet critically important questions as:

- To how much and to what types of healthcare services are which individuals entitled, with how much at their own expense and with how much underwritten by whom?
- To what degree do the potential underwriters have the fiduciary obligation to prescribe lifestyle choices as conditions or disqualifiers of such services?
- What are reasonable and unreasonable expectations of patients?

The systemic disciplines can facilitate those discussions in several ways, including underscoring the unsustainability of present or proposed models, and mediating ideological common ground through polarity management and similar tools and processes. Absent such consensus on the expectations for health care, experiences that fall short of expectations are inescapable.

## 5.2 Intentional Design

Design is the process of intentional craftsmanship toward specific objectives. It may be a combination of analysis and creativity, of linear reasoning and nonlinear inspiration, of function and form. Nonetheless, design starts with a sense of purpose, then proceeds through a course of action that is chosen specifically to maximize the likelihood of actualizing that purpose.

Health care has long lacked intentional, overarching, top-down design. Unfortunately, many within the systemic disciplines assert that such design is not possible, because health care—as a "system of systems"—can only be influenced at best, as it evolves, emerges, and self-organizes.

However, emergent properties of systems are simply the results of deterministic interactions of pre-existing properties of the system's composite elements; any inability to predict such results is based on limited human insight and understanding. As the systemic disciplines mature, they will progressively better understand and predict emergence, even in complex sociotechnical systems of systems such as health care—and design of such systems will be far less daunting.

The success of ant and bee colonies is often used to illustrate the efficacy of self-organization. However, all members of such colonies have the same genetic programming and follow the same blueprint for their behavior, which evidences neither creativity, innovation, nor purpose.

Evolutionary change happens over long periods of time; it seeks no result and accomplishes no purpose other than survival through accommodation of its environment; and it is pitiless toward the myriad individuals who were victims of its failed iterative attempts. Conversely, health care needs to change relatively quickly; it aspires to accomplish purposes in defiance of environmental pressures; the well-being of individuals is valued highly; and as a system that is already in service (literally with lives depending upon it), it cannot afford evolutionary trial and error.

A (re)design of health care will require a collaborative, interdisciplinary effort by doctors, nurses, engineers, psychologists, sociologists, lawyers, economists, ethicists, and scientists of many types. However, a broad base of participants does not demand a purely bottom-up approach; a collaborative approach can produce a high-level, top-down design for health care that includes a coordinating framework for bottom-up innovation.

Systemic disciplines (including communications science and systems engineering) have accomplished feats of staggering complexity, such as mobile cellular telecommunications and space missions to explore Pluto. They have shown that it's possible to be technically sound, financially responsible, yet still responsive to the wants and needs of customers—an equilibrium with which health care still appears to struggle. Such capabilities can and should be brought to a top-down design of health care, to minimize unmet expectations in it.

## 5.3 Scope

Systems engineering is keenly aware of scope: where the "dotted line" is drawn to determine which elements are of primary interest in "the system" under discussion, with surrounding elements abstracted as context or environment. Since everything is connected to everything, this is only for convenience, a concession to the finite limitations of human brainpower.

Inclusion of elements with minimal relevance can complicate the systems analysis unnecessarily, but exclusion of vitally relevant elements can lead to unknowingly incomplete analysis. Many of the seemingly intractable issues in health care may yield more readily to solution when the scope of their "system" is increased, bringing previously neglected elements for inclusion into the analysis for causality and remediation, some examples of which will follow later.

One fundamental scope-extension is the transition from technical to sociotechnical systems. Stakeholder-analysis assumes the validity of a static snapshot of individuals, their requirements, and their constraints. However, people can exhibit highly complex, adaptive, variant, even chaotic behavior; and to build upon any foundation that assumes human invariance is risky at best. Fortunately, people are not totally unpredictable: psychology, sociology, and game theory are but a few of the sciences that characterize human behavior. Such characterizations facilitate expanding the scope of "the system" by relocating stakeholders from being external inputs, outputs, and requirements to being inherent elements. This allows greater anticipation and accommodation of variant and adaptive behavior of stakeholders, substantially improving the ability to manage expectations throughout the system.

## 5.4 Metrics

With scope expanded to realize the sociotechnical nature of a system, metrics can be understood as the input portion of system feedback, the output of which reinforces or compensates certain outputs of the system. In human terms, this incentivizes or disincentivizes certain behaviors and results. Typically, this is intended to seek and to achieve specific objectives within the system.

Unfortunately, the consequences of such feedback can be unintended, even counter-productive. Characteristics of desired objectives may be difficult to quantify or to measure, but readily available or surrogate metrics can be incomplete, irrelevant, misleading, or siloed, thereby incentivizing undesired behaviors.[5]

[5]There have been school systems in the USA that offered financial rewards for teachers whose students scored well on standardized testing. However, while such performance is easily measured, it has uncertain correlation to the actual desired outcome: students who are well equipped to become functioning, contributing adults in society. Furthermore, there arose more than one scandal of teachers improperly coaching students for the test at the expense of the desired instruction and training—exactly counter-productive to the objective of well-educated students.

Health care is transitioning to population health, accountable care organizations, pay for value, and similar concepts that aspire to monitor and to incentivize desired outcomes. Metrics will play an enormous role in those implementations; critical, systemic thinking will be essential to avoid potentially catastrophic unintended consequences of ill-conceived or misconstrued metrics.

For example, some advocates promote tracking and publishing of the "success rates" of doctors, rewarding those whose excellence prompts prospective new patients to seek them out: in theory, thereby incentivizing doctors toward better care. However, other advocates worry that such a process may incentivize doctors to avoid all but the "safest" patients—with the unintended consequences of reducing the availability of health care to those patients who are most in need.

It is far too easy to "win the battle but to lose the war" by optimizing what is visible or easy but not what is needful, by optimizing the localized or immediate at the cost of the big picture or the long term, or simply optimizing past the point of diminishing returns. Proper scope of "the system" lessens the likelihood of invalid metrics setting expectations that will be disappointed.

# 6 Improving Healthcare Experiences

The second stage of investigating the root cause of disappointment includes examining, validating, and possibly improving the experience of both parties. The systemic disciplines can bring innovative and useful perspective to such investigation, both in identifying where to examine and in performing such examination.

## *6.1 Enterprise Model of Healthcare-Delivery Systems*

Every company, hospital, primary or community care center, academic institution, nonprofit organization, or professional society is an enterprise: a complex sociotechnical system that is governed by universal systemic principles, violation of which (even in ignorance) leads ultimately to predictable breakdowns and failures.

Enterprise system engineering is an interdisciplinary methodology that seeks to bring business management, management engineering, organizational behavior, change management, process improvement, psychology, sociology, gaming theory, human factors—as well as systems thinking, complexity science, systems science, and systems engineering—to the domain of enterprises.

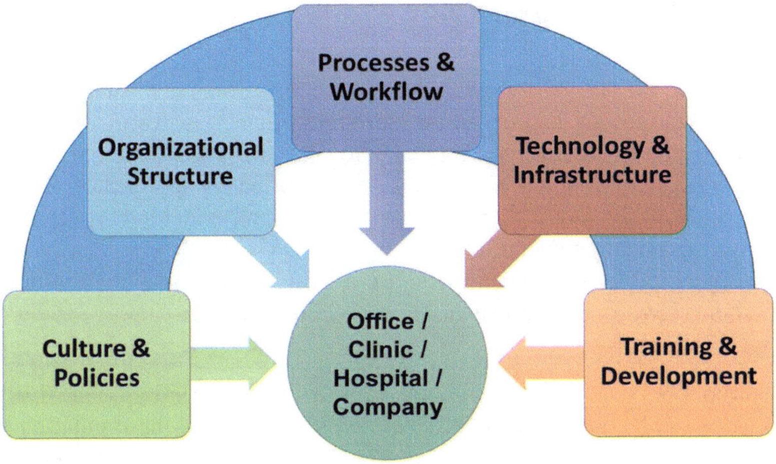


**Fig. 2** One example of an enterprise model. (*Courtesy of Kevin Nortrup / Sugar Creek Solutions*)

Interdisciplinary models of enterprises seek to explain past and present behavior, to predict future behavior, and to facilitate desired change. Their dimensional elements should be orthogonal, yet comprehensive of people, process, and technology (Fig. 2). One such model includes:

- Culture and policies—established first after the vision/mission/objectives, to "set the tone"
- Organizational structure—established next, to distribute the deliverables among workers
- Processes and workflow—established next, to identify and to detail what should happen
- Technology and infrastructure—established next, to provide appropriate means and venue
- Training and development—establish last, to on-board all workers on the above.

Each dimension should be a well-functioning subsystem of the enterprise, with all its dimensions interoperating optimally to achieve its purpose, vision, mission, and objectives.

Hospitals—and their more generalized class, healthcare-delivery systems (or enterprises)—will deliver better experiences that meet or exceed expectations, when they are designed, operated, and maintained as the systems that they are, holistically, through enterprise system engineering.

## 6.2 Organizational Structure

One approach to the design of organizational structure seeks to leverage similarities between system design and software design; arguably, software was the first man-made system of sufficient complexity to mandate a systemic and systematic approach. Structured analysis and design, object-oriented approaches, minimized dependencies between modules: all these lessons that were learned in software have relevance in organizational structure.

Some object to the hierarchical structure of software being applied to organizations: in their view, sociotechnical systems are complex, peer-to-peer networks, not hierarchies. However:

- With arguably beneficial redesign and reprioritization of affinity, most network topologies can be repartitioned into a credibly hierarchical representation.
- Observations of "formal" versus "informal" reporting structures underscore the need for a redesign into a structure where the theoretical and practical affinities correspond.
- Minimized dependencies (or coupling) effectively empower departments and individuals, with less need for "forgiveness or permission."
- Hierarchy is fundamentally about layers of bite-sized abstractions to manage complexity, not about power or worth (historical distortions, abuses, and perversions notwithstanding); higher levels deal more abstractly with wider scope; lower levels deal more concretely with greater depth; every level adds essential value, and none is "more important."
- In a correctly designed hierarchy, every position is an accountable, responsible, and empowered owner (authority, expert, visionary, champion, advocate) of some deliverable, adding value by aggregating, coordinating, prioritizing, and arbitrating the constituent elements of that deliverable (which may be deliverables themselves) (Fig. 3).

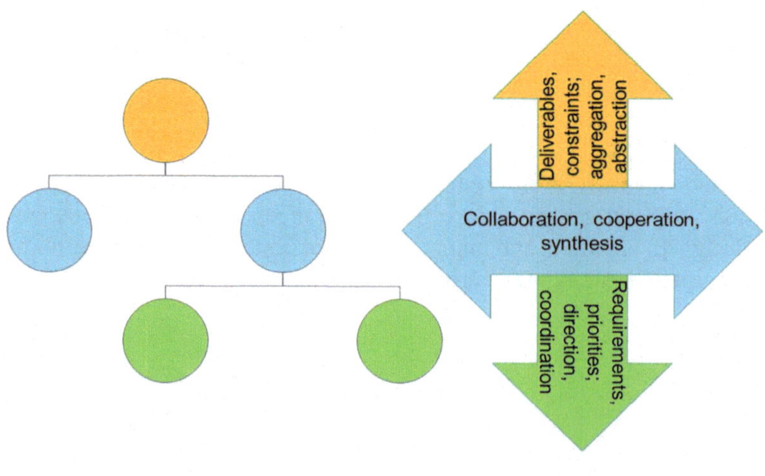


**Fig. 3** 360° added value, responsibility and accountability in hierarchy. (*Courtesy of Kevin Nortrup / Sugar Creek Solutions*)

When designing an organizational structure, one of the applicable lessons from software is the importance of appropriate partitioning. In both worlds, it is preferable to have partitioning that is:

- Highly orthogonal, with mutually exclusive functionalities and mutually exclusive ownership of them (no overlaps or matrixing);
- Highly holistic (minimized silos), with interdisciplinary teams and contributors, with maximal localization of authority, responsibility, and capability;
- Closely parallel to the partitioning of the goods or services being produced, to avoid overlaps or omissions of responsibility for deliverables (objective-oriented organization).

Matrix organizations are the equivalent of "spaghetti code": they can be rather resource-efficient, but as size and complexity grow, their dependencies can cause the very problems that they are intended to solve (silos, territorialism, inflexibility, bottlenecks, resistance to change) as well as new problems (adversarial objectives, conflicting authority, gaps/overlaps of responsibility).

For example, instead of a traditional matrix organization, a hospital could have an interdisciplinary, objective-oriented "Clinical Design and Support" department, comprising:

- Healthcare information technology (applications): EMR, CPOE, EBM, etc.
- Clinical informatics
- Best-practice processes and workflow
- Infection-control and PPC/SRE-avoidance
- Incident-investigation and root-cause analysis
- Training and on-boarding of healthcare staff
- Healthcare purchasing and inventory
- Clinical housekeeping.

Function follows form, and "good fences make good neighbors." A well-designed organizational structure ensures that everyone owns and takes professional pride in a specific, objective-oriented deliverable, resulting in better experiences that meet or exceed expectations.

## *6.3 Technology and Infrastructure*

Technology and infrastructure should enable people and processes by facilitating their existing deliverables and objectives. Too often in health care, technology appears as a "solution looking for a problem": needlessly and negatively disrupting people and processes by creating artificial or intermediate deliverables and objectives.

Lack of interoperability among devices and technology remains a concern in health care today. Its primary cause is ad hoc, bottom-up introduction of new healthcare technology: driven not by meeting an identified need in a master plan and roadmap of facilitating technology, but by how a manufacturer desires to leverage its existing technology, market-position, or reputation (Fig. 4).

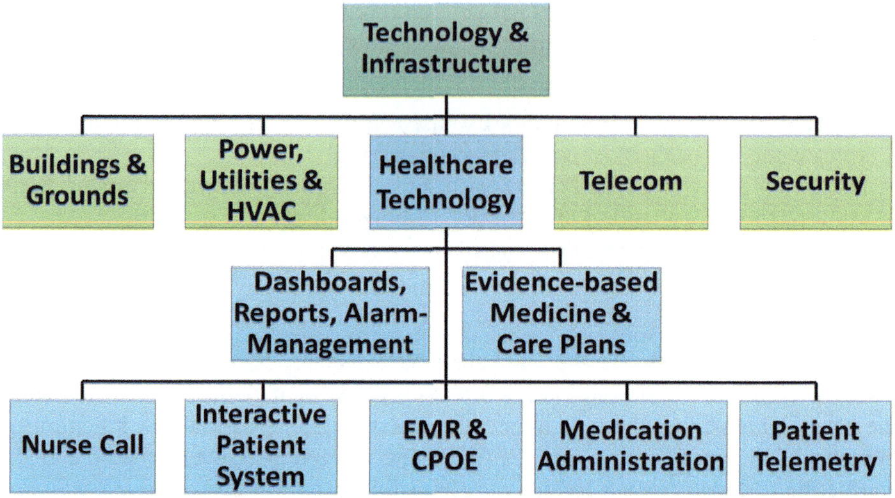


**Fig. 4** Healthcare technology and infrastructure. (*Courtesy of Kevin Nortrup / Sugar Creek Solutions*)

Free-market innovation is the life-blood of healthcare technology, but it must take place within a framework of top-down design of a healthcare technology supersystem, which itself must be driven by clarification and documentation of objectives and needs in health care. Broadly based, industry-driven collaboration can be the architect of system and device specifications that ensure interoperability and other basic requirements without squashing innovation, as demonstrated by the success of cellular mobile communications. Healthcare technology that holistically meets real needs will deliver better experiences that meet or exceed expectations.

## *6.4 Healthcare and Wellness Supersystem*

A hospital (or other healthcare-delivery enterprise) does not exist in a vacuum; its ability to reimagine and to reinvent itself is limited by its interdependence upon the other subsystems in the larger *healthcare and wellness supersystem* of which it is also a subsystem. Indeed, the form and function of hospitals and other healthcare-delivery enterprises today is largely the cumulative result of historic and present forces within this supersystem.

Genuine reform must address issues at this supersystem level, whose complexity reaches all the way to sociopolitical and public-policy issues (Fig. 5). Its subsystems include:

- Healthcare information technology (applications): EMR, CPOE, EBM, etc.
- Healthcare-delivery enterprises
- Other providers
- Payors
- Pharmaceutical companies and device manufacturers
- Agriculture and food system
- Educational system
- Legal system
- Economic and financial system
- Political system
- Patients themselves, whose influencing subsystems include:
  - Genetics and heredity
  - Lifestyle and behavioral choices
  - Family and friends

It is difficult to contemplate analysis, much less remediation, at this level. Nonetheless, without coming to terms with the expectations of and within this supersystem–and without intervening in it to cultivate commensurate experiences throughout it—the ability of healthcare-delivery systems to deliver satisfactory experiences will be limited.

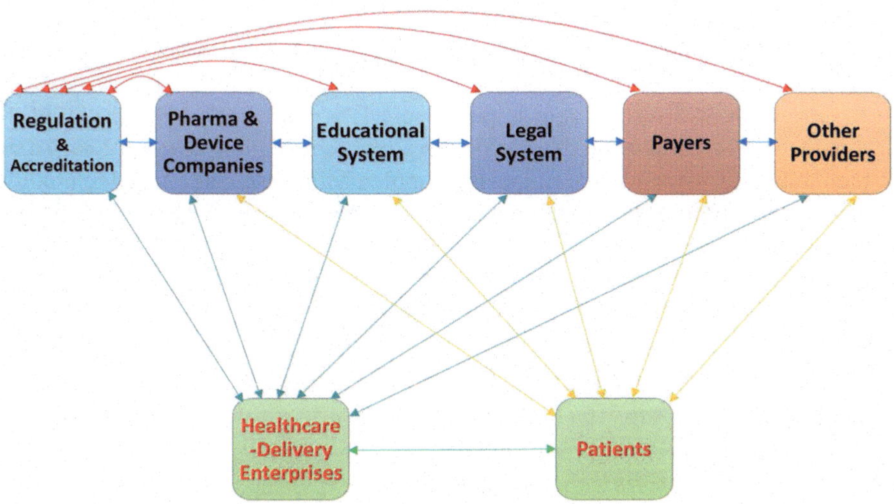


**Fig. 5** Healthcare and wellness supersystem. (*Courtesy of Kevin Nortrup / Sugar Creek Solutions*)

### 6.5 More "Disciplined" Healthcare Workers

Specialization appears to be a logical approach to the mastery of exponentially growing complexity. However, in health care as in other industries, the biggest risks and opportunities exist "between the silos." Skill-set specialists will always be needed, but perhaps they should be the exception instead of the rule, with a greater number of integrative individuals who are categorized by what they deliver and not by any particular skill-set.

This requires health care to demand—and education to produce—more "disciplined" workers, to prepare for the ever-increasing fuzzing and fusing of disciplines (such as informatics, biomechatronics, micro-electro-mechanical systems, enterprise systems):

- ***Multidisciplinary*** = able to change hats as required
- ***Interdisciplinary*** = able to wear more than one hat at a time
- ***Transdisciplinary*** = able to take several hats, rip their seams, and sew them together to make a single hat to wear.

Healthcare workers who are broadly skilled—who can bridge the silos and produce holistic, objective-oriented deliverables—can take the initiative, the responsibility, and the professional pride to ensure that their specific niche within the healthcare-delivery system provides experiences that meet or exceed expectations.

## 7 The Transformative Aspects of This Study

Health care is a complex, sociotechnical system of systems that demands a systemic approach.

Disappointment-driven system improvement is a distributed, holistic approach that mainstreams monitoring, troubleshooting, and remediation to achieve a system of high quality, instead of superimposing supplemental systems to manage quality and to improve processes through oversight and intervention. A handful of simple but powerful concepts can equip everyone throughout the workforce with basic capabilities of quality management and process improvement from a systemic perspective. These concepts utilize the eyes, ears, hands, feet, and minds of everyone throughout the system—not just a few select specialists—to be active, participatory agents of quality and performance improvement:

- ***Qualitative quality***: the degree to which experience meets or exceeds expectations, at interfaces anywhere surrounding or within a system
- ***Harnessing disappointment***: leveraging any experience not meeting expectations (negative qualitative quality) as a trigger and locator for systemic troubleshooting
- ***Managing expectations***: gathering, validating, documenting, utilizing, and managing requirements and specifications

- ***Improving experience***: improving the system (which includes more than just the process) and its deliverables, by investigating the objectives, design, implementation, and operation of the system and its subsystems

Systemic disciplines can facilitate the troubleshooting, remediation, and redesign of systems at all levels of health care, from subsystems of technology, to hospitals, to supersystems of national institutions.

Hospitals (and similar healthcare-delivery systems) can be modeled, remediated, and designed as enterprise systems. One such model includes culture and policies, organizational structure, processes and workflow, technology and infrastructure, and training and development as its dimensional elements.

Health care (as other industries) must demand, and education must provide, a workforce that is far more broadly trained and equipped as transdisciplinary contributors.

**Take Home Message**

- Harness disappointment as a "check-engine" light.
- Internalize and synthesize quality management, management engineering, and process improvement into inherent system improvement.
- Analyze and remediate enterprise systems with models such as "culture and policies, organizational structure, processes and workflow, technology and infrastructure, and training and development."
- Don't forget the fundamentals: documented requirements specification and intentional methodical design.
- Pursue transdisciplinary mindset and capabilities: for yourself, for your organization, and for the next generation.

# Further Readings

1. Complexity Sciences

- Donaldson, William. Simple_Complexity: A Management Book for the Rest of Us: A Guide to Systems Thinking. New York: Morgan James Publishing; 2017.
- Senge, Peter M. The Fifth Discipline: The Art and Practice of the Learning Organization. New York: Doubleday/Currency; 2006.
- Ellis GFR. Top-down causation and emergence: some comments on mechanisms. Interface Focus.2012;2(1):126–40.

2. Improvement

   - Ackoff, Russ. Beyond Continuous Improvement. Conference: The Learning and Legacy of Dr. W. Edwards Deming. 1994.
   - Doerr J. Measure what matters. New York: Portfolio/Penguin; 2018.

3. Leadership

   - Drucker, Peter F. The Effective Executive: The Definitive Guide to Getting the Right Things Done. New York: Harper Collins; 2006.
   - Heifetz R. Leadership Without Easy Answers. Cambridge, Ma: Harvard University Press; 1994.
   - World Health Organization Regional Office for Europe. Governance for health in the 21st century: a study conducted for the WHO Regional Office for Europe. Copenhagen: World Health Organization Regional Office for Europe; 2011.

4. Design Thinking

   - Papanek V. Design for the real world: human ecology and social change. New York: Pantheon Books; 1971.
   - Simon HA. The sciences of the artificial. Cambridge: MIT Press; 1969
   - Brown T. Design thinking. Harv Bus Rev 2008:86(6):84–92.

5. Health System Design

   - President's Council of Advisors on Science and Technology (PCAST). Better Health Care and Lower Costs: Accelerating Improvement through Systems Engineering. May 2014.
   - Sturmberg JP. Health System Redesign. How to Make Health Care Person-Centered, Equitable, and Sustainable. Cham: Springer; 2017.
   - Jones P. Design for Care: Innovating Healthcare Experience. New York: Rosenfeld Media; 2013.
   - Collins B. Intentional whole health system redesign. Southcentral Foundation's 'Nuka' system of care. London: King's Fund; 2015.
   - Hyman DA and Silver C. Overcharged: Why Americans Pay Too Much for Health Care. Washington, DC: Cato Institute; 2018
   - Rouse WB. Health care as a complex adaptive system: implications for design and management. The Bridge. 2008:38(1):17–25.

# A Study on the Modeling of Obesity

**Sung Young Lim, Leticia Mucci da Conceição, and Sergio G. Camorlinga**

## 1 Introduction

According to the World Health Organization (WHO), the number of obese people has almost tripled since 1975. In 2016 more than 1.9 billion adults 18 years and older were overweight. Of these over 650 million were obese. Overall, 39% of adults were overweight in 2016 and 13% were obese. Worldwide, overweight and obesity are linked to more deaths than underweight. Raised body mass index (BMI)—a measure of overweight and obesity—is a major risk factor for common noncommunicable diseases such as cardiovascular diseases, diabetes, musculoskeletal disorders, and some types of cancers [1].

Most of the previous studies have focused on finding a relationship between one risk factor and obesity. In this work, we research a variety of factors affecting obesity by using statistical analysis from a complex adaptive system (CAS) perspective. Our goal is to employ the research outcomes to develop a CAS-based computer model of obesity.

S. Y. Lim (✉) · S. G. Camorlinga
Department of Applied Computer Science, The University of Winnipeg, Winnipeg, MB, Canada
e-mail: lim-s6@webmail.uwinnipeg.ca; s.camorlinga@uwinnipeg.ca

L. M. da Conceição
Department of Nutrition, University of São Paulo, São José dos Campos, São Paulo, Brazil
e-mail: leticia.conceicao@usp.br



J. P. Sturmberg (ed.), *Embracing Complexity in Health*,
https://doi.org/10.1007/978-3-030-10940-0_19

## 2 The Complexity of Obesity

In complex systems research, one of the most powerful tools is the use of computational techniques as they allow a much wider range of exploration of conceptual models. Using computational techniques, we can understand and predict answers to questions arising from our research [2]. Agent-based modeling (ABM) is a simulation approach that consists of an interactive set of agents [3] that represent system components and interactions in a particular environment. ABM offers a theoretical framework from which to explore complex adaptive social systems [2]. Agents interact based on a set of rules and within an environment specified by the researcher [4].

Figure 1 shows our proposed CAS-based obesity model. The complex interrelationship among each of the risk factors which give rise to an individual's obesity (yellow circles $r_1, r_2$, etc.) is shown in the smaller circle. Then, the individuals (orange circles $p_1$, $p_2$, etc.) co-existance and interactions result in the emergence of the obesity rates at the community level. The environment is also an important factor in the emergence of obesity at the individual and community level. For instance, larger entities (e.g., government healthcare organizations, industry, etc.) can have the power to influence the environment either positively or negatively via policies and marketing (e.g., nutrition campaign, junk food marketing, etc.). In this research, we focus on the obesity risk factor interrelationships and interdependencies with the use of statistical analysis. Our final aim is to use the risk factors studied (yellow circles $r_1, r_2$, etc.) to build an obesity model based on CAS principles that will help us to simulate obesity rates for adults in a community.

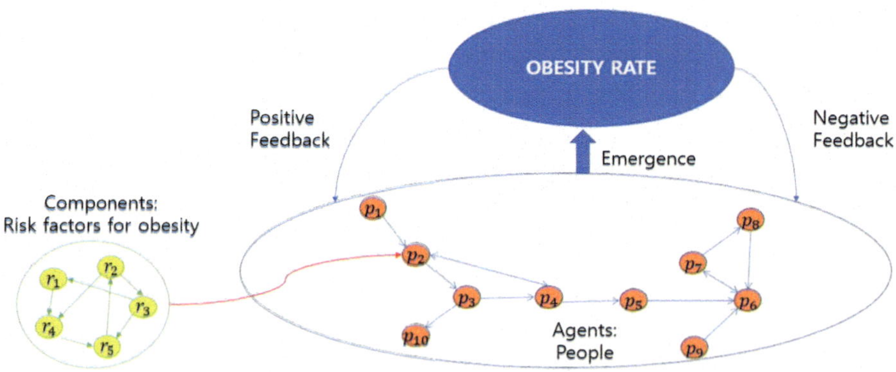


**Fig. 1** CAS-based obesity model

# 3 Obesity Modeling

The data used for this study was provided by Statistics Canada, Canadian Community Health Survey (CCHS), available on the NESSTAR data portal [5]. This survey is a cross-sectional survey that collects *self-reported* information related to health status, healthcare utilization, and health determinants for the Canadian population. It relies upon a large sample of respondents and is designed to provide reliable health estimates at the regional level [6].

## *3.1 CCHS Microdata File Structure*

CCHS provides a microdata file which contains each of person's responses to the survey. The CCHS microdata file is open to researchers from various fields to conduct research to improve health. Table 1 shows an example of the microdata file—each column represents a survey question, and each row represents a participant's answer for a survey item. The numbers represent the answer to a survey item chosen by the participant. For example, in Table 1 the column HWTGISW means body mass index (BMI) classification by a survey participant (underweight, normal weight, overweight, and obese)—the first individual answered "2" to this question, i.e., this survey participant answered: I am of "normal weight."

In addition we obtained data of various health-related risk factors such as chronic conditions, income, age, and sex. Also, each risk factor has sub-factors; e.g., the risk factor chronic conditions has 36 sub-variables such as asthma, diabetes, and heart disease. We only want to include risk factors truly associated with obesity that had been identified by statistical data analyses as described in the next section.

## *3.2 Methodology*

Firstly, a bibliographic search identified human studies of risk factors associated with chronic diseases associated with overweight and obesity [7–11]. These findings allowed us to identify relevant obesity risk factors in the Canadian Community Health Survey.

It was noticed that the survey questions before 2009 were quite different from those in the period 2009–2014. Therefore, we decided to focus on the data from 2009 to 2014 as the survey contained the same factors, variables, questions, and types of answers. Participants with incomplete and missing responses—"not applicable," "don't know," "refusal," and "not stated"—were excluded.

Statistical analysis aimed to identify how the various risk factors contribute to the emergence of an individual's obesity. Ideally, we wanted to obtain a linear mathematical formula that includes the relevant risk factors and their coefficients as shown in Eq. (1).

**Table 1** CCHS microdata file structure

| HWTGISW | FVCDJUI | FVCDFRU | FVCDSAL | FVCDPOT | FVCDCAR | FVCDVEG | … | FVCDTOT |
|---|---|---|---|---|---|---|---|---|
| 2 | 1 | 1 | 1 | 1 | 1 | 1 | 2 | 2 |
| 3 | 1 | 1 | 1 | 1 | 1 | 1 | 1 | 1 |
| 2 | 1 | 1 | 1 | 1 | 1 | 1 | 1 | 1 |
| 4 | 1 | 1 | 1 | 1 | 1 | 1 | 1 | 1 |
| … | … | … | … | … | … | … | … | … |
| 2 | 1 | 1 | 1 | 1 | 1 | 1 | 1 | 1 |

Each column represents a survey question, and each row represents a participant's answer for a survey item.
HWTGISW: body mass index (BMI) classification; FVCDJUI, FVCDFRU, FVCDSAL, FVCDPOT, FVCDCAR, FVCDVEG: daily consumption—other vegetables, FVCDTOT: daily consumption—total fruits and vegetables

$$\text{Individual obesity} = ar_1 + br_2 + cr_3 + \cdots + nr_n \tag{1}$$

where $a, b, c, \ldots n$ are coefficients that represent the risk factor relevance $r_1, r_2, r_3, \ldots r_n$ of the respective obesity risk factor. Risk factors included were alcohol use, chronic conditions, changes made to improve health, depression, food choices, fruit and vegetable consumption, general health, income, mood, physical activities, sedentary activities, and smoking.

## 3.3 *Hypothesis*

We currently do not have a theoretical basis to demonstrate the conversion of the emergence of an individual obesity to a linear relationship of factors as stated in Eq. (1). However, we hypothesize that with computer simulation, we can experimentally demonstrate that Eq. (1) provides relevant results in terms of obesity behaviors for an individual since the individual will have various values for each of the obesity factors $r_i$ as time progresses. An initial empirical evidence for the equation validation can be obtained if the experimental data correlates with the surveyed data.

Then we searched for adequate statistical analyses of the CCHS data. We found that *independent t-test* and *simple linear regression* cannot be used as both tests only apply to up to two independent variables (factors), and this is not applicable for the CCHS data. The CCHS database contains various independent categorical variables (factors).

Our literature review found related work that used *multivariate logistic regression analysis*—Colapinto et al. [12] explored the relationship between BMI and fruit and vegetable intake in the Canadian, and Charlton et al. [13], in the Australian context. These studies differ from our work which is comprehensive as it includes a large range of different risk factors. We also apply correlations among the risk factors into a CAS-based obesity model.

Our aim is to create a mathematical equation for the construction of a model to determine the development of obesity at an individual level. Based on the available datasets good statistical analyses would include *normal test*, *MANOVA* (multivariate analysis of variance), and *multivariate logistic regression analysis.*

## 3.4 *Statistical Analysis*

### 3.4.1 Normal Test

The *normal test* determines if the data distribution presents normality or not. Between 2009 and 2014 all risk factor variables were normally distributed ($p$-value $\leq 0.05$) and these variables can be used to perform a *MANOVA* test.

### 3.4.2 MANOVA Test

*MANOVA* (multivariate analysis of variance) is an extension of *ANOVA* (analysis of variance). *MANOVA* tests whether there is any difference in two or more independent vectors of means on a dependent factor—in our study we have one dependent factor (body weight) and twenty independent vectors. To conduct *MANOVA*, three assumptions must be met [14]:

- Normal distribution: The dependent variable should be normally distributed within groups—the normal test must precede the MANOVA test
- Linearity: MANOVA assumes that there are linear relationships among all pairs of dependent variables. So, when the relationship deviates from linearity, the power of the analysis will be compromised
- Homogeneity of variances and covariances: In multivariate analysis, since there are multiple dependent variables, it is also required that their intercorrelations (covariances) are homogeneous across the variables of the study.

MANOVA test was performed using SPSS [15]. We found that six variables—"daily consumption of fruit juice," "daily consumption of fruit," "daily consumption of green salad," "daily consumption of potatoes," "daily consumption of carrots," and "frequency of drinking alcohol"—showed low or zero variance in relation to the dependent variable "body mass index (BMI classification)" ($p$-value $\leq 0.05$) and thus were removed. We now can execute the *multinomial logistic regression test* on the remaining variables.

### 3.4.3 Multinomial Logistic Regression Test

A regression test explores the relationship between a dependent variable and a set of independent—or predictor—variables [16]. In our study "normal weight" was set as the reference category to compare with the other groups (underweight, overweight, and obesity). At a $p$-value $\leq 0.05$ some variables proved to not be significantly associated with under- or overweight/obesity. Table 2 shows the results of the *multinomial logistic regression test* from the CCHS dataset between 2009 and 2014. The $B$ and Sig. columns represent the logistic constant and the significance value, respectively. Numbers marked in bold indicate numbers that are significant on the 95% confidence limit. For example, in 2014, the logistic constant of "obese" for the variable "leisure and transportation physical activity index" (PACDLTI) is 0.000 and statistically significant since its $p$-value $\leq 0.05$. This means that the risk of obesity increases as the value (1 = active, 3 = inactive) of leisure and transportation physical

**Table 2** *Multinomial logistic regression test* for variables between 2009 and 2014

| BMI | Variables | 2009 | | 2010 | | 2011 | | 2012 | | 2013 | | 2014 | |
|---|---|---|---|---|---|---|---|---|---|---|---|---|---|
| | | *B* | Sig. | *B* | Sig. | *B* | Sig. | *B* | Sig. | *B* | Sig. | *B* | Sig. |
| Under weight | Intercept | −4.025 | 0.000 | −4.012 | 0.000 | −3.404 | 0.000 | −3.815 | 0.000 | −4.215 | 0.000 | −4.205 | 0.000 |
| | FVCDVEG | −0.185 | 0.672 | −0.241 | 0.350 | −0.394 | **0.033** | −0.336 | 0.190 | 0.119 | 0.456 | 0.034 | 0.880 |
| | FVCDTOT | −0.266 | 0.518 | −0.225 | 0.296 | −0.426 | **0.008** | −0.369 | 0.102 | −0.105 | 0.537 | −0.412 | 0.074 |
| | FVCGTOT | 0.289 | 0.440 | 0.305 | 0.101 | 0.380 | **0.006** | 0.350 | 0.075 | 0.042 | 0.782 | 0.371 | 0.067 |
| | PAC_7 | −0.191 | 0.255 | −0.561 | **0.000** | −0.391 | **0.000** | −0.361 | **0.001** | −0.424 | **0.000** | −0.516 | **0.000** |
| | PAC_8 | 0.358 | 0.083 | 0.698 | **0.000** | 0.449 | **0.000** | 0.551 | **0.000** | 0.565 | 0.000 | 0.713 | **0.000** |
| | PACDEE | −0.324 | 0.606 | −0.313 | 0.397 | −0.123 | 0.634 | 0.282 | 0.518 | 0.138 | 0.608 | 0.207 | 0.612 |
| | PACFLEI | 1.146 | **0.033** | −0.235 | 0.546 | 0.299 | 0.210 | 0.623 | **0.048** | −0.175 | 0.535 | −0.145 | 0.726 |
| | PACDFR | 0.218 | 0.057 | 0.283 | **0.000** | 0.183 | **0.000** | 0.181 | **0.010** | 0.229 | **0.000** | 0.188 | **0.007** |
| | PACFD | −0.051 | 0.793 | −0.086 | 0.488 | −0.146 | 0.089 | 0.025 | 0.842 | −0.132 | 0.123 | −0.088 | 0.482 |
| | PACDPAI | 0.125 | 0.683 | −0.149 | 0.459 | 0.221 | 0.076 | 0.290 | 0.105 | 0.356 | **0.004** | 0.043 | 0.829 |
| | PACDLTI | −0.051 | 0.864 | 0.266 | 0.174 | −0.038 | 0.754 | −0.189 | 0.272 | −0.150 | 0.205 | 0.146 | 0.445 |
| | PACDTLE | 0.105 | 0.863 | 0.181 | 0.613 | 0.135 | 0.592 | −0.249 | 0.561 | −0.007 | 0.978 | −0.151 | 0.706 |
| | PACFLTI | −0.753 | 0.180 | 0.464 | 0.247 | −0.166 | 0.511 | −0.588 | 0.083 | 0.220 | 0.457 | 0.152 | 0.724 |

(continued)

**Table 2** (continued)

| BMI | Variables | 2009 | | 2010 | | 2011 | | 2012 | | 2013 | | 2014 | |
|---|---|---|---|---|---|---|---|---|---|---|---|---|---|
| | | *B* | Sig. | *B* | Sig. | *B* | Sig. | *B* | Sig. | *B* | Sig. | *B* | Sig. |
| Over weight | Intercept | 0.285 | 0.194 | −0.352 | 0.011 | −0.067 | 0.494 | −0.160 | 0.250 | −0.097 | 0.316 | −0.135 | 0.329 |
| | FVCDVEG | −0.269 | **0.048** | −0.100 | 0.236 | −0.231 | **0.000** | −0.216 | **0.000** | −0.165 | **0.003** | −0.109 | 0.166 |
| | FVCDTOT | −0.300 | **0.023** | **0.039** | 0.614 | −0.099 | 0.075 | 0.016 | 0.838 | −0.063 | 0.263 | −0.038 | 0.639 |
| | FVCGTOT | 0.093 | 0.444 | −0.213 | **0.002** | −0.085 | 0.091 | −0.205 | **0.005** | −0.115 | **0.026** | −0.147 | **0.049** |
| | PAC_7 | 0.178 | **0.001** | 0.235 | **0.000** | 0.205 | **0.000** | 0.238 | **0.000** | 0.221 | **0.000** | 0.215 | **0.000** |
| | PAC_8 | −0.134 | **0.029** | −0.063 | 0.132 | −0.061 | **0.044** | −0.070 | 0.103 | −0.058 | 0.061 | −0.056 | 0.204 |
| | PACDEE | 0.286 | 0.194 | 0.188 | 0.203 | 0.195 | 0.052 | 0.312 | **0.030** | 0.219 | 0.029 | 0.254 | 0.077 |
| | PACFLEI | 0.145 | 0.643 | −0.109 | 0.531 | −0.181 | 0.149 | −0.239 | 0.200 | −0.113 | 0.377 | −0.184 | 0.318 |
| | PACDFR | −0.042 | 0.246 | −0.018 | 0.419 | −0.030 | 0.066 | −0.034 | 0.147 | −0.042 | **0.010** | −0.099 | **0.000** |
| | PACFD | 0.042 | 0.444 | −0.018 | 0.626 | −0.031 | 0.233 | −0.053 | 0.144 | **0.016** | 0.530 | 0.043 | 0.244 |
| | PACDPAI | −0.216 | **0.046** | −0.101 | 0.154 | −0.087 | 0.077 | 0.036 | 0.613 | −0.058 | 0.241 | −0.085 | 0.228 |
| | PACDLTI | 0.307 | **0.004** | 0.208 | **0.003** | 0.192 | **0.000** | 0.083 | 0.229 | 0.173 | **0.000** | 0.212 | **0.002** |
| | PACDTLE | −0.417 | 0.055 | −0.249 | 0.087 | −0.328 | **0.001** | −0.373 | **0.009** | −0.348 | **0.000** | −0.342 | **0.016** |
| | PACFLTI | −0.193 | 0.547 | 0.147 | 0.410 | 0.266 | **0.039** | 0.299 | 0.119 | 0.085 | 0.520 | 0.124 | 0.516 |

| | | | | | | | | | | | | | |
|---|---|---|---|---|---|---|---|---|---|---|---|---|---|
| Obese | Intercept | −0.836 | 0.002 | −1.297 | 0.000 | −0.924 | 0.000 | −0.981 | 0.000 | −0.960 | 0.000 | −0.729 | 0.000 |
| | FVCDVEG | −0.211 | 0.222 | −0.031 | 0.771 | −0.188 | **0.009** | −0.138 | 0.161 | −0.043 | 0.531 | −0.069 | 0.484 |
| | FVCDTOT | −0.477 | **0.004** | −0.078 | 0.417 | −0.239 | **0.001** | −0.190 | **0.049** | −0.053 | 0.456 | −0.020 | 0.846 |
| | FVCGTOT | 0.193 | 0.204 | −0.154 | 0.077 | 0.004 | 0.949 | −0.042 | 0.631 | −0.187 | **0.005** | −0.253 | **0.009** |
| | PAC_7 | 0.098 | 0.137 | 0.167 | **0.000** | 0.156 | **0.000** | 0.130 | **0.003** | 0.188 | **0.000** | 0.133 | **0.003** |
| | PAC_8 | −0.073 | 0.345 | −0.057 | 0.269 | −0.095 | **0.009** | −0.046 | 0.368 | −0.094 | **0.012** | −0.060 | 0.253 |
| | PACDEE | −0.178 | 0.519 | −0.337 | 0.060 | 0.190 | 0.193 | 0.189 | 0.344 | 0.297 | 0.051 | 0.214 | 0.298 |
| | PACFLEI | 0.074 | 0.829 | 0.015 | 0.932 | −0.028 | 0.824 | −0.166 | 0.382 | −0.200 | 0.145 | −0.150 | 0.421 |
| | PACDFR | 0.073 | 0.070 | 0.092 | **0.000** | 0.046 | **0.010** | 0.053 | **0.037** | 0.085 | **0.000** | 0.052 | **0.036** |
| | PACFD | −0.018 | 0.789 | −0.080 | 0.071 | −0.104 | **0.001** | −0.102 | **0.020** | −0.054 | 0.075 | −0.018 | 0.671 |
| | PACDPAI | −0.294 | **0.039** | −0.064 | 0.476 | 0.022 | 0.715 | 0.073 | 0.395 | −0.127 | **0.044** | −0.189 | **0.031** |
| | PACDLTI | 0.607 | **0.000** | 0.411 | **0.000** | 0.373 | **0.000** | 0.315 | **0.000** | 0.474 | **0.000** | 0.497 | **0.000** |
| | PACDTLE | −0.155 | 0.565 | 0.093 | 0.595 | −0.500 | **0.000** | −0.469 | **0.017** | −0.689 | **0.000** | −0.637 | **0.002** |
| | PACFLTI | 0.142 | 0.683 | 0.115 | 0.533 | 0.190 | 0.148 | 0.275 | 0.159 | 0.350 | **0.013** | 0.317 | 0.098 |

*B*: logistic constant

FVCDVEG: daily consumption—other vegetables, FVCDTOT: daily consumption—total fruits and vegetables; FVCGTOT: grouping daily consumption—total fruits and vegetables; PAC_7: walked to work or school—past 3 months; PAC_8: bicycled to work or school—past 3 months; PACDEE: daily energy expenditure—leisure physical activities; PACFLEI: participant in leisure physical activity; PACDFR: frequency—all leisure physical activity lasting more than 15 min; PACFD: participant in daily leisure physical activity lasting more than 15 min; PACDPAI: leisure physical activity index; PACDLTI: leisure and transportation physical activity index; PACDTLE: daily energy expenditure—transportation and leisure physical activity; PACFLTI: participant in leisure or transportation physical activity

activity index increases. Thus, an inactive person is more likely to be obese than an active person. Significant independent predictors for underweight, overweight, and obese status in 2014 are:

- Underweight—"walked to work or school for past 3 months" (PAC_7), "bicycled to work or school for past 3 months" (PAC_8), and "frequency of all leisure physical activity lasting more than 15 min" (PACDFR)
- Overweight—"grouping of daily consumption - total fruits and vegetables" (FVCGTOT), "walked to work or school for Past 3 months" (PAC_7), "frequency of all leisure physical activity over 15 min" (PACDFR), "leisure and transportation physical activity index" (PACDLTI), and "daily frequency in transportation and leisure physical activity" (PACDTLE)
- Obesity—"daily consumption of total fruits and vegetables" (FVCGTOT), "walked to work or school for past 3 months" (PAC_7), "frequency of all leisure physical activity over 15 min" (PACDFR), "leisure physical activity index" (PACDPAI), "leisure and transportation physical activity index" (PACDLTI), and "daily frequency in transportation and leisure physical activity" (PACDTLE)

## 3.5 *Mathematical Relationship Among Factors*

Based on the statistical data analysis carried out, the main *factors* and *variables* for obesity and overweight were identified and their respective mathematical relationship obtained. The mathematical formula indicates how the relevant factors contribute to the emergence of overweight and obesity. Table 3 shows the main *factors* and *variables* found to contribute to obesity. For example, the factor, fruit and vegetable consumption (FVC), has three variables (daily consumption of other vegetables (FVCDVEG), daily consumption of total fruits and vegetables (FVCD-TOT), and grouping daily consumption - total fruits and vegetables (FVCGTOT)). Then, the variable daily consumption of other vegetables (FVCDVEG) has two different answers (behaviors) which are less than five times (Answer 1) or five times and more (Answer 2).

One advantage of logistic regression analysis is its ability to directly estimate the probability of the occurrence of an event. In the case of the dependent variable $Y$ with only two possible states (1 or 0) and a set of the independent variables, $x_1, x_2, \ldots x_P$, the multiple logistic regression function can be written as [17]:

$$logit(P)(Y = 1) = \frac{1}{1 + e^{-g(x)}}, g(x) = B_0 + B_1 x_1 + \cdots + B_P x_P \qquad (2)$$

To determine the equation for each weight category, the constants "$B_n$" of the regression function "$g(x) = B_0 + B_1 x_1 + \cdots + B_P x_P$" should be replaced by the factors' variable logistic constants obtained from the *multinomial logistic regression* analysis as summarized in Table 2, where $B_0$ equals the "intercept" value.

**Table 3** Multinomial logistic regression test for variables between 2009 and 2014

| Factors | Variable | Code | Behaviors | | |
|---|---|---|---|---|---|
| FVC: Fruit and vegetable consumption | Daily consumption—other vegetables | FVCDVEG | Less than five times | Less than five times | |
| | Daily consumption—total fruits and vegetables | FVCDTOT | Less than five times | Less than five times | |
| | Grouping daily consumption—total fruits and vegetables | FVCGTOT | Eats fruits and vegetables less than five times per day | Eats fruits and vegetables between five and ten times per day | Eats fruits and vegetables more than ten times per day |
| PAC: Physical activities | Walked to work or school—past 3 months | PAC_7 | Yes | No | Does not work or go to school |
| | Bicycled to work or school—past 3 months | PAC_8 | Yes | No | Does not work or go to school |
| | Daily energy expenditure—leisure physical activities | PACDEE | Less than five times | Five times or more | |
| | Participant in leisure physical activity | PACFLEI | Yes | No | |
| | Frequency—all leisure physical activity lasting more than 15 min | PACDFR | Regular | Occasional | Infrequent |
| | Participant in daily leisure physical activity lasting more than 15 min | PACFD | Yes | No | |
| | Leisure physical activity index | PACDPAI | Active | Moderate active | Inactive |
| | Leisure and transportation physical activity index | PACDLTI | Active | Moderate active | Inactive |
| | Daily energy expenditure—transportation and leisure physical activity | PACDTLE | Less than five times | Five times or more | |
| | Participant in leisure or transportation physical activity | PACFLTI | Yes | No | |

For example, for the category "Obese in 2014" the equation is

$$\begin{aligned} g(x) = & -0.729 - 0.069x_1 - 0.020x_2 - 0.253x_3 + 0.133x_4 \\ & - 0.60x_5 + 0.214x_6 - 0.150x_7 + 0.052x_8 - 0.018x_9 \\ & + 0.189x_{10} + 0.497x_{11} - 0.637x_{12} + 0.317x_{13} \end{aligned} \quad (3)$$

The standard interpretation of the logistic constant is that for a unit change in the independent variable ($x_1, x_2, \ldots x_{13}$), the logit outcome relative to the reference group (normal weight) is expected to change by its respective parameter estimate if all the other variables are held fixed [18]. For instance, if the agent's daily consumption of other vegetables ($x_1$) increases by one unit, the risk of the occurrence of obesity to normal weight would be expected to decrease by 0.069 while holding all other variables in the model constant. Intercept ($B_0$) is the multinomial logit estimate for obesity relative to normal weight when the independent variables in the model are evaluated at zero. If $x_1, x_2, \ldots, x_{13} = 0$, the intercept is simply the expected mean value of $Y$ at that value (in this case, $-0.729$).

As the absolute value of the constant "$B_n$" is larger, its influence is larger too (positively or negatively). For example, Eq. (3) implies that the obese state is affected more strongly by "daily frequency in transportation and leisure physical activity ($x_{12}$)" which has the biggest absolute value among the constants. In contrast, the obese state is affected less strongly by "participant in daily leisure physical activity lasting more than 15 min ($x_9$)" which has the smallest absolute value among the constants.

Our next step is to build the CAS-based obesity model by using the set of equations obtained for the four weight states (underweight, normal weight, overweight, and obese). First, we need to set the BMI status of agents representing a population. In 2009–2010, the ratio of underweight, normal weight, overweight, and obese is 1.79%, 43.23%, 35.22%, and 19.76%, respectively. We will use this ratio as an initial value of the BMI states in the population. Second, we will set rules and factors for the agents. Each of the agent has 13 different obesity factors. To define the rules in the time series for the agent, we will use the obesogenic state equations each year in the period. For example, in 2014, we can set the agents in the obese state by using Eq. (3). Thus, agents have four different equations (underweight, normal weight, overweight, and obese) available each year for calculating their obesogenic state. The original dataset contains the person's perception of their own obesogenic state. This information is used to guide the suitable equation for an individual.

Each of the agents (individuals) have different conditions on factor values (Table 3). Thus, with the computer model using the equations and datasets, we will carry out a year-to-year statistical data analysis simulation of people in a community. In other words, we will evaluate people changing behaviors in terms of the relevant obesity factors identified and see how obesogenic state rates arise in the community as a consequence of people's actions (Fig. 1).

## 4 Conclusion and Future Work

Over the past 20 years, the percentage of adult's being overweight and obese has increased considerably. To solve this problem, we conducted a CAS-based statistical data analysis to understand its causes. Based on the statistical results, the main factors for obesity were "fruit and vegetable consumption" and "frequency of physical activities." Also, the equations that show how the factors relate to the emergence of obesity are achieved. Moreover, we found that variables show distinctive characteristics for BMI status. For instance, one of the independent variables, "grouping daily consumption - total fruits and vegetables (FVCGTOT)," shows a different impact in each group (underweight, overweight, and obese). In 2014, the daily consumption total fruits and vegetables has a negative relationship with the risk of the occurrence of both overweight and obesity whereas it has a positive effect on the risk of the occurrence of underweight. That is, a person who is overweight or obese consumes less fruit and vegetable than a normal weight person while an underweight person tends to consume more fruits and vegetables.

Our future work is to build and validate our CAS-based model to simulate obesity rates by using the equations obtained from the data analysis. With our model, we aim to build a tool to assist obesity management by providing capabilities to evaluate various policies and getting insights about how obesity emerges in our communities.

**Acknowledgements** This work was supported in part by the University of Winnipeg Applied Computer Science Department, Mitacs Globalink program, and a Natural Sciences and Engineering Research Council of Canada Discovery Development Grant.

## The Transformative Aspects of This Study

Most of the previous studies are focused on the relationship between one risk factor and obesity; however, our study approach uses various risk factors and demonstrates their interrelationships. Thus, we can conduct sophisticated analysis of obesity in different time periods. Also, we obtained obesity factor correlation equations that can be applied to the development of a CAS-based population obesity model for different communities.

**Take Home Message**

- Statistical analysis of the Canadian Community Health Survey (CCHS) identified two main factors associated with obesity—fruit and vegetable consumption and frequency of physical activities.
- There are independent variables that define distinctive characteristics for each BMI state.

## References


1. World Health Organization (WHO). Obesity and overweight fact-sheets. WHO Press; 2018. Available from: http://www.who.int/news-room/fact-sheets/detail/obesity-and-overweight. Accessed 9 Aug 2018.
2. Miller J, Page S. Complex adaptive systems: an introduction to computational models of social life. Princeton studies in complexity. Princeton: Princeton University Press; 2009.
3. Wooldridge M. An introduction to multiagent systems. 2nd ed. Chichester: Wiley; 2009.
4. Bruch E, Atwell J. Agent-based models in empirical social research. Sociol Methods Res. 2015;44(2):186–221.
5. Statistics Canada. Canadian Community Health Survey (CCHS). NESSTAR data portal. Available from: http://libproxy.uwinnipeg.ca/login?url=http://dli-idd-nesstar.statcan.gc.ca/webview/. Accessed 9 Aug 2018.
6. Health Statistics Division. Statistic Canada, Canadian Community Health Survey 2014 - Annual Component (CCHS); 2018.
7. World Health Organization. Noncommunicable diseases country profiles 2014. Geneva: WHO Press; 2014.
8. Mayo Clinic. Obesity. Available from: https://www.mayoclinic.org/diseases-conditions/obesity/symptoms-causes/syc-20375742. Accessed 9 Aug 2018.
9. US Department of Health and Human Services. What causes obesity & overweight? Last updated: 2016. Available from: https://www.nichd.nih.gov/health/topics/obesity/conditioninfo/cause. Accessed 9 Aug 2018.
10. Centers for Disease Control and Prevention. Adult obesity causes & consequences. Last updated: 2018. Available from: https://www.cdc.gov/obesity/adult/causes.html. Accessed 9 Aug 2018.
11. Remedy Health Media. Risk factors and causes of obesity. Last updated: 2015. Available from: http://www.healthcommunities.com/obesity/causes.shtml. Accessed 9 Aug 2018.
12. Colapinto CK, Graham J, St-Pierre S. Trends and correlates of frequency of fruit and vegetable consumption, 2007 to 2014. Health Rep. 2018;29(1):9–14.
13. Charlton K, Kowal P, Soriano MM, Williams S, Banks E, Vo K, Byles J. Fruit and vegetable intake and body mass index in a large sample of middle-aged Australian men and women. Nutrients. 2014;6(6):2305–19.
14. French A, Macedo M, Poulsen J, Waterson T, Yu A. Multivariate analysis of variance (MANOVA). San Francisco: San Francisco State University; 2008.
15. IBM SPSS Statistics. IBM SPSS software. Available from: https://www.ibm.com/analytics/spss-statistics-software. Accessed 9 Aug 2018.
16. Bewick V, Cheek L, Ball J. Statistics review 7: Correlation and regression. Crit Care. 2003;7(6):451–9.
17. Pohar M, Blas M, Turk S. Comparison of logistic regression and linear discriminant analysis: a simulation study. Metodoloski Zvezki. 2004;1(1):143–61.
18. UCLA: Statistical Consulting Group. Multinomial logistic regression. Available from: https://stats.idre.ucla.edu/spss/output/multinomial-logistic-regression/. Accessed 9 Aug 2018.

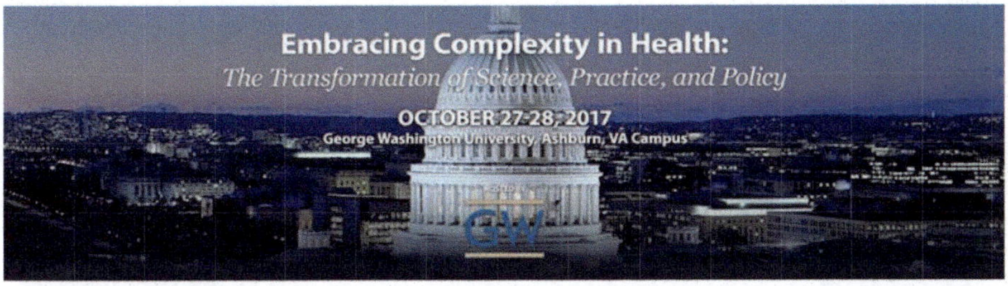
Embracing Complexity in Health:
The Transformation of Science, Practice, and Policy
OCTOBER 27-28, 2017
George Washington University, Ashburn, VA Campus
GW

# The Program

## Friday, October 27

| | |
|---|---|
| 8:00–8:30 | Impromptu networking |
| | Welcome and opening remarks |

| | | |
|---|---|---|
| 8:30–9:30 | Mini-TED talks | Five 5-minute highlights of each presentation followed by small group session |
| | Joachim P. Sturmberg | If You Change the Way You Look at Things, Things You Look at Change. Clinical Disease: Cause or Consequence? |
| | Jennifer Potts | Complexity of Being a Millennial |
| | Paige L. McDonald, Curt Lindberg, and Robert Hausmann | Is the learning health system a complex adaptive system or a complex responsive process? |
| | Curt Lindberg | Positive deviance: a novel process for optimizing antibiotic use |
| | Tilo Winkler | A puzzling question: how can different phenotypes possibly have indistinguishable disease symptoms? |
| | James Palmer | Complexity sciences dramatically improve biomarker research and use |

Panel Discussion

## Advances in Medicine, Policy, and Leadership Inspired by Complexity Science
## Moderator: Paige McDonald

| | |
|---|---|
| James K. Hazy | What Leaders Should Know About Complexity (And Why Knowing This Will Make You a More Effective Leader) |
| Jesse Pines and Brendan G. Carr | Complex Systems Thinking in Acute and Emergency Care |

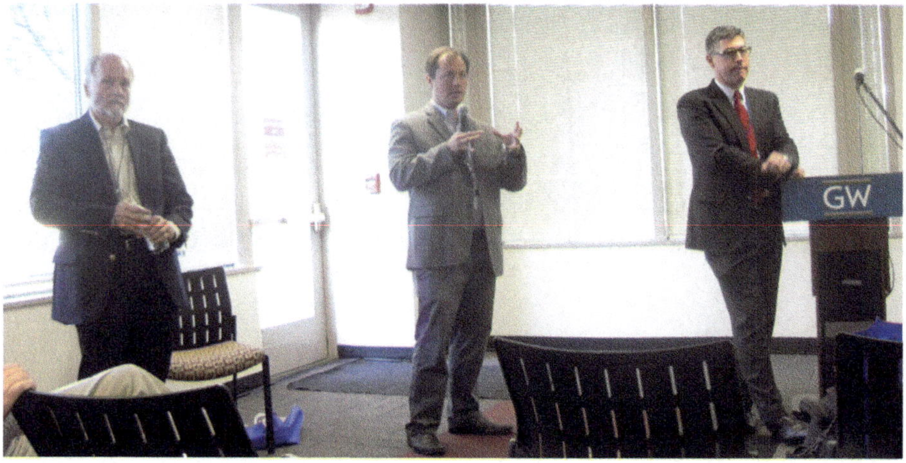


Jim Hazy (l), Jesse Pines (c), and Bredon Carr (r)

| | | |
|---|---|---|
| 11:00–12:00 | Mini-TED talks | Five 5-minute highlights of each presentation followed by small group session |
| | Paul Harper | OR saves lives! |
| | Alonzo Jones | Can salutogenesis work in the US? |
| | Carmel Martin | Resilience as a Preliminary Exploration of a Theoretical Framework of Nonlinear Stability. Individual Health Journeys and Health Systems |
| | Gaetano R. Lotrecchianoa, Mary Kane, Mark S. Zocchi, Jessica Gosa, Danielle Lazar, and Jesse M. Pines | Bringing voice in policy building: a cross population multi-stakeholder conceptual model or management of acute unscheduled care in the united states using group concept mapping |
| | Guo Liu, Christine Ye, Zachary Armstrong and Henry H Heng | Stress-Induced Variants Through Genome-Environment Interaction: The General Mechanism of Diseases |
| | Stefan Topolski | Health Complexity Loss in Addiction |

| | | |
|---|---|---|
| 13:00–14:15 | Graduate student presentations | 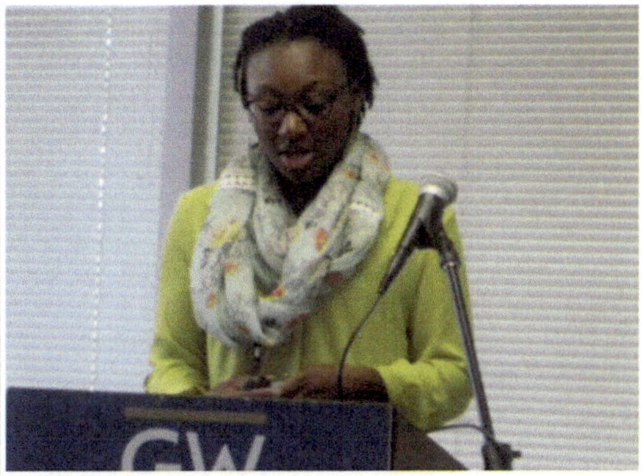  Romiya Barry |
| | Sasmira Matta and Ligia Paina | OR using simulations as teaching tools to better understand complex health systems |
| | Junqiao Chen | Impact analysis of complexity science modelling techniques in health care: a mixed-method research proposal |
| | Surio Priyanka, Vaishali Joshi, and Elizabeth Ciemins | Hypertension (HTN) prevalence disparities for predicted and diagnosed HTN in African Americans and Caucasians: a longitudinal ecological epidemiology study |
| | Jennifer Weaver | Complexity Science and Cognitive Interventions for TBI |
| | Romiya G. Barry, Landria Sheffey, and Anab Mohamed | Understanding the complexity of stakeholder needs: ethical conduct prioritizations for clinical trials in low-middle-income countries |
| | Sung Young Lim, Shi Wenting, and Sergio G. Camorlinga | A Study on the Modeling for Childhood Obesity |

| Posters | | |
|---|---|---|
| | Russell Gonnering and William Riley | The paradoxical "hispanic paradox": the dark side of acculturation |
| | Michael Reens | Optimising operating room efficiency |

| 15:30–16:45 | Mini-TED talks physiology stream | Five 5-minute highlights of each presentation followed by small group session |
|---|---|---|
| | Nicolas Rohleder | OR Mechanisms of Habituation of Inflammatory Responses to Repeated Acute Stress and Its Role in Health and Disease |
| | Andrew Seely | Origins of Degree and Complexity of Variation Inherent to Complex Systems |
| | Bela Suki | Elastic Network Models of Tissue Failure: Implications for Treatments of Emphysema |
| | Henry H. Heng, Guo Liu, Sarah Alemara and Christine J. Ye | The Mechanisms of How Genomic Heterogeneity Impacts Bio-emergent Properties: The Challenges for Precision Medicine |
| | Sergio G. Camorlinga | Complex Adaptive Systems in the Brain |
| | Douglas P. Barnaby | Predictive Modeling with Heart Rate Variability, Clinical and Laboratory Measures to Predict Future Deterioration in Patients Presenting with Sepsis |

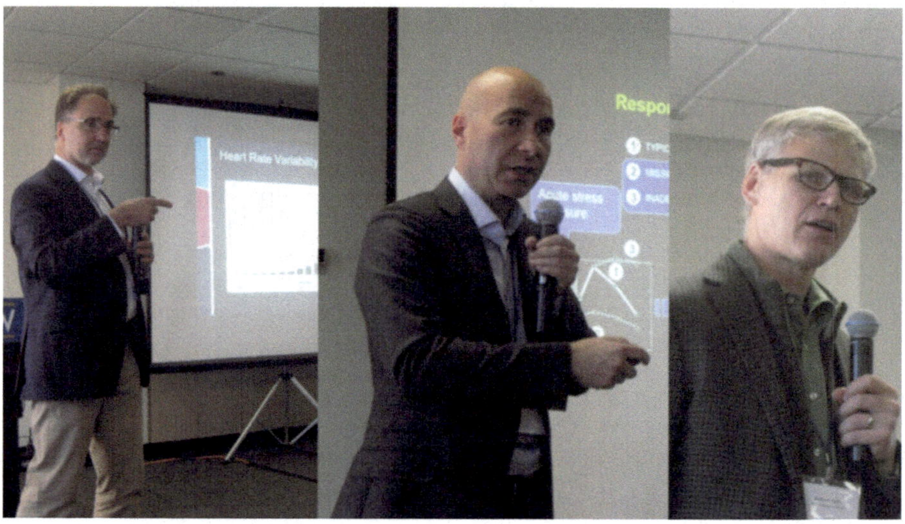

Douglas Barnaby (l), Nicolas Rohleder (c), and Andrew Seely (r)

| | | |
|---|---|---|
| 15:30–16:45 | Mini-TED talks patient care stream | Five 5-minute highlights of each presentation followed by small group session |
| | Diane Finegood | Complex Is Not the Same as Complicated: Frameworks and Tools Are Needed to Support Application of Systems Thinking to Complex Health-Related Challenges |
| | David C. Aron, Chin-Lin Tseng, Orysya Soroka, and Leonard M. Pogach | Balancing Measures: Identifying Unintended Consequences of Diabetes Quality Performance Measures |
| | Suzie Carmack | Physician Burnout: A Public Health Crisis in Need of a Socio-ecological Solution |
| | Susanne Reventlow | Coordinated Co-produced Care for Patients with Complex Health Problems: An Example from Denmark |
| | Carmel Martin | Complex Adaptive Systems Approaches to Potentially Avoidable Hospitalizations. Implementing the Patient Journey Record System (PaJR) in Ireland and Australia |
| | David Katerndahl, Sandra K. Burge, Robert L. Ferrer, RL, John Becho, and Robert Wood | Is Perceived Need-for-Action Among Women in Violent Relationships Nonlinear and, If So, Why? |

# Launch of ISSCSH

## International Society for Systems and Complexity Sciences for Health

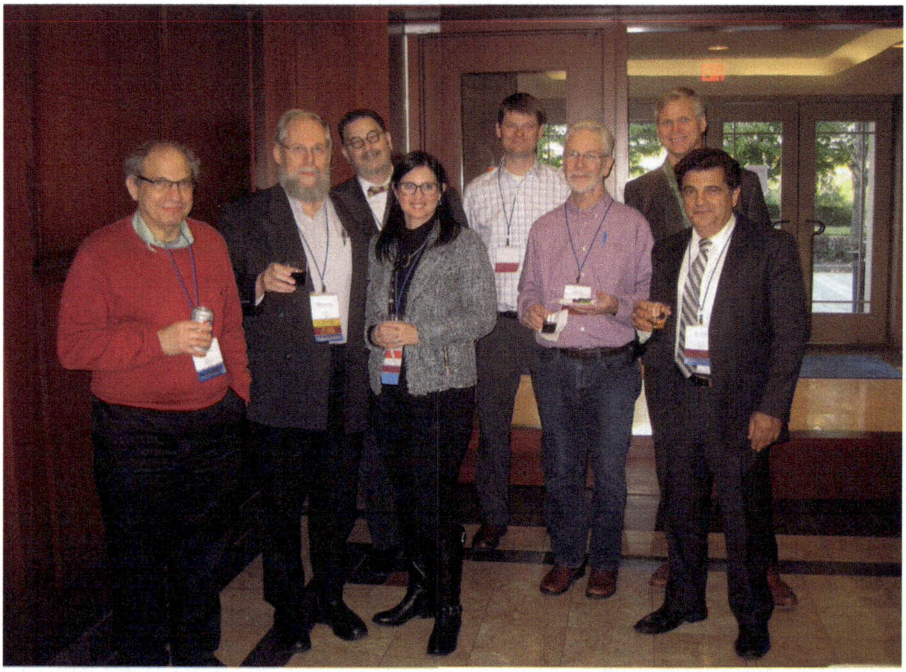

The Foundation Board of the Society David Aron, Joachim Sturmberg (Foundation President), Gaetano Lotrecchiano (Foundation Vice-President), Paige McDonald (Foundation Secretary), Chad Swanson, John Scott, Andrew Seely, Peter Tsasis absent: Curt Lindberg (Foundation Treasurer), Randy Thompson

A dream has come true—after more than 20 years, 23 August 2017 has become the official launching date of the *International Society for Systems and Complexity Sciences for Health.*

The Society is the result of the large and diverse group of people who all believe that the problems facing the health and well-being of our patients and communities can only be solved by addressing the interconnected nature of their problems.

Our Society aims to be an umbrella organization that links all those interested in promoting systems and complexity thinking for the benefit of the health and well-being of patients and communities. The Society also aims to educate the wider professional and lay community about the interconnected nature of health and disease, and to become the lead advocacy voice in relation to the health and disease impacts of policy settings.

The Society provides its members with three principal benefits—educational activities, support to implement systems and complexity science-informed approaches for research and health professional practice, and cross-disciplinary collaboration. In time, the Society aims to be recognized as the preeminent body to provide systems and complexity science input to policy and decision-makers working for health.

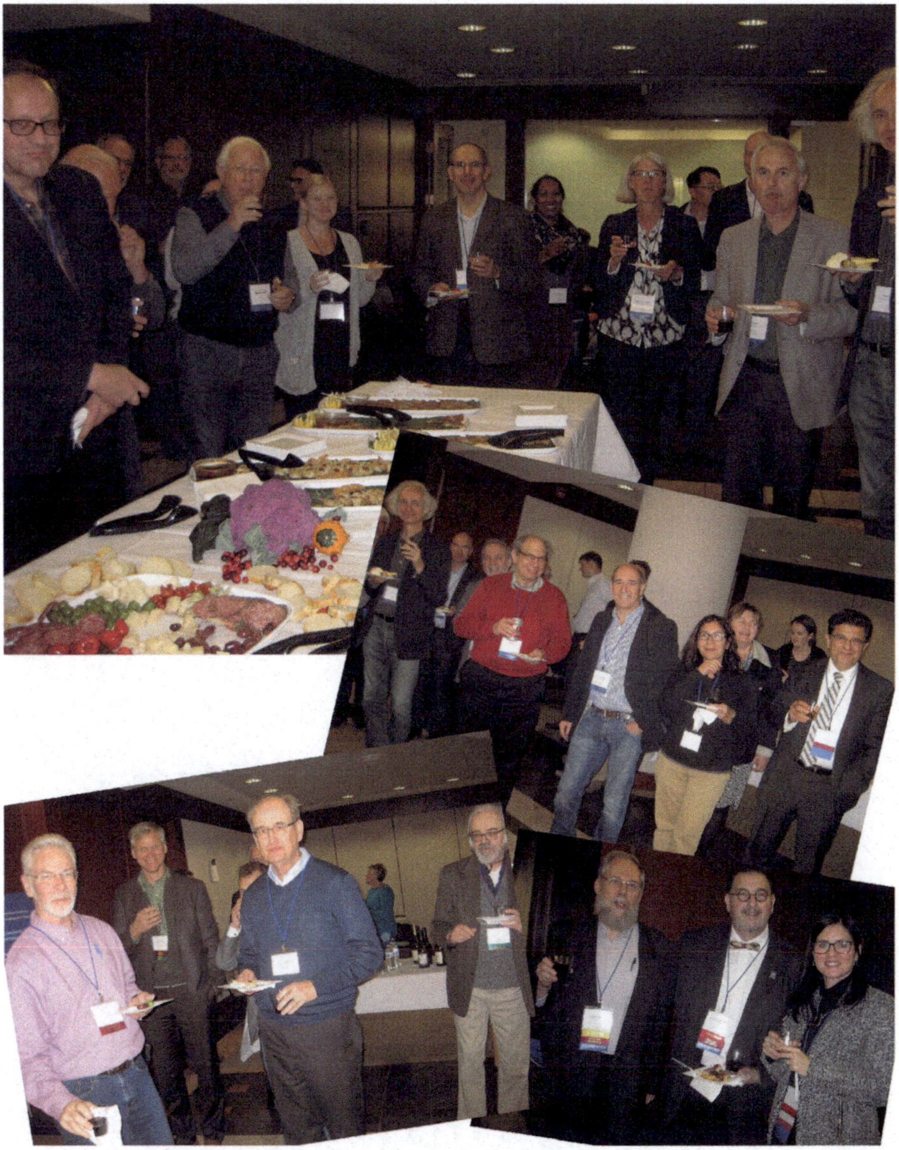

## Saturday, October 28

| | | |
|---|---|---|
| 8:15–9:15 | Mini-TED talks | Five 5-minute highlights of each presentation followed by small group session |
| | Joachim P. Sturmberg | Linking the Environmental and Physiological Components of Health and Disease |
| | Elena A. Doty, C. Matthew Kinsey, and Jason H.T. Bates | Analyzing Complex Medical Image Information: Convolution Versus Wavelets in a Neural Net |
| | Roseanne Moore, Marsha Hertzberg, and Junqiao Chen | Assessment Framework on the Complexity in Primary Care Practice |
| | Eric Sarriot | Call an Agent-Based Modeler Stat! Bringing Evidence to Global Health Blind Spots |
| | John Watkins | Organisational Relativity: Changing Our Perspective on Health and Healthcare |

## Keynote Addresses

Advances in Medicine, Policy, and Leadership Inspired by Complexity Science
Moderator: Paige McDonald

| | |
|---|---|
| Bruce West | Fail Small, Fail Often |
| Andrew Seely | Variability-Derived Clinical Decision Support to Improve Care |

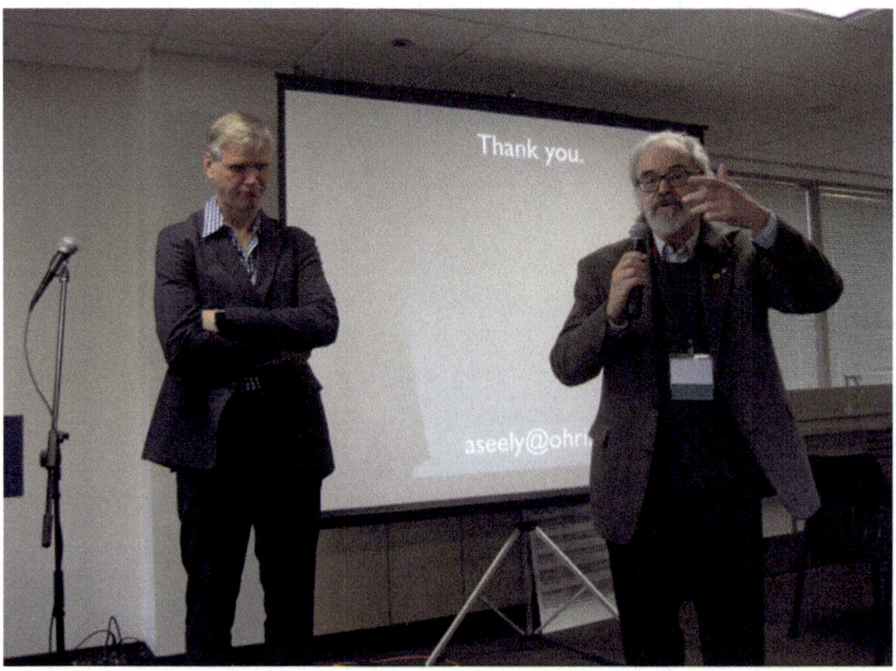


Andrew Seely (l) and Bruce West (r)

| 10:30–11:30 | Mini-TED talks | Five 5-minute highlights of each presentation followed by small group session |
|---|---|---|
| | Andrew Seely | Monitoring Adverse Events and Using Positive Deviance to Improve Surgical Care |
| | Joachim P. Sturmberg | Deviant Behaviour Is Neither Irrational nor Ignorant |
| | Junqiao Chen and Milesh Patel | The Challenge in Quality Measurement: The Complex Interplay of Technical Difficulties, Social Construct, and Business Enterprise |
| | Kevin Nortrup | Quality and Value in Healthcare: Simple Goals for a Complex System |
| | John Scott | The Healing Journey: Healing as an Emergent Property of Complex Social Interactions |

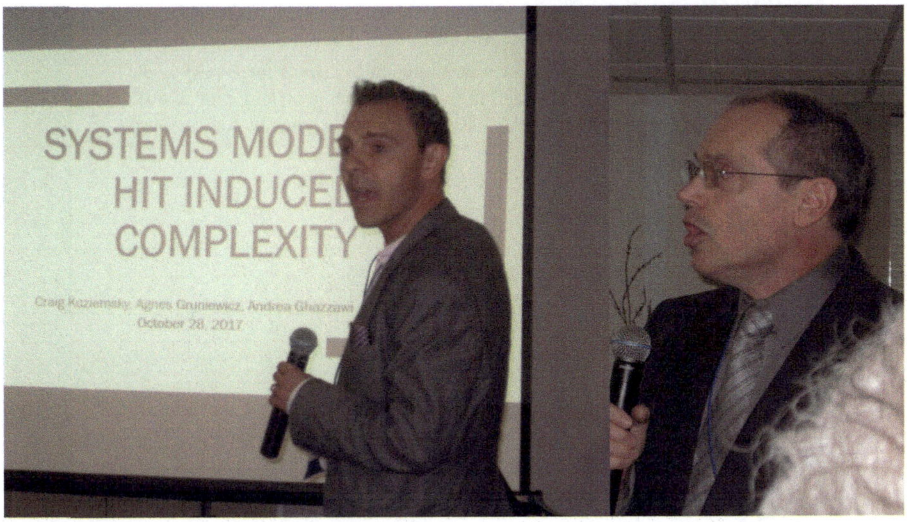


Craig Kuziemsky (l) and Kevin Nortrup (r)

| 14:30–15:30 | Mini-TED talks health systems stream | Five 5-minute highlights of each presentation followed by small group session |
|---|---|---|
| | Eddie Price | Complexity Medicine Now. Transforming Medicine from the Biomedical Model to a Systems and Complexity Model |
| | Joao Costa | Strengthening Health Systems, How Can This Be Done? |
| | Jan van der Kamp | Positive Cooperation for Sustainable Health |
| | Craig Kuziemsky, Agnes Gruniewicz, and Andrea Ghazzawi | Systems Model of HIT-Induced Complexity |
| | Kaja Abbas | Systems Thinking to Improve Effectiveness, Efficiency, and Equity in Health |

| | | |
|---|---|---|
| 14:30–15:30 | Mini-TED talks education and improvement stream | Five 5-minute highlights of each presentation followed by small group session |
| | Gaetano R. Lotrecchiano and S. Misra | Features of Transdisciplinary Knowledge Producing Teams (TD KPTS): A Systems Perspective |
| | Cheryl Miller and Kelsey A. Hanson | A Relational Coordination Theory Informed Nurse Residency Program |
| | Chad Swanson and Matthew Widmer | Arizona State University: An Example of a Complex Systems Approach to University Transformation |
| | Robert Hausmann and Jennifer Nelson | Capitalizing on Complexity: The Stories Behind the Numbers in a Global Health Initiative |
| | Paige L. McDonald, Kenneth J. Harwood, and Jennifer Weaver | Scoping Reviews: A Mechanism for Conveying the Value of a Complexity Approach to Problem Exploration and Knowledge Generation |
| | Rick Botelho | Cultivate Open Mindsets for Equity and Planetary Health: How Can Leaders and Change Makers Close the Advocacy-Action Gap? |

| | |
|---|---|
| 15:30–16:00 | Closing reflections<br>Moderator: Joachim Sturmberg |

# Index




J. P. Sturmberg (ed.), *Embracing Complexity in Health*,
https://doi.org/10.1007/978-3-030-10940-0

Printed by Printforce, the Netherlands